Pediatric PET Imaging

Guest Editors

HONGMING ZHUANG, MD, PhD
ABASS ALAVI, MD,
MD (Hon), PhD (Hon), DSc (Hon)

PET CLINICS

www.pet.theclinics.com

Consulting Editor
ABASS ALAVI, MD,
MD (Hon), PhD (Hon), DSc (Hon)

October 2008 • Volume 3 • Number 4

SAUNDERS an imprint of ELSEVIER, Inc.

W.B. SAUNDERS COMPANY
A Division of Elsevier Inc.

1600 John F. Kennedy Boulevard ● Suite 1800 ● Philadelphia, Pennsylvania 19103-2899

http://www.theclinics.com

PET CLINICS Volume 3, Number 4
October 2008 ISSN 1556-8598, ISBN 10: 1-4160-6112-6, ISBN-13: 978-1-4160-6112-0

Editor: Barton Dudlick
Developmental Editor: Theresa Collier

PET Clinics (ISSN 1556-8598) is published quarterly by W.B. Saunders, 360 Park Avenue South, New York, NY 10010-1710. Months of publication are January, April, July, and October. Business and Editorial Offices: 1600 John F. Kennedy Blvd., Suite 1800, Philadelphia, PA 19103-2899. Accounting and Circulation Offices: 11830 Westline Industrial Drive, St. Louis, MO 63146. Periodicals postage paid at New York, NY, and additional mailing offices. Subscription prices per year are $196.00 (US individuals), $274.00 (US institutions), $97.00 (US students), $223.00 (Canadian individuals), $306.00 (Canadian institutions), $118.00 (Canadian students), $237.00 (foreign individuals), $306.00 (foreign institutions), and $118.00 (foreign students). To receive student and resident rate, orders must be accompanied by name of affiliated institution, date of term, and the signature of program/residency coordinator on institution letterhead. Orders will be billed at individual rate until proof of status is received. Foreign air speed delivery is included in all Clinics subscription prices. All prices are subject to change without notice. POSTMASTER: Send address changes to PET Clinics, Elsevier Periodicals Customer Service, 11830 Westline Industrial Drive, St. Louis, MO 63146. **Customer service: 1-800-654-2452 (US). From outside of the United States, call 314-453-7041. Fax: 314-453-5170. E-mail: JournalsCustomerService-usa@elsevier.com (for print support); JournalsOnlineSupport-usa@elsevier.com (for online support).**

Reprints. For copies of 100 or more of articles in this publication, please contact the Commercial Reprints Department, Elsevier Inc., 360 Park Avenue South, New York, NY 10010-1710. Tel.: 212-633-3812; Fax: 212-462-1935; E-mail: reprints@elsevier.com.

Contributors

CONSULTING EDITOR

ABASS ALAVI, MD,
MD (Hon), PhD (Hon), DSc (Hon)
Professor of Radiology, Department
of Radiology, Division of Nuclear Medicine,
Hospital of the University of Pennsylvania,
Philadelphia, Pennsylvania

GUEST EDITORS

HONGMING ZHUANG, MD, PhD
Chief, Nuclear Medicine Division, Department
of Radiology, Children's Hospital of Philadelphia;
Associate Professor of Radiology, Hospital of the
University of Pennsylvania, Philadelphia,
Pennsylvania

ABASS ALAVI, MD,
MD (Hon), PhD (Hon), DSc (Hon)
Professor of Radiology, Department
of Radiology, Division of Nuclear Medicine,
Hospital of the University of Pennsylvania,
Philadelphia, Pennsylvania

AUTHORS

ABASS ALAVI, MD,
MD (Hon), PhD (Hon), DSc (Hon)
Professor of Radiology, Department
of Radiology, Division of Nuclear Medicine,
Hospital of the University of Pennsylvania,
Philadelphia, Pennsylvania

WICHANA CHAMROONRAT, MD
Department of Radiology, Division of Nuclear
Medicine, The Children's Hospital
of Philadelphia, Pennsylvania

WEI CHEN, MD, PhD
Associate Clinical Professor, Department
of Molecular and Medical Pharmacology,
David Geffen School of Medicine, University of
California, Los Angeles; Chief, Nuclear Medicine,
Kaiser Permanente Woodland Hills Medical
Center, Woodland Hills, California

GANG CHENG, MD
Department of Radiology, Children's Hospital of
Philadelphia, Philadelphia; Department of
Radiology, Hospital of the University of
Pennsylvania; Philadelphia, Pennsylvania

HARRY T. CHUGANI, MD
Professor, Departments of Pediatrics and
Neurology, School of Medicine, Wayne State
University, Children's Hospital of Michigan;
Chief, Division of Pediatric Neurology,
Children's Hospital of Michigan; Director,
PET Center, Children's Hospital of Michigan,
Detroit, Michigan

MICHAEL J. FISHER, MD
Assistant Professor of Pediatrics,
Department of Pediatrics, University of
Pennsylvania School of Medicine; Attending
Physician, Division of Oncology, Children's
Hospital of Philadelphia, Philadelphia,
Pennsylvania

MICHAEL J. GELFAND, MD
Professor of Radiology and Pediatrics,
University of Cincinnati; Chief, Section
of Nuclear Medicine, Department of Radiology,
Cincinnati Children's Hospital Medical Center,
Cincinnati, Ohio

MIGUEL HERNANDEZ-PAMPOLINI, MD
Department of Radiology, Division of Nuclear
Medicine, The Children's Hospital of Philadelphia;
Department of Radiology, Hospital of the
University of Pennsylvania, Philadelphia,
Pennsylvania

MOHAMED HOUSENI, MD
Division of Nuclear Medicine, Department of
Radiology, The Children's Hospital of Philadelphia,
Pennsylvania; Department of Radiology, National
Liver Institute, Egypt

ROLAND HUSTINX, MD, PhD
Chargé de Cours, Department of Medicine,
Division of Nuclear Medicine, University Hospital
of Liège, Campus Universitaire du Sart Tilman,
Belgium

AJAY KUMAR, MD, PhD, DNB
Assistant Professor, Departments of Pediatrics
and Neurology, Wayne State University, Children's
Hospital of Michigan, Detroit, Michigan

EDOUARD LOUIS, MD, PhD
Chargé de Cours, Department of Medicine,
Division of Gastroenterology, University Hospital
of Liège, Campus Universitaire du Sart Tilman,
Belgium

M. BETH McCARVILLE, MD
Associate Member, Department of Radiological
Sciences, St. Jude Children's Research Hospital,
Memphis, Tennessee

SABAH SERVAES, MD
Assistant Professor of Radiology,
Department of Radiology, Division
of Nuclear Medicine, Children's Hospital of
Pennsylvania, Philadelphia, Pennsylvania

SUSAN E. SHARP, MD
Assistant Professor of Radiology,
University of Cincinnati; Staff Radiologist,
Department of Radiology, Cincinnati Children's
Hospital Medical Center, Cincinnati, Ohio

BARRY L. SHULKIN, MD, MBA
Chief, Nuclear Medicine Division,
Department of Radiological Sciences,
St. Jude Children's Research Hospital,
Memphis, Tennessee

AMOL TAKALKAR, MD
Associate Medical Director, PET Imaging
Center, Biomedical Research Foundation
of Northwest Louisiana; Assistant Professor
of Clinical Radiology, Department of
Radiology, LSUHSC-S, Shreveport,
Louisiana

HONGMING ZHUANG, MD, PhD
Chief, Nuclear Medicine Division, Department of
Radiology, Children's Hospital of Philadelphia;
Associate Professor of Radiology, Hospital of
University of Pennsylvania, Philadelphia,
Pennsylvania

Contents

> Appropriate patient preparation is necessary for high-quality PET and PET/CT imaging in children and adolescents. Standard adult protocols and techniques will sometimes give suboptimal results, so attention to specific pediatric protocols is important. Additionally, attempts should be made to limit radiation doses, as pediatric patients are more sensitive to the effects of radiation. Administered [F-18]2-fluoro-2-deoxyglucose activities may be reduced using weight based protocols, and CT parameters should be reduced to appropriate pediatric levels, with low-dose localization settings used when diagnostic-quality CT images are not needed. Complicating factors, such as patient motion and brown adipose-tissue uptake, are more commonly encountered in pediatric patients, and appropriate measures should be taken to limit their impact on imaging.

> This article discusses and reviews the role and contribution of PET in understanding the structural and functional changes that occur during brain development, and how these changes relate to behavioral and cognitive development in the infant and child. Data regarding various aspects of brain development, such as glucose metabolism, protein synthesis, and maturation and development of neurotransmitter systems will help in understanding the pathogenesis and neurologic basis of various developmental and neurologic disorders. This may help in following disease evolution and progression, planning and development of various therapeutic interventions, timing these interventions and monitoring their responses, and rendering long-term prognostication.

> While rare in adults, central nervous system tumor is the most common solid tumor in childhood and is the leading cause of cancer death in children. Childhood brain tumors are different from those in adults in epidemiology, histologic features, and responses to treatment. Gliomas make up over one-half of all childhood brain tumors. Clinical application of PET imaging in brain tumors has demonstrated that it is helpful in tumor grading, establishing prognosis, defining targets for biopsy, and planning resection. This article emphasizes PET applications in childhood brain tumors, focusing on mainly gliomas with regard to tumor-grading and prognosis, distinguishing tumor recurrence from radiation necrosis, and PET guided diagnosis and treatment.

> Neurofibromatosis type 1 (NF1) is one of the most common tumor predisposition disorders. The role of PET for distinguishing tumor from non-malignant processes,

detecting and grading tumors, evaluating tumor margins, predicting prognosis, directing biopsy, planning treatment, and evaluating response to therapy has been established for a wide variety of benign and malignant tumors. Children with NF1 are particularly at risk for the development of tumors of the peripheral and central nervous system, such as neurofibromas, malignant peripheral nerve sheath tumors, and low-grade astrocytomas of the optic pathway and other brain regions. This article reviews the role of PET in the management of these NF1-associated tumors of childhood.

I-123–metaiodobenzylguanidine (MIBG) is the most commonly used functional imaging agent in patients with neuroblastoma, but use of [F-18]- FDG PET is increasing. MIBG is useful for defining the extent of disease at diagnosis, following response to treatment, and localizing residual and recurrent disease. In early-stage disease, FDG is often better concentrated in tumor sites than MIBG. In all stages, disease extent in the chest, abdomen, and pelvis and local metastases may be better delineated by FDG. In advanced-stage disease, MIBG is superior for following the treatment response of metastatic tumor in the marrow and bone. Several C-11– and F-18–labeled tracers may be equal to or superior to I-123-MIBG if supply problems can be resolved.

Because of the rarity of pediatric bone and soft tissue malignancies, it is difficult to validate the role of emerging imaging technologies in their management. The growing body of literature regarding the use of PET and PET/CT in children supports the continued investigation of this modality in the management of pediatric sarcomas. This article reviews the current literature regarding FDGPET imaging in the management of pediatric sarcomas and presents important pitfalls in PET/CT imaging of these patients that the author, her colleagues, and others have encountered.

Congenital hyperinsulinism is the principle cause of hypoglycemia during infancy but successful treatment is difficult and persistent hypoglycemia carries the risk of neurologic damage. Focal and diffuse abnormalities are the common forms of hyperinsulinism. Identification and localization of focal hyperinsulinism can be cured by partial pancreatectomy. It has been shown that affected pancreatic areas utilize LDOPA in a higher rate than normal pancreatic tissue and, thus, labeling L-DOPA with fluorine-18 (FDOPA) allows functional mapping of hyperinsulinism using PET. This article presents a fundamental overview of the genetics background, pathology, management, and the role of FDOPA-PET imaging in hyperinsulinism.

Cardiac PET imaging can play a significant role in assessing and managing children with congenital and acquired heart disorders but remains largely underused for multiple reasons, not related to the accuracy or usefulness of the modality. Current work focusing on evaluation of cardiac innervation, cardiac receptor function and noninvasive cardiac gene therapy assessment with PET imaging has tremendous potential to revolutionize cardiac evaluation. Awareness and widespread availability of PET systems is expected to increase use of cardiac PET applications in the pediatric population. The advent of integrated PET/CT systems with advanced CT technology and the possible integrated PET/MR imaging systems opens even more promising future possibilities for cardiac evaluation in a one-stop approach.

Ulcerative colitis and Crohn's disease are chronic immune-mediated inflammatory diseases that affect the digestive tract. Major progresses have been made in our comprehension the underlying molecular substrate of these diseases, and therapeutic algorithms have greatly changed over the past decade. In this article, we review the various methods for monitoring the activity of inflammatory bowel disease, with a particular emphasis on [F-18]2-fluoro-2-deoxyglucose PET and PET/CT imaging.

Fever of unknown origin (FUO) is a challenging problem. In children, FUO is critical, as it may hide a life threatening disease. One of the main difficulties in managing patients with FUO is the absence of a universal diagnostic approach. There are many impending causes for FUO. Most cases are attributable to atypical presentations of common diseases. The key to establishing the diagnosis is through comprehensive clinical data and targeted investigations. Despite all efforts, the underlying cause remains undiagnosed in many cases. PET/CT is a powerful modality that has been proven to be useful in many common causes that could emerge as FUO. This article reviews the utility of PET/CT imaging in children with FUO.

Fluorodeoxyglucose (FDG) PET has an ever-increasing role in the management of Hodgkin's and non-Hodgkin's lymphomas, which has been demonstrated in numerous studies in the adult population. In children and adolescents, however, only a limited number of studies have investigated the role of FDG PET in lymphoma. This article reviews the currently available literature on the clinical application of FDG PET in the management of childhood lymphoma. The authors believe that FDG PET (and especially PET/CT) is a valuable imaging modality in the initial diagnosis, response assessment, and post-therapy residual evaluation of Hodgkin's and FDG-avid non-Hodgkin's lymphomas in children and adolescents, and will have a significant impact on the clinical management of pediatric lymphoma.

PET Clinics

THE CLINICS ARE NOW AVAILABLE ONLINE!

Access your subscription at:
www.theclinics.com

GOAL STATEMENT
The goal of the *PET Clinics* is to keep practicing radiologists and radiology residents up to date with current clinical practice in positron emission tomography by providing timely articles reviewing the state of the art in patient care.

ACCREDITATION
PET Clinics is planned and implemented in accordance with the Essential Areas and Policies of the Accreditation Council for Continuing Medical Education (ACCME) through the joint sponsorship of the University of Virginia School of Medicine and Elsevier. The University of Virginia School of Medicine is accredited by the ACCME to provide continuing medical education for physicians.

The University of Virginia School of Medicine designates this educational activity for a maximum of 60 *AMA PRA Category 1 Credits*™. Physicians should only claim credit commensurate with the extent of their participation in the activity.

The American Medical Association has determined that physicians not licensed in the US who participate in this CME activity are eligible for *AMA PRA Category 1 Credits*™.

Category 1 credit can be earned by reading the text material, taking the CME examination online at http://www.theclinics.com/home/cme, and completing the evaluation. After taking the test, you will be required to review any and all incorrect answers. Following completion of the test and evaluation, your credit will be awarded and you may print your certificate.

FACULTY DISCLOSURE/CONFLICT OF INTEREST
The University of Virginia School of Medicine, as an ACCME accredited provider, endorses and strives to comply with the Accreditation Council for Continuing Medical Education (ACCME) Standards of Commercial Support, Commonwealth of Virginia statutes, University of Virginia policies and procedures, and associated federal and private regulations and guidelines on the need for disclosure and monitoring of proprietary and financial interests that may affect the scientific integrity and balance of content delivered in continuing medical education activities under our auspices.

The University of Virginia School of Medicine requires that all CME activities accredited through this institution be developed independently and be scientifically rigorous, balanced and objective in the presentation/discussion of its content, theories and practices.

All authors/editors participating in an accredited CME activity are expected to disclose to the readers relevant financial relationships with commercial entities occurring within the past 12 months (such as grants or research support, employee, consultant, stock holder, member of speakers bureau, etc.). The University of Virginia School of Medicine will employ appropriate mechanisms to resolve potential conflicts of interest to maintain the standards of fair and balanced education to the reader. Questions about specific strategies can be directed to the Office of Continuing Medical Education, University of Virginia School of Medicine, Charlottesville, Virginia.

The faculty and staff of the University of Virginia Office of Continuing Medical Education have no financial affiliations to disclose.

The authors/editors listed below have identified no professional or financial affiliations for themselves or their spouse/partner:
Abass Alavi, MD, MD (Hon), PhD(Hon), DSc(Hon) (Consulting and Guest Editor); Wichana Chamroonrat, MD; Wei Chen, MD, PhD; Gang Cheng, MD; Harry T. Chugani, MD; Barton Dudlick (Acquisitions Editor); Michael J. Fisher, MD; Michael J. Gelfand, MD; Miguel Hernandez-Pampaloni, MD; Mohamed Houseni, MD; Roland Hustinx, MD, PhD; Ajay Kumar, MD, PhD, DNM; Edouard Louis, MD, PhD; M. Beth McCarville, MD; Patrice Rehm, MD (Test Author); Sabah Servaes, MD; Susan E. Sharp, MD; Barry L. Shulkin, MD, MBA; Amol M. Takalkar, MD; and Hongming Zhuang, MD, PhD (Guest Editor).

Disclosure of Discussion of Non-FDA Approved Uses for Pharmaceutical Products and/or Medical Devices.
The University of Virginia School of Medicine, as an ACCME provider, requires that all faculty presenters identify and disclose any off-label uses for pharmaceutical and medical device products. The University of Virginia School of Medicine recommends that each physician fully review all the available data on new products or procedures prior to clinical use.

TO ENROLL
To enroll in the PET Clinics Continuing Medical Education program, call customer service at 1-800-654-2452 or visit us online at www.theclinics.com/home/cme. The CME program is available to subscribers for an additional fee of $175.00.

Preface

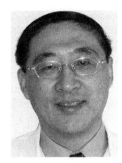
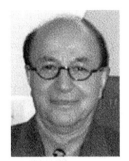

Hongming Zhuang, MD, PhD   Abass Alavi, MD,
                        MD (Hon), PhD (Hon), DSc (Hon)
                        Guest Editors

In the past few years, PET/CT imaging has become an indispensable modality in the evaluation of a variety of pathological processes in the adult population. In particular, PET/CT has played a vital role in the management of patients with a substantial members of malignancies.[1,2] PET imaging is also increasingly playing a major role in the detection of many neurological disorders, such as Alzheimer disease and seizure disorders.[3-5] FDG PET findings have become the gold standard in the determination of myocardial viability.[6] Mismatch between decreased blood flow and increased glucose metabolism demonstrated by FDG, an indicator of myocardial viability, can predict postrevascularization improvement in heart function and long-term survival.[7] Furthermore, PET/CT is emerging as a very valuable modality in the management of many infectious and inflammatory processes.[8]

Compared to the adult population, the literature regarding PET/CT in the management of pediatric patients is just emerging. The role and the importance of PET/CT and PET are becoming clear in the field of pediatrics as more experience is gained in regards to this population. Since pediatric patients are distinct biologically from the adults, many issues that are specific to this population need to be taken into consideration. First, the protocols for PET/CT imaging in pediatric patients differ from adults. Sedation and anesthesia are frequently necessary to achieve optimal diagnostic images. Also, a reduction in radiation dose, an issue which is of concern in the adult population,[9] is ever more critical in pediatric patients. In addition, the tracer biodistribution in pediatric patients is not the same as in adults. For example, thymic uptake is more common and brown adipose tissue activity is more widespread in the pediatric population. More importantly, the types of disease present in the pediatric population differ substantially from those in adults.

Nuclear medicine procedures, including PET and PET/CT, are relatively underutilized in the field of pediatrics. In this issue of *Positron Emission Tomography Clinics*, the current applications of PET and PET/CT in the pediatric population are reviewed. Although most reviews have focused on the applications of PET and PET/CT in the evaluation of pediatric malignancies such as sarcomas and lymphomas, other potential applications of FDG PET in the pediatric population, such as detection of the source of fever of unknown origin, are also discussed. Finally, the high sensitivity and accuracy of F-DOPA PET/CT imaging in the identifying and localizing focal lesion in child suffering congenital hyperinsulinism are discussed. It is our belief that the list of applications of PET and PET/CT for probating diseases and disorders will surely increase in the coming years.

Hongming Zhuang, MD, PhD
Associate Professor or Radiology
University of Pennsylvania School of Medicine
Chief of Division of Nuclear Medicine
Department of Radiology
The Childrens Hospital of Philadelphia
Philadelphia, PA, USA

PET Clin 3 (2009) xi–xii
doi:10.1016/j.cpet.2009.06.002
1556-8598/09/$ – see front matter © 2009 Elsevier Inc. All rights reserved.

Abass Alavi, MD,
MD (Hon), PhD (Hon), DSc (Hon)
Professor of Radiology
Director of Research Education
Department of Radiology
Hospital of the University of Pennsylvania
Philadelphia, PA, USA

E-mail addresses:
zhuang@email.chop.edu (H. Zhuang)
abass.alavi@uphs.upenn.edu (A. Alavi)

REFERENCES

1. Bockisch A, Freudenberg LS, Schmidt D, et al. Hybrid imaging by SPECT/CT and PET/CT: proven outcomes in cancer imaging. Semin Nucl Med 2009;39(4):276–89.
2. De Wever W, Coolen J, Verschakelen JA. Integrated PET/CT and cancer imaging. Jbr-Btr 2009;92(1):13–9.
3. Foster NL, Heidebrink JL, Clark CM, et al. FDG-PET improves accuracy in distinguishing frontotemporal dementia and Alzheimer's disease. Brain 2007; 130(Pt 10):2616–35.
4. Coleman RE. Positron emission tomography diagnosis of Alzheimer's disease. Neuroimaging Clin N Am 2005;15(4):837–46, x.
5. Alavi A, Hirsch LJ. Studies of central nervous system disorders with single photon emission computed tomography and positron emission tomography: evolution over the past 2 decades. Semin Nucl Med 1991;21(1):58–81.
6. Chacko GN. PET imaging in cardiology. Hell J Nucl Med 2005;8(3):140–4.
7. Ghesani M, Depuey EG, Rozanski A. Role of F-18 FDG positron emission tomography (PET) in the assessment of myocardial viability. Echocardiography 2005; 22(2):165–77.
8. Zhuang H, Alavi A. 18-fluorodeoxyglucose positron emission tomographic imaging in the detection and monitoring of infection and inflammation. Semin Nucl Med 2002;32(1):47–59.
9. Brenner DJ, Hall EJ. Computed tomography–an increasing source of radiation exposure. N Engl J Med 2007;357(22):2277–84.

Patient Preparation and Performance of PET/CT Scans in Pediatric Patients

Michael J. Gelfand, MD[a,b,*], Susan E. Sharp, MD[a,b]

KEYWORDS
- Patient preparation • Artifacts • PET/CT
- Imaging protocols • Dose reduction

PET/CT has had a significant impact on the diagnosis and treatment of oncologic diseases in children and adolescents. [F-18]2-fluoro-2-deoxy-glucose (FDG) PET/CT imaging has been useful in lymphoma, neuroblastoma, and many sarcomas, including osteogenic sarcoma, Ewing sarcoma, and rhabdomyosarcoma.[1–5] FDG-PET has also been useful in the evaluation of children with intractable epilepsy who are being considered for surgical ablation of their seizure focus.[6]

If adult techniques and protocols are used for PET/CT scans in pediatric patients, some of the scans that are acquired will be of suboptimal quality. With appropriate attention to the imaging needs of children and adolescents, optimal quality PET/CT imaging can almost always be achieved. This article reviews patient preparation and appropriate design of pediatric PET/CT protocols.

CREATING A SAFE CLINICAL ENVIRONMENT FOR IMAGING

Pediatric emergency equipment and supplies must be provided and maintained wherever pediatric examinations are performed. This is especially important if PET/CT scanners are located in adult hospitals or imaging centers. Available equipment and supplies must include pediatric resuscitation equipment (including airway and intubation supplies), intravenous supplies, and suction supplies. Personnel should have appropriate training in pediatric resuscitation. Emergency drugs should be supplied, with charts of appropriate pediatric doses. If a mobile imaging trailer is used, pediatric supplies and equipment must be taken to the mobile unit. Oxygen and suction must also be immediately available, if not already supplied, in the mobile imaging trailer.

PATIENT PREPARATION

For FDG-PET/CT body imaging, pediatric patients should have nothing by mouth for 4 hours before administration of FDG. In addition, no glucose should be infused during the 4-hour period before FDG administration if the study is performed to evaluate patients with suspected or known malignancies. When oral contrast is part of the preparative regimen for CT, only artificially sweetened contrast should be used. If the patient eats, receives intravenous glucose, or is given sugar containing oral contrast during this 4-hour period, the patient will secrete insulin; this will increase the amount of FDG entering skeletal muscle and therefore degrade image quality.

Plasma glucose should be tested before the study. However, in contrast to adult patients, elevated fasting-glucose levels are very uncommon in pediatric oncology patients. If the patient has type I diabetes, the patient's physician

[a] Nuclear Medicine Section, Department of Radiology, Cincinnati Children's Hospital Medical Center, MLC 5031, 3333 Burnet Avenue, Cincinnati, OH 45229-3039, USA
[b] Department of Radiology, University of Cincinnati, 231 Albert Sabin Way, Cincinnati, OH 45267-0761, USA
* Corresponding author. Department of Radiology, University of Cincinnati, 231 Albert Sabin Way, Cincinnati, OH 45267-0761, USA.
E-mail address: michael.gelfand@cchmc.org (M.J. Gelfand).

PET Clin 3 (2009) 473–485
doi:10.1016/j.cpet.2009.04.001

should be consulted for appropriate management of oral intake and insulin administration. For cardiac imaging with FDG, a different approach is followed to enhance cardiac-muscle FDG uptake, as described in the section, "FDG Myocardial Imaging." FDG brain imaging protocols are also discussed separately in the subsection "FDG brain imaging for intractable epilepsy," later in this article.

At the authors' institution, PET body imaging is begun 50 to 60 minutes after FDG injection. The time when imaging is started is based on available adult tumor uptake data, but unfortunately these data are based on adult tumors that are quite dissimilar to pediatric solid tumors.[7]

If the patient is too young to hold still and cooperate with imaging, sedation will be needed. When sedation is given, it is administered immediately before imaging. Sedation protocols vary from hospital to hospital, and sedation practice should conform to the individual hospital's regulations. Oral intake is restricted for up to 8 hours before sedation. However, some sedation protocols permit intake of clear liquids up to 2 hours before sedation in infants; in this case, the more stringent 4-hour restriction on glucose intake should be followed as closely as possible.

As with adults, patients should not engage in strenuous exercise for 48 hours before the PET/CT scan; muscles that have been heavily exercised may continue to have increased glucose utilization for at least 24 hours. Patients should also lie still during the period from FDG injection until imaging is started to avoid uptake in skeletal muscle. Even nonstrenuous activity during the uptake period can result in FDG activity in muscle.

Patients should void immediately before imaging. If there is high activity of FDG in the bladder at the time of imaging, "star artifacts" may be seen on axial images through the bladder. Protocols exist in adults that minimize the amount of bladder activity, but these have not been evaluated in children. If part of the injected activity is infiltrated at the intravenous site or if more than a trivial amount of activity is left behind in an injection port, a similar "star artifact" will be seen on axial images at the level of the infiltration site.

TIMING OF FDG IMAGING IN RELATION TO CHEMOTHERAPY

Multidrug chemotherapy in pediatric oncology usually involves multiple courses of chemotherapeutic agents separated by rest periods that allow the patient's marrow elements to recover. For example, in a commonly used protocol for pediatric intermediate-risk Hodgkin's disease, a course of chemotherapy consists of six drugs that are given over 8 days; then there is then a rest period of 13 days before the next course of chemotherapy is administered. A total of four cycles of chemotherapy are given. Successful therapy of Hodgkin's disease will often result in complete disappearance of all FDG tumor uptake during the first course of chemotherapy, with no reappearance of tumor uptake during the remainder of treatment or during the follow-up period.[8]

Whenever possible, it is suggested that FDG-PET/CT be performed shortly before a course of chemotherapy is scheduled to begin. FDG uptake during the first days of a course of chemotherapy may underestimate disease extent before the course of chemotherapy, and may not give an accurate picture of the amount of tumor that remains viable after the course of the chemotherapy. In an adult study, FDG uptake at 20 days after chemotherapy gave a more accurate representation of the effectiveness of chemotherapy than FDG uptake shortly after the onset of chemotherapy.[9] In some pediatric chemotherapy protocols, there are no rest periods in-between courses of chemotherapy, with some chemotherapy given every week. In these protocols, FDG-PET/CT imaging should be performed shortly before the next weekly round of chemotherapy. In tumors that respond slowly, the effect of chemotherapy on FDG uptake is usually less dramatic, and FDG imaging is clinically effective even if performed between two closely spaced rounds of chemotherapy.

Cell stimulating factors, including granulocyte cell stimulating factor (G-CSF), will cause a marked increase in FDG localization in normal bone marrow, as demonstrated in **Fig. 1**. Unfortunately, if there is a focal metastasis in bone marrow, it may be obscured by confluent-intense marrow stimulated by G-CSF. This is rarely a problem with lymphoma, as focal metastases in areas that contain hematopoetic marrow are uncommon after initial treatment, but it may be a problem in patients with other tumors, such as neuroblastoma.[10] This potential problem often can be avoided by scheduling FDG imaging just before the next scheduled course of chemotherapy. Unfortunately, at this time the PET imaging literature does not indicate how many days should elapse between the last dose of a cell stimulating factor and attempted FDG imaging. Experimental work in animals indicates that the amount of FDG uptake in bone marrow increases with both increasing doses and repeated administration of cell stimulating factors.[11,12]

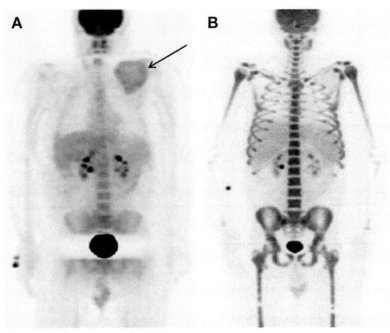

Fig. 1. FDG-PET maximum-intensity projection (MIP) images in an adolescent boy with Ewing sarcoma. (A) Image obtained at diagnosis shows uptake in the primary left scapular tumor (arrow.) (B) Image obtained after chemotherapy and G-CSF administration shows a reduction in tumor uptake of FDG and markedly increased uptake throughout the bone marrow related to G-CSF.

PREVENTION OF FDG UPTAKE IN BROWN ADIPOSE TISSUE

FDG uptake in brown adipose tissue on PET and PET/CT has been recognized since 2002. In 1996, FDG uptake in brown adipose tissue was first noted adjacent to the costovertebral junctions, but at that time the uptake was attributed to muscle tension.[13] In 2002, Hany and colleagues[14] used PET/CT to demonstrate that the FDG uptake sometimes seen in the supraclavicular regions and adjacent to the costovertebral junctions corresponded to fat density. In the same year, uptake of I-123-metaiodobenzylguanidine, sometimes seen in the neck and shoulders, was also demonstrated to be related to cold exposure, and autoradiography in mice demonstrated that this uptake was in brown adipose tissue.[15] Prior to FDG-PET/CT, brown adipose tissue was believed to completely involute during infancy. PET/CT has shown this belief to be incorrect, with FDG uptake in brown adipose tissue seen as late as the sixth decade of life. Prominent brown adipose-tissue uptake has been observed in 25% to 30% of pediatric patients in both cold and warm climates, not only in winter but also in summer.[16,17] The intensity of cold stress seems to determine which regions of brown adipose tissue are activated. FDG uptake first appears in the posterior cervical and supraclavicular regions, followed by appearance of activity in the costovertebral regions. With the greatest levels of cold stress, activity appears in the suboccipital regions and mediastinum.[16] The typical distribution of brown-fat activity in an adolescent or young adult is shown in Fig. 2. However, the brown-fat distribution in the pediatric patient is generally more extensive.

Many sites of brown-fat uptake occur in areas that are rich in lymph nodes. This is a particular problem in children and adolescents with lymphoma, as lymph nodes that are frequently involved in lymphoma are found in very close proximity to sites where brown adipose-tissue activation occurs; and this is particularly true in the posterior cervical regions, supraclavicular regions, and mediastinum. Some have argued that PET/CT can be used to differentiate FDG uptake in brown adipose tissue from FDG uptake in lymph nodes. Although PET/CT can be useful in differentiating between FDG uptake in lymph nodes and brown adipose tissue, this approach has significant limitations. Small amounts of patient movement (as little as 2 mm–3 mm) between the CT and PET acquisitions will result in misplacement of foci of FDG uptake on the fused, coregistered CT images, with possible misplacement of FDG uptake over lymph nodes on fused images. FDG-PET images

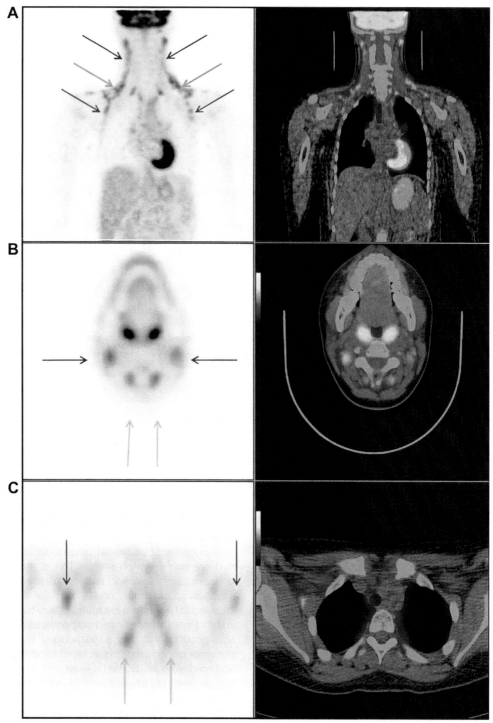

Fig. 2. FDG uptake in brown adipose tissue. (*A*) On coronal images, there is FDG uptake in brown adipose tissue in the posterior cervical (*blue arrows*), supraclavicular (*green arrows*), and axillary (*red arrows*) regions. (*B*) On axial images, there is FDG uptake in brown adipose tissue in posterior cervical (*blue arrows*) and suboccipital (*orange arrows*) regions. (*C*) On axial images, there is FDG uptake in brown adipose tissue in axillary (*red arrows*) and cost-overtebral junction (*orange arrows*) regions. On all fused PET/CT images, there is slight misregistration of PET and CT because of patient movement.

also have lower resolution than CT images, resulting in FDG foci appearing somewhat larger than they actually are; FDG uptake in brown adipose tissue may, therefore, appear to overlap uninvolved lymph nodes.

There is often uncertainty about the significance of a focus of FDG uptake that appears to correspond to a lymph node that measures less than 1 cm (below the size threshold that raises clinical concern for malignancy on CT). An important aspect of the increased sensitivity of PET over conventional imaging in lymphoma is its ability to detect involved lymph nodes that measure less than 1 cm. If there is apparent FDG uptake in a subcentimeter lymph node, the question is whether the FDG uptake is because of neoplastic involvement or because of a tiny rest of brown adipose tissue adjacent to the lymph node. There is much less uncertainty if FDG uptake in brown adipose tissue is well blocked by appropriate patient preparation. If FDG uptake in brown adipose tissue is adequately blocked, the risk of false-negative and false-positive observations is reduced. Finally, PET and PET/CT scans are much easier and faster to read if there is no brown-fat uptake on the scan. An example of complicating brown-fat activity is shown in **Fig. 3**.

Two approaches have been used to successfully block cold stimulation of brown adipose tissue. The simplest approach is to warm the patient and avoid cold stimulation. Patients can be asked to dress warmly (more warmly than required by the outside temperature) and to turn down the automobile air conditioning on the way to the hospital or PET center. Patients can then be held in a warm room or warmed with preheated blankets for 30 to 60 minutes before FDG injection. One study kept patients in a 25°C (77°F) holding room for 30 to 60 minutes, with a marked decrease in the frequency of significant brown adipose-tissue uptake on subsequent FDG-PET scans.[17] It is important to remember that patients must be warmed before FDG injection; warming after FDG injection is ineffective.

The second approach is to pharmacologically block FDG uptake in brown adipose tissue. Several drugs block transmission of cold-receptor impulses through the hypothalamus and abolish postoperative shivering; these drugs are potentially useful as blocking agents of cold-induced FDG uptake in brown adipose tissue. The initial report in 1996 suggested that oral diazepam can be used to block FDG uptake in brown adipose tissue, and diazepam and other benzdiazopines have been used in adults.[13] Opiates are considered to be more effective blockers of cold-induced impulse transmission through the hypothalamus than benzdiazopines. Fentanyl has been used successfully in school-aged children and adolescents.[16] Another approach that has been validated in animals and described in adults is pretreatment with the beta-blocker propranolol.[18–20] Of interest, one report states that nicotine and ephedrine enhance uptake of FDG in brown adipose tissue, so these drugs should be avoided.[21]

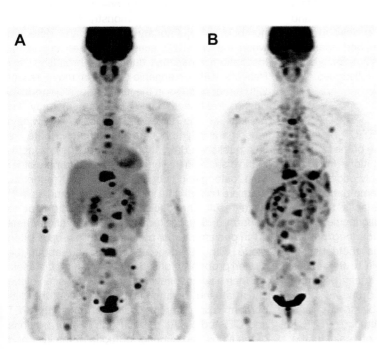

Fig. 3. FDG-PET MIP images in a young woman with multiple metastases. (*A*) Initial image shows uptake in multiple metastatic foci within the spine, pelvis, and proximal long bones. (*B*) Follow-up image again shows uptake in multiple metastatic foci, but interpretation is complicated by significant amounts of FDG uptake in mediastinal, costovertebral, retroperitoneal (perinephric), lateral abdominal wall, and diaphragmatic brown adipose tissue.

Almost all of the studies that describe blockade of FDG uptake in brown adipose tissue by prewarming or pharmacologic means suffer from serious design deficiencies. In most studies, patients with FDG uptake in brown adipose tissue were studied again after prewarming or pharmacologic intervention. This study design introduces obvious biases. Subsequently it was observed that patients, in the absence of intervention, will have FDG uptake in brown adipose tissue on one study and no FDG uptake on another study, in either order.[22] Two studies in pediatric patients, mentioned above, used a different design, and looked at separate cohorts of patients who either received an intervention or no intervention before FDG administration. In one study, the intervention was pretreatment with fentanyl 10 minutes prior FDG injection.[16] In the other, the intervention was warming the patient for 30 to 60 minutes in a temperature-controlled room at 25°C.[17] In both cases, the frequency of significant FDG uptake in brown adipose tissue was decreased from a range of 25% to 30% to a range of 5% to 10%.

DESIGN OF IMAGING PROTOCOLS

CT and PET are complex imaging modalities. Bringing the two technologies together in a single scanner keeps the complexity of each modality and adds a number of additional complexities that are uniquely related to the fusion of the two technologies. Design of imaging protocols must take in account, not only the usual protocol design considerations of PET and CT, but also artifact prevention in the combined PET/CT study and minimization of absorbed radiation dose in children and adolescents who are imaged. Many of the PET/CT protocol design questions have been discussed in adults by Beyer and colleagues.[23]

SCOPE OF THE EXAMINATION

In adult nuclear medicine, most PET/CT examinations image the body from the base of the brain to the upper thighs; PET/CT examinations from the base of the brain to the feet are only occasionally performed, for example, in melanoma patients. In children and adolescents, metastases to bone occur in a large number of malignancies. The metastases are often located in the long bones, occurring most frequently in the metaphyses. Imaging from the base of the brain to the ankles should be performed routinely in many pediatric malignancies, particularly those prone to bone metastases, such as neuroblastoma and sarcomas. At the authors' institution PET/CT scans are performed from base of brain to the thighs only in selected oncology patients with lymphoma, limited to patients who have had negative PET/CT scans of the lower extremities in the past. Other oncology patients receive PET/CT scans from the base of the brain to the ankles.

AVOIDING ARTIFACTS RELATED TO ATTENUATION CORRECTION AND MISREGISTRATION OF PET AND CT IMAGES

Misregistration and attenuation-correction artifacts occur when an organ or body part is not in the same position during the CT and PET acquisitions, or when the radiodensity of an organ or body part changes significantly between the CT and PET acquisitions. If the patient cannot hold still from the start of the CT acquisition through the end of PET acquisition, appropriate sedation or general anesthesia must be arranged; appropriate no-oral-intake status for sedation or general anesthesia must also be anticipated, as previously discussed. Nothing-taken-by-mouth instructions must be clearly communicated to the patient's parents so that the PET/CT study and sedation or general anesthesia do not have to be rescheduled because of prohibited oral intake.

Artifacts related to respiratory motion are often difficult to eliminate. A multidetector CT scan can be acquired rapidly during a breath-hold. In contrast, a PET acquisition must be acquired during normal tidal respiration because of the long imaging time. A diagnostic-quality CT scan of the chest is best acquired during full inspiration. Several studies, including one in pediatric and adolescent patients, demonstrate that larger numbers of pulmonary nodules are detected when the chest CT scan is acquired during full inspiration rather than during free breathing.[24–29] Patients with osteogenic sarcoma may present with tumor nodules in the lung or develop nodules during treatment. Lung involvement may be present at the time of diagnosis in Ewing's sarcoma and lymphoma. Unfortunately, there are little published data about the frequency of metastatic disease in the lung at relapse of tumors other than osteogenic sarcoma. Even in lymphoma, there are limited data in only two adult studies.[30,31] As a result, the decision of whether or not to perform a diagnostic-quality full-inspiration chest CT in pediatric tumor patients at follow-up is often made without adequate information about the a priori probability of finding new lung metastases.

When a full-inspiration diagnostic CT scan of the chest is used for attenuation correction, the diaphragm is in different positions during the PET and CT studies. As a result, the inferior portions of the lungs and superior portions of the liver and spleen will be in different positions on the PET and CT scans. In an adolescent patient, the position of the diaphragm may be up to 4-cm lower on the full-inspiration CT scan than on the PET scan obtained during tidal respiration. If the CT scan is used for attenuation correction, the most superior portions of the liver will "disappear" on the attenuation correction PET scan because "incorrect" attenuation correction values corresponding to the radiodensity of the lungs are being used for portions of the liver near the diaphragm. Lesions with increased FDG uptake may become difficult to see or disappear on attenuation-corrected PET images, as shown in **Fig. 4**. Artifacts may occur along the diaphragm. For these reasons, a full-inspiration CT scan cannot be used for attenuation correction of PET images acquired at tidal respiration.[32–34]

The best match in the position of the diaphragm between CT and PET occurs when the CT is acquired during end-tidal respiration.[35] A breath-hold at end-tidal inspiration has been suggested as the optimal breath-hold maneuver during CT acquisition; however, in the authors' institution, there has been limited success with pediatric patients holding the diaphragm and chest in end-tidal respiration during the CT portion of the study. Even with practice before the study, some patients try to sneak in a quick breath and a full-inspiration

CT scan is inadvertently acquired. As a result, the authors' have chosen to image patients throughout the entire PET/CT study during normal tidal respiration.

Because of attenuation-correction artifacts, if the PET/CT scan is used to generate optimal diagnostic-quality CT images for anatomic diagnosis, the chest must be imaged twice, once during tidal respiration in conjunction with the PET scan and again during full inspiration to maximize nodule detection. The amount of increased radiation exposure from the second acquisition of the chest CT can be limited to a relatively low additional dose, because the volume that is reimaged is considerably less than the entire CT acquisition and because some reduction in exposure settings is possible for the repeat diagnostic CT of the air containing lungs.[36–39] A review of the problems associated with respiratory motion was recently published by Daou.[40]

If the CT scan used for attenuation correction is obtained immediately after bolus-contrast injection, there may be incorrect attenuation correction over the path of the intravenous contrast. Dense contrast in a vascular structure during CT acquisition (later to be used to calculate the attenuation-correction matrix) will have dissipated by the time of the PET scan. There will be over-correction of the actual amount of attenuation and an

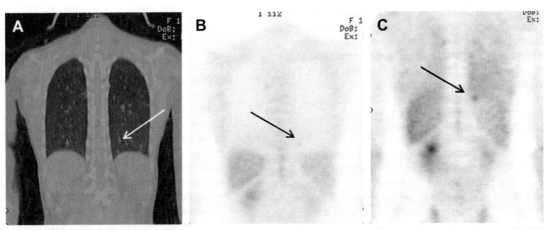

Fig. 4. Mismatch of diaphragmatic position on PET and CT. (*A*) Localization CT scan of the chest fused with PET images demonstrates a nodule in the left lower lobe (*small faint area of reddish color at the tip of the white arrow*). The nodule appears to lie above the diaphragm. The patient was asked to hold end-tidal expiration during acquisition, but instead held partial to full inspiration. (*B*) The same attenuation-corrected PET acquired during tidal respiration displayed without fused CT images. Because PET and CT images were acquired at different phases of respiration (CT at partial to full inspiration, and PET during tidal breathing), uptake in the nodule and nearby liver on nonattenuation-corrected images is artifactually decreased and the nodule is misplaced (*black arrow*) with respect to the diaphragm. (*C*) Nonattenuation-corrected PET. The nodule is now more clearly seen at the level of the diaphragm (*black arrow*). The entire liver is now visualized. (*Reprinted from* Gelfand MJ. Dosimetry of FDG PET/CT and other molecular imaging applications in pediatric patients. Pediatr Radiol 2009;39(S1):S46–56; with permission.)

artifactual hot-spot will appear on attenuation-corrected PET images corresponding to the location of the vessel. When this occurs, the nonattenuation-corrected images should be reviewed, as they will not have this artifact. Some people feel that intravenous contrast does not affect the PET imaging qualitatively, nor does it have a very significant quantitative effect on the measurement of standardized uptake value. Artifacts because of oral soluble contrast are also possible, but they are rarely clinically significant.[41,42] However, this opinion has not been uniformly accepted at the present time.

RADIATION DOSE AND ADMINISTERED ACTIVITY FOR PET

A recent survey indicated that there is a little variation in administered FDG activities at North American children's hospitals. Typical administered activities in children and adolescents were 0.14 mCi/kg to 0.15 mCi/kg (5.18 MBq/kg–5.55 MBq/kg). An administered activity of 0.14 mCi/kg (5.18 MBq/kq) corresponds to an administered activity of 9.8 mCi (363 mBq) in a 70-kg adult. The effective dose to the patient from this administered activity varies with age from 0.50 rem (5 mSv) in a 1 year old to 0.87 rem (8.7 mSv) in a 15 year old.[43–45] PET/CT scanners sold today are capable of three-dimensional (3D) imaging, which provides much greater sensitivity than 2D imaging, but at a somewhat increased noise level. For 2D PET scanners, typical imaging times are 5 minutes per bed position. With a 3D scanner, imaging time can be decreased. An alternative that may be considered to reduce radiation dose is keeping the time per bed position at 5 minutes and reducing the administered activity for studies acquired in 3D mode.

RADIATION DOSIMETRY AND DESIGN OF THE CT-IMAGING PROTOCOL

Prior to 2000, pediatric diagnostic CT studies were usually performed with adult CT exposure settings and were not modified for patient size. CT exposure settings were based on the X-ray flux needed to obtain the highest quality imaging study in adults. CT imaging settings did not take into account a number of important factors in children:

- Infants, children, and to a lesser extent adolescents, are more susceptible to the carcinogenic effects of radiation than middle-aged or elderly adults.[46,47]
- Data published in 1996 from atom bomb survivors who were exposed as children indicated the risks of radiation exposure were larger than previously estimated,

because the increased risk of cancer from exposure to ionizing radiation was found to persist into middle age.[46,47]
- If CT imaging parameters are kept constant, the amount of radiation absorbed by the patient increases as patient size decreases.[48–50]

With a moderate reduction in CT imaging parameters, the diagnostic utility of the images is not affected by the small amounts of image noise that are introduced.[36,39,51–53] As these factors were recognized, particularly during the first few years of this decade, a major effort was made to educate the radiology community about the need to use the lowest radiation dose for CT in children and adolescents that was consistent with quality imaging.[54–57] Subsequent surveys have indicated that education led to more appropriate practice, with widespread reduction in CT-exposure parameters used in clinical practice.[58]

PET/CT scanners use CT data to calculate the attenuation-correction matrix for each axial section. The needed CT data can be obtained with any of the following three approaches:

- A diagnostic quality CT scan is acquired. Appropriate pediatric CT exposure parameters are used for the diagnostic CT scan, instead of adult exposure parameters very often used before 2000.
- A localization-CT scan is acquired. The CT images are adequate for localization of abnormal areas of radiopharmaceutic uptake, but the images are of lower quality than the diagnostic quality images obtained in the first alternative. Although a considerable amount of anatomic pathology can be recognized on these images, it is important to repeatedly caution clinicians that localization-CT images should not be considered to be a substitute for diagnostic-quality CT images.
- A very low-dose attenuation-only scan is acquired. No diagnostic information can be obtained from the CT images because of extremely poor image quality, but the X-ray flux is large enough to create attenuation-correction matrices for all axial sections.

A typical effective dose for a diagnostic CT scan of the neck, chest, abdomen, and pelvis using appropriate pediatric CT exposure parameters is about 1.2 rem to 1.4 rem (12 mSv–14 mSv) (see Appendix I). Dose modulation, which adjusts the mA to the thickness of the patient along the direction of the X-ray beam as the CT tube rotates, can reduce radiation exposure without a reduction in image quality. The reduction in effective dose when dose modulation is used is usually about 25% to 35%.

For localization-CT scans, CT-exposure parameters are deliberately reduced. Image quality may be reduced, particularly when the CT scan is viewed at soft-tissue windows. If arms or shoulders are in the field, they may create streak artifact, as demonstrated in **Fig. 5**. Dose modulation may be effective in preserving image quality at lower exposure settings, as well as reducing effective dose and reducing streak artifact. CT-exposure parameters should be kept high enough that lymph nodes and other small structures are clearly identified. Reduction of effective dose of 50% to 65% is possible when compared with appropriate, already reduced pediatric diagnostic-CT parameters. In addition, streak artifacts may also be significantly reduced by imaging from the base of the brain to the shoulders with the arms down, and separately imaging the chest, abdomen, and pelvis with the arms up, with enough overlap to ensure the shoulders and proximal humerii are within the field of view of one of the scans.

The localization scan should not be considered to be a replacement for a high quality diagnostic-CT scan. As stated earlier, a tidal respiration diagnostic-CT scan can be performed in conjunction with the PET scan, but if a full-inspiration diagnostic-CT scan is needed to detect pulmonary nodules, the chest CT will need to be repeated at full inspiration.

Fahey and colleagues[59] determined the minimal CT settings needed to obtain attenuation correction data without imaging. For infants and school-aged children, the required CT exposure parameters were very low: for example, 80 kVp, 5 mAs, 1.5:1 pitch. For larger teenagers, the voltage potential was increased to 120 kVp.

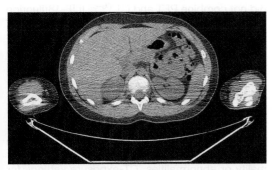

Fig. 5. Axial localization CT image acquired with low-dose technique. Streak artifact is seen from the patient's arms. (*Reprinted from* Gelfand MJ, Lemen LC. PET/CT and SPECT/CT Dosimetry in children: the challenge to the pediatric imager. Semin Nucl Med 2007;37(5): 394; with permission.)

When exposure settings were further reduced, some noise was introduced into the attenuation-corrected images.

Table 1 indicates some possible PET/CT protocols and the absorbed radiation doses associated with these protocols.

FDG-PET STUDIES LESS COMMONLY PERFORMED IN CHILDREN AND ADOLESCENTS
FDG Myocardial Imaging

Preparation for PET imaging of the myocardium uses a glucose load to stimulate insulin production and increase myocardial uptake of FDG. In the authors' experience, complicated protocols that involve administration of both glucose and insulin do not appear to be necessary in children and adolescents. In a limited number of patients, the authors have used a simple protocol to increase insulin levels and "force" FDG into viable myocardium. In the authors' experience to date, an appropriate glucose load 2 hours before FDG injection has been all that was needed to adequately enhance FDG uptake in myocardium.

FDG Brain Imaging for Intractable Epilepsy

FDG brain imaging has been useful in the evaluation of patients with intractable seizures. Use of multiple imaging modalities, including interictal FDG-PET, ictal and interictal SPECT using Tc-99m cerebral-blood flow agents, quantitative analysis of these methods, MR imaging, PET/MR imaging fusion, and functional MR imaging all have an important role in the identification of the epileptogenic zone and in surgical planning.[60,61]

At the authors' institution, 0.10 mCi/kg of F-18-FDG (3.7 MBq/kg) is injected, although larger administered activities of 0.14 mCi/kg of F-18-FDG (5.2 MBq/kg) are used at many institutions.[61,62] Typical waiting time from injection to the start of imaging is 40 minutes. During this time interval, the patient should lie quietly in a partially darkened quiet room. Imaging is generally performed for 5 to 10 minutes in 3D mode.[62]

FDG Imaging for Inflammatory Bowel Disease in Children and Adolescents

FDG imaging of inflammatory bowel disease in children and adolescents has been described by Loeffler and colleagues.[63] In a retrospective analysis of 26 FDG-PET scans from 23 pediatric patients with suspected inflammatory bowel disease, Loeffler and colleagues found that FDG-PET showed a sensitivity, specificity, and accuracy of 98%, 68%, and 83%, respectively, as

Table 1
Estimated effective dose for PET/CT protocols

Protocol	Effective Dose
Protocol 1: Diagnostic CT followed by PET/localization CT	
Diagnostic CT with contrast (full inspiration, neck to pubis) followed by PET/CT (with localization CT) without contrast (tidal breathing, base of brain to pubis)	1.35 rem–2.16 rem
Protocol 2: PET/diagnostic CT	
PET/CT (with diagnostic CT) with contrast (tidal breathing, base of brain to pubis)	1.0 rem–1.6 rem
Protocol 3: PET/diagnostic CT, repeat full-inspiration diagnostic-chest CT	
PET/CT (with diagnostic CT) with contrast (tidal breathing, neck to pubis) followed by Diagnostic CT (full inspiration, chest only)	1.25 rem–2.0 rem
Protocol 4: PET/attenuation correction only CT	
PET/CT (attenuation correction only; that is, no imaging) without contrast (tidal breathing, any field of view, for example, brain)	0.35 rem–0.56 rem

Assumptions used in calculations:
1. Diagnostic exposure CT settings are those used at the authors' hospital.[56]
2. For the localization-CT scan, the pediatric diagnostic CT-exposure settings were reduced by 65%.
3. The assumed administered activity of FDG is 0.14 mCi/kg (5.18 MBq/kg).
Data from Gelfand MJ, Lemen LC. PET/CT and SPECT/CT Dosimetry in children: the challenge to the pediatric imager. Semin Nucl Med 2007;37(5):391–8; and ImPACT. Available at: impactscan.org. London.

compared with endoscopy (90%, 75%, and 82%, respectively) and ultrasound (56%, 92%, and 75%, respectively). For the small bowel, FDG-PET was even more reliable (100%, 86%, and 90%, respectively). The investigators concluded that, because of its high sensitivity and accuracy, FDG-PET is an excellent, noninvasive diagnostic tool for inflammatory bowel disease, especially in the pediatric patient population.[63]

[F-18] Fluoride Bone Imaging

[F-18] Fluoride was the first radiopharmaceutic used to image bone, but with the development or the Tc-99m-phosphate and diphosphonate radiopharmaceutics and improvements in gamma-camera technology, [F-18]fluoride fell into disuse. The recent growth of FDG-PET imaging in oncology has led to wide availability of high-quality PET imaging equipment. Studies that compared [F-18]fluoride PET bone imaging with Tc-99m-diphosphonate imaging in adults have demonstrated improved spatial resolution and improved sensitivity for the detection of metastases when [F-18]fluoride PET was used.[64,65]

Lim and others investigators[66–68] demonstrated the utility of [F-18]fluoride PET bone imaging in children and adolescents with back pain not associated with malignancy. Very high-resolution images were obtained, aided by the inherently tomographic nature of the technique. They determined some of the study parameters appropriate for [F-18]fluoride PET bone imaging, as follows:

> An administered activity of [F-18]sodium fluoride of 0.055 mCi/kg (2.1 Mbq/kg) has been suggested, which yields an effective dose of 0.31 mrem to 0.35 mrem (3.1 mSv–3.5 mSv), comparable to the effective dose of bone scintigraphy.
>
> Imaging can begin at 30 minutes after injection.

These investigators had a PET-only scanner and did not combine PET and CT.[66–69] If [F-18]fluoride PET bone imaging is performed on a PET/CT scanner, it is possible to obtain PET imaging information with an effective dose that is close to the effective dose of [F-18]fluoride PET alone, when the [F-18]fluoride PET bone scan can be performed with attenuation-only non-imaging CT scan. If needed, areas that are abnormal on [F-18]fluoride PET bone imaging can be reimaged with coregistered PET/CT imaging, limiting the volume reimaged to the region of the PET abnormality or abnormalities. CT-exposure settings for this limited repeat imaging can be at localization settings, or at pediatric diagnostic when precise anatomic information about adjacent soft tissue is required. If only bone anatomic information is needed, the low-dose localization-CT scan viewed at bone windows may be of adequate quality for CT bone imaging.

APPENDIX I: CHANGES IN ABSORBED-RADIATION DOSE ASSOCIATED WITH CHANGES IN CT IMAGING PARAMETERS

kVp: If 120 kVp is assigned a relative dose level of 100 and other exposure parameters are kept constant, at other kVp settings, the relative absorbed-radiation doses will be: The relationship between kVp and absorbed-radiation dose is exponential.

mA: There is a linear relationship between mA and absorbed-radiation dose. A 100% increase

kVp	Relative absorbed radiation dose
80	32
100	63
120	100
140	143

in mA will result in a 100% increase absorbed-radiation dose.

mAs: mAs is the product of time per rotation (in seconds) and mA. A 100% increase in mAs will result in a 100% increase in absorbed-radiation dose.

Rotation time: There is a linear relationship between time per rotation and absorbed-radiation dose. For PET/CT, usually 0.5 or 0.8 seconds per rotation is used.

Pitch: The tightness of the spiral of the CT scanner is called pitch; a lower pitch implies a tighter spiral and a higher absorbed-radiation dose if all other parameters are kept constant. The absorbed-radiation dose is also dependent upon the characteristics of the individual model of CT scanner and slice thickness.

Data from Refs; with permission.[59,70,71]

REFERENCES

1. Kushner BH, Yeung HW, Larson SM, et al. Extending positron emission tomography scan utility to high-risk neuroblastoma: fluorine-18 fluorodeoxyglucose positron emission tomography as sole imaging modality in follow-up of patients. J Clin Oncol 2001;19(14):3397–405.

2. McCarville MB, Christie R, Daw NC, et al. PET/CT in the evaluation of childhood sarcomas. Am J Roentgenol 2005;184(4):1293–304.

3. Miller E, Metser U, Avrahami G, et al. Role of 18F-FDG PET/CT in staging and follow-up of lymphoma in pediatric and young adult patients. J Comput Assist Tomogr 2006;30(4):689–94.

4. Shulkin BL, Hutchinson RJ, Castle VP, et al. Neuroblastoma: positron emission tomography with 2-[fluorine-18]-fluoro-2-deoxy-D-glucose compared with metaiodobenzylguanidine scintigraphy. Radiology 1996;199(3):743–50.

5. Tatsumi M, Miller JH, Wahl RL. 18F-FDG PET/CT in evaluating non-CNS pediatric malignancies. J Nucl Med 2007;48(12):1923–31.

6. Dietrich RB, el Saden S, Chugani HT, et al. Resective surgery for intractable epilepsy in children: radiologic evaluation. Am J Neuroradiol 1991;12(6): 1149–58.

7. Beaulieu S, Kinahan P, Tseng J, et al. SUV varies with time after injection in (18)F-FDG PET of breast cancer: characterization and method to adjust for time differences. J Nucl Med 2003; 44(7):1044–50.

8. Kostakoglu L, Goldsmith SJ, Leonard JP, et al. FDG-PET after 1 cycle of therapy predicts outcome in diffuse large cell lymphoma and classic Hodgkin disease. Cancer 2006;107(11):2678–87.

9. Yamane T, Daimaru O, Ito S, et al. Decreased 18F-FDG uptake 1 day after initiation of chemotherapy for malignant lymphomas. J Nucl Med 2004;45(11): 1838–42.

10. Sharp S, Shulkin B, Furman W, et al. I-123-MIBG scintigraphy and [F-18]FDG PET in neuroblastoma. J Nucl Med 2008;49:84P [abstract].

11. Jacene HA, Ishimori T, Engles JM, et al. Effects of pegfilgrastim on normal biodistribution of 18F-FDG: preclinical and clinical studies. J Nucl Med 2006; 47(6):950–6.

12. Sugawara Y, Fisher SJ, Zasadny KR, et al. Preclinical and clinical studies of bone marrow uptake of fluorine-1-fluorodeoxyglucose with or without granulocyte colony-stimulating factor during chemotherapy. J Clin Oncol 1998;16(1):173–80.

13. Barrington SF, Maisey MN. Skeletal muscle uptake of fluorine-18-FDG: effect of oral diazepam. J Nucl Med 1996;37(7):1127–9.

14. Hany TF, Gharehpapagh E, Kamel EM, et al. Brown adipose tissue: a factor to consider in symmetrical tracer uptake in the neck and upper chest region. Eur J Nucl Med Mol Imaging 2002;29(10):1393–8.

15. Okuyama C, Sakane N, Yoshida T, et al. (123)I- or (125)I-metaiodobenzylguanidine visualization of brown adipose tissue. J Nucl Med 2002;43(9): 1234–40.

16. Gelfand MJ, O'Hara SM, Curtwright LA, et al. Premedication to block [(18)F]FDG uptake in the brown adipose tissue of pediatric and adolescent patients. Pediatr Radiol 2005;35(10):984–90.

17. Zukotynski KA, Fahey FH, Laffin S, et al. Constant ambient temperature of 24 degrees C significantly reduces FDG uptake by brown adipose tissue in children scanned during the winter. Eur J Nucl Med Mol Imaging 2009;36(4):602–6.

18. Parysow O, Mollerach AM, Jager V, et al. Low-dose oral propranolol could reduce brown adipose tissue F-18 FDG uptake in patients undergoing PET scans. Clin Nucl Med 2007;32(5):351–7.

19. Soderlund V, Larsson SA, Jacobsson H. Reduction of FDG uptake in brown adipose tissue in clinical patients by a single dose of propranolol. Eur J Nucl Med Mol Imaging 2007;34(7):1018–22.

20. Tatsumi M, Engles JM, Ishimori T, et al. Intense (18)F-FDG uptake in brown fat can be reduced pharmacologically. J Nucl Med 2004;45(7):1189–93.

21. Baba S, Tatsumi M, Ishimori T, et al. Effect of nicotine and ephedrine on the accumulation of 18F-FDG in brown adipose tissue. J Nucl Med 2007;48(6):981–6.

22. Rousseau C, Bourbouloux E, Campion L, et al. Brown fat in breast cancer patients: analysis of serial (18)F-FDG PET/CT scans. Eur J Nucl Med Mol Imaging 2006;33(7):785–91.

23. Beyer T, Antoch G, Muller S, et al. Acquisition protocol considerations for combined PET/CT imaging. J Nucl Med 2004;45(Suppl 1):25S–35S.

24. Allen-Auerbach M, Yeom K, Park J, et al. Standard PET/CT of the chest during shallow breathing is inadequate for comprehensive staging of lung cancer. J Nucl Med 2006;47(2):298–301.

25. Aquino SL, Kuester LB, Muse VV, et al. Standard PET/CT of the chest during shallow breathing is inadequate for comprehensive staging of lung cancer. Eur J Nucl Med Mol Imaging 2006;33:692–6.

26. Karabulut N, Toru M, Gelebek V, et al. Comparison of low-dose and standard-dose helical CT in the evaluation of pulmonary nodules. Eur Radiol 2002;12(11):2764–9.

27. Rusinek H, Naidich DP, McGuinness G, et al. Pulmonary nodule detection: low-dose versus conventional CT. Radiology 1998;209(1):243–9.

28. Sharp SE, Helton KJ, Gelfand MJ, et al. Detection of pulmonary nodules on localization CT scans acquired during PET/CT imaging. Pediatr Radiol 2007;37(Suppl 1):S60.

29. Weng MJ, Wu MT, Pan HB, et al. The feasibility of low-dose CT for pulmonary metastasis in patients with primary gynecologic malignancy. Clin Imaging 2004;28(6):408–14.

30. Cobby M, Whipp E, Bullimore J, et al. CT appearances of relapse of lymphoma in the lung. Clin Radiol 1990;41(4):232–8.

31. Hwang GL, Leung AN, Zinck SE, et al. Recurrent lymphoma of the lung: computed tomography appearance. J Comput Assist Tomogr 2005;29(2):228–30.

32. Beyer T, Antoch G, Blodgett T, et al. Dual-modality PET/CT imaging: the effect of respiratory motion on combined image quality in clinical oncology. Eur J Nucl Med Mol Imaging 2003;30(4):588–96.

33. Osman MM, Cohade C, Nakamoto Y, et al. Clinically significant inaccurate localization of lesions with PET/CT: frequency in 300 patients. J Nucl Med 2003;44(2):240–3.

34. Osman MM, Cohade C, Nakamoto Y, et al. Respiratory motion artifacts on PET emission images obtained using CT attenuation correction on PET-CT. Eur J Nucl Med Mol Imaging 2003;30(4):603–6.

35. Goerres GW, Kamel E, Heidelberg TN, et al. PET-CT image co-registration in the thorax: influence of respiration. Eur J Nucl Med Mol Imaging 2002;29(3):351–60.

36. Ambrosino MM, Genieser NB, Roche KJ, et al. Feasibility of high-resolution, low-dose chest CT in evaluating the pediatric chest. Pediatr Radiol 1994;24(1):6–10.

37. Brody AS. Thoracic CT technique in children. J Thorac Imaging 2001;16(4):259–68.

38. Lucaya J, Piqueras J, Garcia-Pena P, et al. Low-dose high-resolution CT of the chest in children and young adults: dose, cooperation, artifact incidence, and image quality. Am J Roentgenol 2000;175(4):985–92.

39. Rogalla P, Stover B, Scheer I, et al. Low-dose spiral CT: applicability to paediatric chest imaging. Pediatr Radiol 1999;29(8):565–9.

40. Daou D. Respiratory motion handling is mandatory to accomplish the high-resolution PET destiny. Eur J Nucl Med Mol Imaging 2008;35(11):1961–70.

41. Antoch G, Freudenberg LS, Stattaus J, et al. Whole-body positron emission tomography-CT: optimized CT using oral and IV contrast materials. AJR Am J Roentgenol 2002;179(6):1555–60.

42. Groves AM, Kayani I, Dickson JC, et al. Oral contrast medium in PET/CT: should you or shouldn't you? Eur J Nucl Med Mol Imaging 2005;32(10):1160–6.

43. Stabin MG. Internal dosimetry. In: Treves ST, editor. Pediatric nuclear medicine/PET. New York: Springer; 2007. p. 513–20.

44. Stabin MG, Gelfand MJ. Dosimetry of pediatric nuclear medicine procedures. Q J Nucl Med 1998;42(2):93–112.

45. Treves ST, Davis RT, Fahey FH. Administered radiopharmaceutical doses in children: a survey of 13 pediatric hospitals in North America. J Nucl Med 2008;49(6):1024–7.

46. Pierce DA, Preston DL. Radiation-related cancer risks at low doses among atomic bomb survivors. Radiat Res 2000;154(2):178–86.

47. Preston DL, Pierce DA, Shimizu Y. Age-time patterns for cancer and noncancer excess risks in the atomic bomb survivors. Radiat Res 2000;154(6):733–4 [discussion: 734–5].

48. Brasch RC, Boyd DP, Gooding CA. Computed tomographic scanning in children: comparison of radiation dose and resolving power of commercial CT scanners. Am J Roentgenol 1978;131(1):95–101.

49. Brasch RC, Cann CE. Computed tomographic scanning in children: II. An updated comparison of radiation dose and resolving power of commercial scanners. Am J Roentgenol 1982;138(1):127–33.

50. Fearon T, Vucich J. Pediatric patient exposures from CT examinations: GE CT/T 9800 scanner. Am J Roentgenol 1985;144(4):805–9.

51. Kamel IR, Hernandez RJ, Martin JE, et al. Radiation dose reduction in CT of the pediatric pelvis. Radiology 1994;190(3):683–7.

52. Robinson AE, Hill EP, Harpen MD. Radiation dose reduction in pediatric CT. Pediatr Radiol 1986; 16(1):53–4.

53. Vade A, Demos TC, Olson MC, et al. Evaluation of image quality using 1:1 pitch and 1.5:1 pitch helical CT in children: a comparative study. Pediatr Radiol 1996;26(12):891–3.

54. Brenner D, Elliston C, Hall E, et al. Estimated risks of radiation-induced fatal cancer from pediatric CT. Am J Roentgenol 2001;176(2):289–96.

55. Brenner DJ. Estimating cancer risks from pediatric CT: going from the qualitative to the quantitative. Pediatr Radiol 2002;32(4). 228–3 [discussion: 242–4].

56. Donnelly LF, Emery KH, Brody AS, et al. Minimizing radiation dose for pediatric body applications of single-detector helical CT: strategies at a large Children's Hospital. Am J Roentgenol 2001;176(2): 303–6.

57. Paterson A, Frush DP, Donnelly LF. Helical CT of the body: are settings adjusted for pediatric patients? Am J Roentgenol 2001;176(2):297–301.

58. Arch ME, Frush DP. Pediatric body MDCT: a 5-year follow-up survey of scanning parameters used by pediatric radiologists. AJR Am J Roengenol 2008; 191(2):611–7.

59. Fahey FH, Palmer MR, Strauss KJ, et al. Dosimetry and adequacy of CT-based attenuation correction for pediatric PET: phantom study. Radiology 2007; 243(1):96–104.

60. Lee JJ, Kang WJ, Lee DS, et al. Diagnostic performance of 18F-FDG PET and ictal 99mTc-HMPAO SPET in pediatric temporal lobe epilepsy: quantitative analysis by statistical parametric mapping, statistical probabilistic anatomical map, and subtraction ictal SPET. Seizure 2005;14(3):213–20.

61. Muzik O, Pourabdollah S, Juhasz C, et al. Application of an objective method for localizing bilateral cortical FDG PET abnormalities to guide the resection of epileptic foci. IEEE Trans Biomed Eng 2005; 52(9):1574–81.

62. Williams G, Fahey FH, Treves ST, et al. Exploratory evaluation of two-dimensional and three-dimensional methods of FDG PET quantification in pediatric anaplastic astrocytoma: a report from the Pediatric Brain Tumor Consortium (PBTC). Eur J Nucl Med Mol Imaging 2008;35(9):1651–8.

63. Loffler M, Weckesser M, Franzius C, et al. High diagnostic value of 18F-FDG-PET in pediatric patients with chronic inflammatory bowel disease. Ann N Y Acad Sci 2006;1072:379–85.

64. Even-Sapir E, Metser U, Flusser G, et al. Assessment of malignant skeletal disease: initial experience with 18F-fluoride PET/CT and comparison between 18F-fluoride PET and 18F-fluoride PET/CT. J Nucl Med 2004;45(2):272–8.

65. Schirrmeister H, Guhlmann A, Elsner K, et al. Sensitivity in detecting osseous lesions depends on anatomic localization: planar bone scintigraphy versus 18F PET. J Nucl Med 1999;40(10):1623–9.

66. Drubach LA, Sapp MV, Laffin S, et al. Fluorine-18 NaF PET imaging of child abuse. Pediatr Radiol 2008;38(7):776–9.

67. Lim R, Fahey FH, Drubach LA, et al. Early experience with fluorine-18 sodium fluoride bone PET in young patients with back pain. J Pediatr Orthop 2007;27(3):277–82.

68. Ovadia D, Metser U, Lievshitz G, et al. Back pain in adolescents: assessment with integrated 18F-fluoride positron-emission tomography-computed tomography. J Pediatr Orthop 2007;27(1):90–3.

69. Grant FD, Fahey FH, Packard AB, et al. Skeletal PET with 18F-fluoride: applying new technology to an old tracer. J Nucl Med 2008;49(1):68–78.

70. Setty B, Kalra M, Liu B, et al. Optimazation of radiation doses for pediatric head and neck CT protocols. Pediatr Radiol 2007;37(Suppl 1):S81 [abstract].

71. Gelfand MJ, Lemen LC. PET/CT and SPECT/CT Dosimetry in children: the challenge to the pediatric imager. Semin Nucl Med 2007;37(5):391–8.

PET in the Assessment of Pediatric Brain Development and Developmental Disorders

Ajay Kumar, MD, PhD, DNB[a], Harry T. Chugani, MD[a,b,c],*

KEYWORDS

- Alpha methyl tryptophan (AMT)
- Brain development • Developmental disorder • FDG
- Flumazenil (FMZ) • Functional imaging • Pediatric
- Positron emission tomography (PET)

Positron emission tomography (PET), along with various molecular imaging agents in its arsenal, can play an invaluable role in understanding the structural and functional changes that occur during brain development, and how these changes relate to behavioral and cognitive development in the infant and child. Although the application of PET technology has had an important impact in the study of human brain functional maturation, it is important and appropriate to begin with a brief review of the salient features of developmental neuroanatomy. In this regard, the contribution of MR imaging has been equally important and complementary to PET studies.

SOME BASICS ON DEVELOPMENTAL NEUROANATOMY

The human brain remains structurally and functionally immature at the time of birth and continues to undergo multiple complex and dynamic processes consisting of anatomic, molecular, functional, and organizational changes. In fact, brain development is orchestrated through the interaction of numerous synchronized processes, some of which continue even after birth, while some others start postnatally and take different courses, depending upon the specific brain region. For example, the neural tube is formed by 4 weeks of gestation, with neurogenesis taking place between 4 and 20 weeks and neuronal migration to their cortical destination from 12 to 20 weeks.[1] Although neurogenesis and migration was previously believed to be completed by birth, it is now known that some degree of neurogenesis continues into adulthood in the hippocampus and probably in other structures.[2] Neurogenesis is followed by apoptosis, peaking after neuronal migration, and reducing the number of neurons by half from 24 weeks of gestation to 4 weeks after birth.[3]

Although neocortical dendritic growth takes place between the third trimester of pregnancy and 2 years of age,[4] some regions, such as the calcarine cortex, show earlier dendritic growth (as compared with the prefrontal cortex), with about one-third of the growth completed by birth followed by some decline between 2 and 7 years of age.[5] Dendritic growth and synaptogenesis are

---

[a] Departments of Pediatrics and Neurology, School of Medicine, Wayne State University, Children's Hospital of Michigan, 3901 Beaubien Boulevard, Detroit, MI 48201, USA
[b] Division of Pediatric Neurology, Children's Hospital of Michigan, 3901 Beaubien Boulevard, Detroit, MI, USA
[c] PET Center, Children's Hospital of Michigan, Detroit, MI 48201, USA
* Corresponding author. Department of Pediatrics, School of Medicine, Wayne State University, PET Center, Children's Hospital of Michigan, 3901 Beaubien Boulevard, Detroit, MI 48201.
E-mail address: hchugani@pet.wayne.edu (H.T. Chugani).

PET Clin 3 (2009) 487–515
doi:10.1016/j.cpet.2009.04.006
1556-8598/09/$ – see front matter © 2009 Elsevier Inc. All rights reserved.

closely linked and have a similar time course.[6] Synaptogenesis also begins around the twentieth week of gestation, increases rapidly after birth, and reaches peak synaptic density, 50% more than adult levels, by 2 years of age.[7] However, the peak in synaptic density depends upon the brain region; the peak is earliest in the primary sensory areas, followed by the prefrontal cortex.[8] In the visual cortex, it is almost 90% of the maximum at birth, reaches the maximum number by 8 months of age, and then decreases to about half the maximum between 1 and 5 years of age.[9] It reaches the peak in the auditory cortex at 3 months, but only at about 15 months in the prefrontal cortex.[8] Synaptic density starts decreasing around 7 years of age, reaching adult values by 12 years of age in the auditory cortex and by mid-adolescence in the prefrontal cortex.[8]

Myelination starts prenatally at around 28 weeks in the brain stem and generally proceeds from inferior to superior and posterior to anterior.[10] Myelination of the optic radiation and occipital white matter begins 1 to 2 months after birth and gradually extends to the frontal lobe by 9 months postnatally.[11,12] Myelination appears to follow the maturational pattern of functional circuitries; sensory fibers myelinate first, followed by motor fibers and associations fibers.[13] The surface of the growing brain begins to fold into sulci and gyri around 15 weeks of gestational age with all major gyri, except for the occipital lobe, formed by 28 weeks.[3,14] All gyri are present by birth, though relatively immature in terms of their inter- and intraregional connectivity.

Average brain weight at birth is about 370 g and increases rapidly to achieve 80% of adult weight by 2 to 3 years and 90% by 5 to 6 years of age.[15] Total cerebral volume peaks at 14.5 years in males and 11.5 years in females, with approximately 50% variation of brain volume in normal children of the same age.[16] One cubic millimeter of adult brain may contain between 35 and 70 million neurons and up to twice as many glial cells,[17] and about 500 billion synapses[18] in the cortical gray matter, or up to 20 miles of myelinated fibers in white matter.[19]

Although human brain development closely follows the sequence of events observed in other primates, it proceeds on a slower timescale. According to the model that predicts the timing of different neural developmental events in various mammalian species,[20,21] a delayed developmental time course leads to a relatively larger volume of the later developing structures, which may be the reason for the larger frontal cortex in human beings. Brain growth is further underscored by various remodeling processes, all undergoing simultaneously, and leading to variable growth of gray and white matter in a region-specific fashion. Cortical gray-matter volume peaks differently in different brain regions, peaking in the frontal lobe at 11 years in girls and 12 years in boys, in the parietal lobe at 10 years in girls and 12 years in boys, and in the temporal lobe at 17 years in girls and 16 years in boys, followed by a gradual decrease.[3,16] It seems that primary sensorimotor areas attain their peak thickness before secondary areas, followed by higher-order association areas.[22,23] Caudate size peaks at age 7.5 years in girls and 10 years in boys.[3] While total temporal lobe volume appears relatively stable from 4 to 18 years of age, the amygdala, which contains a high number of androgen receptors, increases in size in males and the hippocampus, having a higher number of estrogen receptors, significantly increases in size in females only, although no direct relationship between receptor density and growth patterns has been found.[24–26] The volume and density of white matter, including corpus callosum, usually increases with age until the fifth decade, with an almost similar pattern of change seen in all the lobes.[16,27–29] Although brain size is approximately 9% larger in males, the volume of frontal gray matter is higher in females, and the volume of occipital white matter is higher in males across all ages and after adjusting for the different overall brain sizes.[30]

Maturation of different parts of the brain also proceeds differently and is usually associated with thinning of gray matter and thickening of white matter. Longitudinal MR imaging studies have shown that cortical thickness generally decreases throughout late childhood and adolescence, with thinning of gray matter occurring first in sensorimotor areas, followed by parietal, superior temporal, and dorsolateral prefrontal cortices.[27,28,31,32] Regions subserving primary functions, such as motor and sensory systems, mature earliest, with temporal and parietal association cortices associated with basic language skills and spatial attention maturing next. Higher-order association areas, such as the prefrontal and lateral temporal cortices, which integrate primary sensorimotor processes and modulate basic attention and language processes, seem to mature last.[27,33] The cortical thinning may be a consequence of the pruning of neural connections that has been documented in animal models,[34] or may be related to increased myelination of axons within the cortical gray matter, leading to apparent thinning of gray matter.[28,33] Increase in white-matter volume appears to be associated with myelination. Both these regressive and progressive processes, occurring simultaneously, strengthen and fine tune the relevant neuronal circuitries, leading to behavioral and cognitive maturation.

Concurrent with the structural development and maturation, functional (behavioral and cognitive) development also takes place. However, not much is known about the relationship between the two and it is not only a matter of scientific and academic interest but also of huge clinical and social interest to understand and explain this relationship. The human brain is highly structurally and functionally specialized, with different cortical regions supporting different components of various cognitive functions, such as language, memory, and so forth. We still do not fully understand how these specializations arise. One view is that functional specialization of various cortical regions is the result of intricate genetic and epigenetic interactions, with experience having only a fine-tuning effect. In this model, the human infant is born with "innate modules" and "core knowledge" relevant to the physical and social world.[35] According to this maturational viewpoint, the anatomic maturation of specific regions of the brain, usually cortical regions, is related to newly emerging sensory, motor, and cognitive functions. Thus, in this model, visually guided behavior in an infant is controlled by subcortical structures, but with brain development, posterior followed by anterior cortical regions start to have an influence on this behavior.[36,37] For example, during the first few months of life, an infant is unable to reach for objects and cannot accurately retrieve a hidden object after a short delay period if the object's location is changed. This behavior is similar to those made by human adults with frontal lesions and monkeys with dorsolateral prefrontal lesions, suggesting that the maturation of this region is necessary to retain information over space and time.[38] However, it seems too simplistic to assume that any particular cognitive function can be assigned to a certain cortical region. It is more likely that postnatal functional brain development results from interregional interactions and the onset of new behaviors during infancy should be associated with changes in activity over several brain regions.

Furthermore, during infancy, patterns of cortical activation in different behavioral tasks might differ from, and be more extensive than, those observed in adults, and even similar behaviors may involve different patterns of cortical activation in infants and adults. Indeed, recent evidence indicates that the same behavior in infants and adults can be mediated by different cortical regions and neuronal circuitries. Developmental disorders like autism, which seems to involve different cortical regions and their networks, also support this mode of cortical development.[39] On other hand, functional brain development may be largely shaped by postbirth experiences and the behavioral changes are the result of continuous learning and plasticity. This notion of an extended period during childhood, when activity-dependent synaptic stabilization occurs, may help in designing early intervention to provide environmental enrichment and the optimal educational curricula, as learning is perhaps more efficient and easily retained in this biologic window of opportunity.

FUNCTIONAL ASPECTS OF BRAIN DEVELOPMENT

The measurement of progressive metabolic changes, particularly energy production, in various brain regions during development is one of the various strategies employed to study structural and functional brain development and to delineate their relationship, as the process of neuronal growth, dendritic and synaptic proliferation, their maintenance, myelination, and various other processes involved require considerable energy expenditure. Ontogeny of these maturational changes should be reflected by changes in energy requirements in different regions of the brain. Because glucose and oxygen are the main substrates used in energy production in the brain, measurements of their consumption rates may provide a means whereby regional energy demand can be related to structural and behavioral maturation. Because energy requirement and local blood flow are closely related,[40] local cerebral blood flow (CBF) rates can also be used as a surrogate measure of local energy need. Functional brain maturation is also related to change in various receptor densities, such as gamma-aminobutyric acid (GABA) receptors, neurotransmitter levels, and cerebral protein synthesis.[41,42]

PET is a powerful imaging modality, which can be used for the noninvasive in vivo measurement of these functional changes and has been used to measure various regional biochemical and physiologic processes, including the mapping of brain regions involved in the processing of various sensory, motor, and other stimuli in normal adults. However, PET cannot be performed in normal children because of ethical considerations, as there is an associated radiation exposure, albeit low. For example, in studies of local cerebral metabolic rates for glucose (LCMRglc) with 2-deoxy-2[F-18] fluoro-D-glucose (FDG), the whole-body radiation dose to the child is only about 0.3 cGy and to the brain 0.5 cGy, in comparison to about 1 cGy to 3 cGy radiation dose from a CT scan.[43] Although these doses are well within guidelines used for common diagnostic radiologic procedures in children, it is ethically unacceptable to subject entirely normal children to even these low doses. On the other hand, brain development data should ideally come from normal children, so that besides understanding the various aspects and nuances of true structural and functional brain development, they can be reliably and confidently compared with children with various neurologic and developmental disorders. Therefore, various strategies and protocols have to be devised to acquire normative brain development data from apparently not completely healthy children. Data from children undergoing brain PET scan because of suspected neurologic problem, but later turning out to be normal, or children who underwent whole-body PET scan for some specific problem (eg, tumor) outside of the brain can be used with some caution and deliberation.

Animal Studies of Brain Development and Maturation

Maturational changes of local cerebral blood flow (LCBF) and LCMRglc have been determined in a number of animals, providing important information about the relationship of change in local cerebral substrate use and behavioral maturation. Kennedy and colleagues[44] used [C-14]-deoxyglucose autoradiography for quantitative determination of LCMRglc in newborn macaque monkeys. They found that the rates for structures in the lower neuraxis were equal to or exceeded those reported for the mature animal, while those above the midbrain were generally lower. The auditory system was found to have rates equal to, or exceeding, its mature levels in all parts of the pathway including the cortex. In the visual system, subcortical structures were at their mature levels while rates in the cortical areas were found to be variably low. They also found a high correlation between glucose use and local blood flow. This pattern of substrate use correlated well with the behavioral state of the neonatal monkey, whose auditory and tactile functions are more advanced than visual function. Gregoire and colleagues[45] determined LCMRglc in 2- to 8-day-old beagle dogs by the quantitative [C-14]-deoxyglucose autoradiographic method and found highest glucose consumption values in brain stem nuclei (inferior olivary nucleus, vestibular nucleus, and red nucleus) and in selected deep-cerebral structures (subthalamic nucleus and ventrolateral thalamic nucleus), whereas consistently lower glucose consumption were found in the cerebral cortex. Duffy and colleagues[46] measured LCMRglc in 36 neuroanatomic structures of normal newborn puppies and found that LCMRglc was highest in the vestibular nucleus and in other gray matter nuclei of the brainstem, and declined in a caudal-to-rostral progression through the neuraxis. Lowest rates of glucose metabolism were detected in white-matter structures. In another study of cerebral energy metabolism during development, Abrams and colleagues[47] found that LCMRglc in sheep was low in most brain structures during the perinatal period. The postnatal changes of LCBF in freely moving rats were measured by means of the quantitative autoradiographic [C-14]-iodoantipyrine method by Nehlig and colleagues.[48] At 10 days after birth, rates of blood flow were very low and quite homogeneous in most cerebral structures except in a few posterior areas, and rose notably to reach a peak at 17 days in all brain regions studied. Rates of blood flow decreased between 17 and 21 days after birth and then increased from weaning time to reach the known characteristic distribution of the adult rat.

Chugani and colleagues[49] measured LCMRglc in kittens at various stages of postnatal development and in adult cats using quantitative [C-14]-2-deoxyglucose autoradiography. In the kitten, very low LCMRglc levels were seen during the first 15 days of life, with phylogenetically older brain regions being generally more metabolically mature than newer structures. After 15 days of age, many brain regions (particularly telencephalic structures) underwent sharp increases of LCMRglc to reach, or exceed, adult rates by 60 days. This developmental period (15–60 days) corresponded to the time of rapid synaptic proliferation known to occur in the cat. During the immediate newborn period, synapses in area 17 of the visual system are sparse[50] and showed low LCMRglc. Subsequently, there is a rapid rise in synaptic density, with a peak occurring by about 70 days postnatally,[51] which matched well with the period of rapid LCMRglc increase seen in the visual cortex, reaching an initial peak at about 60 days. The investigators also found good correlation between the metabolic maturation of various neuroanatomic regions and the emergence of behaviors mediated by the specific region, and the "critical period" of development of visual cortex corresponded to the portion of the LCMRglc maturational curve surrounding the 60-day metabolic peak.

From these animal studies, it appears that phylogenetically older brain structures (ie, brain stem, cerebellum, and thalamus) are structurally and functionally more mature at the time of birth, compared with telencephalic structures, as manifested in the primitive and low level of function and behavior at or immediately after birth. Gradual activation and maturation of various phylogenetically newer brain regions leads to greater behavioral complexity. On the basis of these metabolic-behavioral relationships, Kennedy and colleagues[44] hypothesized that the developmental increase in the metabolic rate of a particular brain region heralds its contribution to the behavioral manifestation.

Human Studies of Brain Development and Maturation

Cerebral perfusion studies

In a study of cerebral blood flow and oxygen use in nine normal children, aged 3 to 11 years, Kennedy and Sokoloff[52] demonstrated that the average global cerebral blood flow was approximately 1.8 times that of normal adults. Similarly, they found that average cerebral oxygen use was approximately 1.3 times higher in children compared with adults. Chiron and colleagues[53] studied regional cerebral blood flow (rCBF) in 42 children, aged 2 days to 19 years and considered as neurologically normal. They found that cortical rCBFs were lower than those for adults at birth, but subsequently increased until 5 or 6 years of age to values 50% to 85% higher than those for adults and thereafter decreased, reaching adult levels between 15 and 19 years. They found that the neonatal values of rCBF in the cerebellum and thalamus were slightly higher than adult levels, but not significantly. They also reported that cortical rCBFs, expressed in percent-global CBF, were lower at birth, then increased and reached a plateau corresponding to the adult value before the second year of age, with different cortical regions requiring different times to reach normal adult values. The shortest time was found for primary cortical regions and the longest for the associative cortex. Cognitive development appeared to be related to blood flow changes of the corresponding brain regions. Takahashi and colleagues[54] evaluated functional developmental changes of the brain in children in relation to CBF and oxygen metabolism. They measured rCBF, regional cerebral metabolic rate for oxygen (rCMRO$_2$), and regional oxygen extraction fraction (rOEF) with PET in 24 children aged 10 days to 16 years (9 boys, 15 girls), using a steady inhalation method with $^{15}CO_2$, $^{15}O_2$, and ^{15}CO to measure rCBF, rCMRO$_2$, and rOEF, respectively. They found that rCBF and rCMRO$_2$ was lower in the neonatal period than in older children and adults, and increased significantly during early childhood. No difference in rCBF was observed between the basal ganglia and the primary cerebral cortex; however, it was prominent in the occipital lobe in every age bracket. No significant changes in rOEF were found during childhood.

FDG-PET studies

Chugani and colleagues[55,56] studied developmental changes of LCMRglc in 29 children, aged 5 days to 15.1 years, who had suffered transient neurologic events not significantly affecting normal neurodevelopment. They found highest LCMRglc in the sensorimotor cortex, thalamus, brain stem, and cerebellar vermis in infants less than 5 weeks old. By 3 months, LCMRglc increased in the parietal, temporal, and primary visual cortex (medial occipital or calcarine cortex), basal ganglia, and cerebellar cortex. Lateral and inferior prefrontal regions and the dorsolateral occipital cortex displayed a maturational rise in LCMRglc by approximately 6 to 8 months, with the medial and dorsal frontal cortex becoming active between 8 and 12 months of age (**Fig. 1** and **Table 1**). Although an adult pattern was seen by 1 year of age, brain maturation was far from complete. Subsequent studies showed that limbic structures, such as the amygdala and hippocampus, were also functionally active at birth, with the anterior cingulate cortex showing a maturational rise of glucose metabolism soon after.[57] Absolute values of LCMRglc for various gray-matter regions were low at birth (about 30% less than adult values).[56] Mean LCMRglc for cerebral cortical regions in the first year of life was found to range from 65% to 86% of the corresponding adult values. The LCMRglc for the sensorimotor cortex, which was the earliest cortical region to display its maturational rise, was found to be closest to the adult rates during the first year, compared with other cortical structures (93% of adult value). The basal ganglia and thalamus were found to have developmental increases of LCMRglc earlier than most areas of the cerebral cortex. The thalamus was one of the earliest structures to show a maturational rise in LCMRglc and mean LCMRglc for the thalamus, lenticular nuclei, and caudate were found to be 84%, 79%, and 71%, respectively, of the adult rates during the first year. Although LCMRglc for the cerebellum as a whole was found to be closest to adult rates than any other area of brain (93% of adult value), the maturational pattern within the cerebellum was heterogeneous, with vermis, a phylogenetically older structure, showing higher maturation at birth. The brain stem was also found to have relatively advanced maturation at birth, with mean LCMRglc 89% of the adult value in the first year of life. However, LCMRglc rapidly rose to reach adult values by the second year of life and continued to rise until, by 3 to 4 years, it

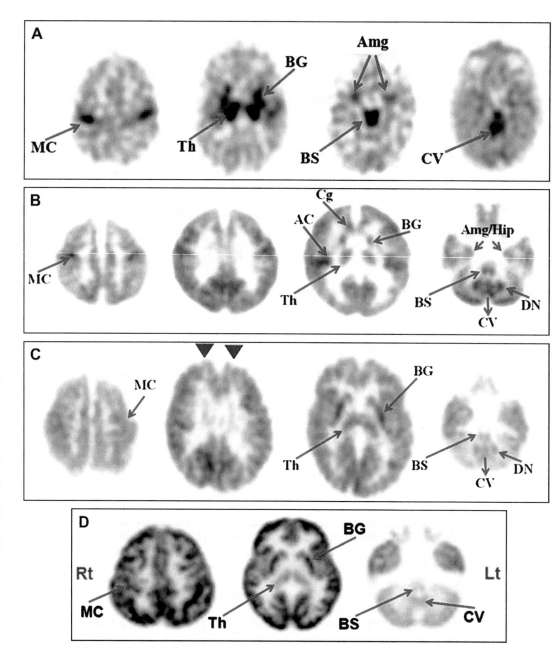

Fig. 1. Normal FDG-PET scan in (*A*) a 7-day-old newborn, (*B*) 3-month-old infant, (*C*) 7-month-old child, and (*D*) 1-year-old child (Amg, amygdala; BG, basal ganglia; BS, brain stem; CV, cerebellar vermis; DN, dentate nucleus; Hip, hippocampus; MC, motor cortex; Th, thalamus). Note that besides motor cortex, thalamus more than basal ganglia, brain stem, and cerebellar vermis, the amygdale is also quite active at birth. With increasing age, cortical glucose metabolism increases and becomes higher than cerebellar and other subcortical glucose metabolism. Even at 7 to 8 months of age, medial frontal glucose metabolism is less than lateral frontal lobe (*arrowheads*) and is the last to mature.

reached almost twice the adult value. These high rates were maintained until approximately 9 years of age, when they began to decline, reaching the adult rates again by the latter part of the second decade (**Fig. 2**). They found that highest increases of LCMRglc over adult values occurred in cerebral cortices (190%–226%), followed by the cerebellum and brain stem (about 170%), and basal ganglia and thalamus (155%–160%). This transient increase in LCMRglc in brain is consistent with the transiently increased CBF and cerebral oxygen use, shown by Kennedy and Sokoloff

Table 1
Rank order of adult brain regions with highest to lowest uptake/binding for various PET tracers

Fluorodeoxyglucose (FDG)[56]	Flumazenil (FMZ)[119]	Alpha Methyl Tryptophan (AMT)[208]
Putamen and pallidum	Primary visual cortex	Cerebellum
Caudate (head)	Temporal cortex	Occipital cortex
Thalamus	Frontal cortex	Parietal cortex
Calcarine cortex	Hippocampus/amygdala	Temporal cortex
Transverse temporal cortex	Cerebellum	Putamen
Anterior cingulate	Basal ganglia	Frontal cortex
Frontal cortex	Thalamus	Thalamus
Occipital cortex	—	Pallidum and caudate
Parietal cortex	—	Midbrain
Temporal cortex	—	Amygdala and hippocampus
Brain stem	—	—
Cerebellum	—	—

both in human beings (1957) and in dogs (1972).[52,58]

Kinnala and colleagues[59] also reported similar findings for LCMRglc during the first 6 months of life in 20 children. LCMRglc for various cortical brain regions and the basal ganglia was reported to be low at birth. Within the first 2 months of age, LCMRglc was found to be highest in the sensorimotor cortex, thalamus, and brain stem. By 5 months, LCMRglc was found to increase in the frontal, parietal, temporal, occipital, and cerebellar cortical regions. In general, they found

good positive correlation between whole-brain LCMRglc and postconceptional age. Van Bogaert and colleagues[60] analyzed FDG-PET studies of 42 subjects, ages 6 to 38 years, using statistical parametric mapping to identify age-related changes in regional distribution of glucose metabolism adjusted for global activity, and found that adjusted glucose metabolism varied very significantly in the thalamus and the anterior cingulate cortex, and to a lesser degree in the basal ganglia, the mesencephalon, and the insular, posterior cingulate, and frontal and postcentral cortices.

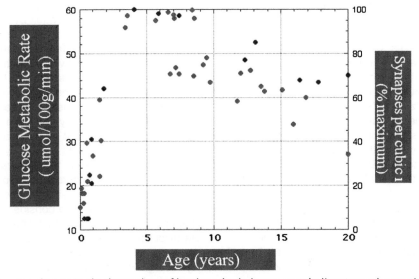

Fig. 2. Plot showing change in absolute values of local cerebral glucose metabolic rates and synaptic density with age.

Adjusted glucose metabolism increased mainly before the age of 25 years and then remained relatively stable. They suggested that brain maturation from the age of 6 years gives rise to a relative increase of synaptic activities in the thalamus, possibly as a consequence of improved cortico-thalamic connections and the increased metabolic activity in the anterior cingulate cortex was probably related to these thalamic changes.

Relationship between LCMRglc ontogeny and functional brain development

FDG-PET studies have shown that the pattern of LCMRglc in human neonates is markedly different from that of normal young adults.[55,56] The sequence of functional development of the brain during the first year of life, shown by the ontogeny of glucose metabolic pattern, correlates well with the maturation of behavioral, neurophysiologic, and neuroanatomic events in the infant. Low cortical LCMRglc—along with typically active brain-stem structures, such as the thalamus, brainstem, and cerebellar vermis, and phylogenetically older structures—appears to be related to limited behavioral functions of neonates, dominated by brain stem reflexes, such as Moro, root, and grasp response. There is relatively limited higher cortical function, such as visuomotor integrative activity. The prominent metabolic activity in the sensorimotor cortex is also consistent with its relatively early morphologic maturation compared with other cortical areas.[61] Comparisons between the neonatal pattern of cerebral glucose use and those seen in various pathologic states provide some information on the structure-function relationship. For example, older infants and children who have suffered perinatal brain insult, such as hypoxic-ischemic encephalopathy, and have persistence of the primitive newborn reflexes, presumably because of a persisting immature cortex, show the newborn pattern of LCMRglc in FDG-PET scans. A neonatal or infantile pattern of LCMRglc is also seen in very advanced Alzheimer's disease where, along with dementia, the patient also manifests some brain stem reflexes. At around 1 month of age, infants have difficulty in shifting their gaze from one stimulus to another, similar to that seen in adults with Balint's syndrome, where patients with bilateral parietal cortical damage find difficulties in disengaging from one stimulus to saccade to another, indicating that immaturity of the parietal cortex in the infant has a similar behavioral outcome.

As visuospatial and visuosensorimotor integrative functions are acquired in the second and third months of life, and primitive reflexes become organized,[62–64] increases in LCMRglc are observed in parietal, temporal, and primary visual cortical regions, basal ganglia and cerebellar hemisphere. It is interesting to note that, because the frontal lobe is still hypometabolic at this time, cortical suppression of brain stem reflexes probably does not seem to be exclusively related to frontal cortex inputs. By 2 to 3 months of age, infants will look toward the object and will open their hands while reaching for an object.[65] This increasing refinement of their reaching maneuver is because of the maturation of the primary visual cortex by this time, compared with neonatal vision, which is largely mediated by subcortical visual structures.[63] Later maturation of the dorsolateral occipital region, compared with the calcarine cortex (as shown by many anatomic studies[61]) also corresponds to the low glucose-metabolic activity in this region during the first few months of life. Similarly, LCMRglc remains relatively low in the frontal cortex during the first 6 months of life. Maturation of large cortical areas during the first few months of life, as shown by FDG-PET, also coincides with the maturation of EEG activity seen during this period.[66] Functional maturation of the frontal cortex, lateral frontal at 6 to 8 months, followed by dorsolateral prefrontal at 8 to 12 months, coincides with the appearance of higher cortical and cognitive abilities, such as more purposeful interaction with the surroundings and development of stranger anxiety.[67,68] The child also shows marked improvement in the performance on the delayed-response task, a commonly used neuropsychologic paradigm to evaluate prefrontal lobe integrity.[69]

Neurobiologic correlates of LCMRGlc changes

Although LCMRglc patterns qualitatively resemble those of the normal young adult by 1 year of age, absolute measurement of LCMRglc indicates that cortical maturation is far from complete, which is also reflected by relatively immature cognitive development. By 2 years of age, LCMRglc for most brain areas becomes equal to adult values, but these rates continue to increase, and in some cortical regions they reach more than twice the adult value by 3 to 4 years of age and then remain at a plateau until 9 to 10 years of age, decreasing subsequently to adult values by late second decade. To understand the possible neurobiologic events responsible for these LCMRglc changes, it is important to consider some fundamental changes during postnatal brain maturation. As discussed earlier, brain development in most species, including human beings, is characterized by overgrowth followed by elimination.[61] This general rule applies to neurons as well as to their processes and synaptic contacts. Whereas proliferation of neurons takes place prenatally, their elimination starts prenatally and continues until the second postnatal year.[61] However, the overproduction and subsequent elimination (pruning) of neuronal processes and synaptic contacts mostly occur after birth, with a protracted and variable time course, depending upon the brain region.[6] For example, at 7 years of age, when the brain has almost attained adult weight and volume, average synaptic density in the frontal cortex is about 1.4 times the adult value.[7] As the major portion of glucose metabolism is expended to maintain the resting membrane potential,[70] it is reasonable to assume a direct relationship between the cerebral energy demand (reflected by LCMRglc and indirectly by LCBF) and total membrane surface area. Therefore, it seems that the ascending portion of the rapid LCMRglc increase corresponds to the period of synaptic overproduction, whereas the plateau phase of higher-than-adult value corresponds to the period of increased energy demand as a result of transiently increased connectivity, and subsequent decline to the normal adult values may reflect the selective elimination or pruning of excessive connectivity. Indeed, a similar profile of LCMRglc changes was seen in the kitten, corresponding to changes in synaptic densities.[49] Another cause for the LCMRglc pattern seen in children could be increased energy demand by oligodendrocytes during myelination, which is high during the first decade of life. Conversely, inefficient transmission by incompletely myelinated neuronal circuitries may result in higher energy demand.

LCMRGlc profile and brain plasticity

The developing brain shows remarkable plasticity; it can sustain extensive damage without much functional deficit. Particularly, the developmental phase of increased synaptic connectivity is characterized by considerable plasticity, and it starts to decline—both in terms of recovery and sparing of function—around 9 to 10 years of age, which coincides to the time when LCMRglc starts to decrease. Similar relationships have been seen in other species as well. In the kitten, it has been shown that the period of excessive connectivity and higher LCMRglc (from 15–30 days to 60–90 days) is also associated with a high degree of brain plasticity.[49,71] Various experimental manipulations (such as monocular deprivation by suturing one eyelid) can cause neuroanatomic changes, resulting in altered connectivity during this time period.[72] To understand and evaluate this critical time period, Timney and colleagues[73] deprived monocular vision at different ages in cats. Their experiment indicated that a brief period of monocular deprivation between 30 and 80 days effectively prevented the normal development of binocular depth perception. This time period corresponds to the plateau phase of increased LCMRglc in kittens and implies its relationship with higher brain plasticity. The experiment also suggests the critical role and importance of external stimuli in the development and stabilization of corresponding cortical networks. Similarly, the anatomic representation of the sensorimotor cortex in kittens has been shown to alter, with external stimulation, during this critical period of development.[74] Kittens, trained for 4 to 10 weeks to avoid a mild electrical shock simply by flexing one foreleg, were found to have not only an expanded electrophysiologic representation, but also increased dendritic arborization in the somatosensory cortex contralateral to the trained foreleg. Such changes could not be induced after 10 weeks of age,[74] the age that corresponds to the downward trend of LCMRglc in sensorimotor areas in the kittens.[49]

Language acquisition and reorganization in response to dominant hemisphere damage has been found to be maximal during early childhood, when this window of increased plasticity exists. For example, in children who have been isolated since birth from all civilization and exposure to language ("feral" children), the subsequent ability to acquire language is greatest if intervention is started in early childhood and decreases significantly if it is started after 10 years of age.[75] Similarly, string instrument players, who start playing in childhood demonstrate greater cortical representation for left than right digits.[76] The decline of LCMRglc in visual cortex, beginning at about 8 to 10 years, coincides with a significant decrease in visual plasticity, as shown by the fact that enucleation before 8 years of age results in better depth perception than after 8 years.[77] Significant reorganization in sensory processing occurring in blind and deaf subjects appears to have an age-at-lesion effect. In contrast to subjects with late-onset blindness (after 13 years of age) who show lower glucose use in the visual cortex compared with normal subjects studied with their eyes closed,[78] in subjects with early blindness (onset before 3 years of age), glucose metabolism is maintained at a higher rate in the striate and prestriate visual cortex, with even higher activity than in blindfolded subjects with normal vision.[79,80] Interestingly, the occipital cortex of early-onset blind subjects can be activated during Braille reading.[81] Similarly, early-onset (before 2 years of age) deaf subjects show higher glucose use in the auditory and auditory association cortex than normal subjects with their ears plugged.[82] These interesting observations support earlier suggestions of intermodal competition and cortical reorganization in subjects with early sensory deprivation.[83,84]

Young children undergoing resective brain surgery for epilepsy or other reasons, or sustaining brain injury, show remarkable functional recovery. In a O-15 water cerebral blood perfusion study, Muller and colleagues[85] showed that while there was normal left rolandic activation with movement of the right hand, hemiplegic left hand movement was accompanied by rCBF increases in the supplementary motor area, premotor area, insula, and inferior frontal cortex of the left hemisphere in a child following right hemispherectomy.[85] In another study, the same group reported that patients with early-onset (before 4 years) unilateral primary motor cortex lesions showed greater activation in the secondary motor and frontoparietal nonmotor cortical regions, compared with patients with late lesions (after 10 years), suggesting a greater potential for reorganization during early development.[86] It seems that some additional or seemingly unrelated brain region may also participate in functional organization, particularly early in life. Children with congenital hemiplegia, a unilateral form of cerebral palsy, often show significantly less functional and cognitive deficits in comparison to their extensive unilateral cortical damage, believed to be related to brain plasticity.[87,88] Now it is well known that even higher cortical functions and cognitive skills can be sustained by a single hemisphere.[89,90] However, the compensation for early unilateral brain damage may not be always complete and may depend on various neurologic factors, including the side of injury. One group reported that early right hemisphere injury may have a more detrimental overall effect on intellectual outcome than early left hemispheric injury.[91]

Subcortical structures, such as the basal ganglia, thalamus, and cerebellum also show variable extents of plasticity. Initial loss of glucose metabolism in the ipsilateral basal ganglia and thalamus and contralateral cerebellum, seen 3 to 6 months after hemispherectomy, is usually followed by reappearance of glucose metabolic activity in the caudate after 1 to 2 years if the surgery was done early in life.[92] Partial restoration of glucose metabolism in hypometabolic ipsilateral caudate has been shown after unilateral ablation of Brodman areas 4 and 6 in young macaque monkeys.[93] Restoration of caudate metabolism in the monkeys appears to be related to the remaining intact ipsilateral corticostriatal pathways or to increased influence from crossed corticostriatal pathways, described in a number of species, as in the case of hemispherectomy.[94,95] In fact, basal ganglia may play a role in motor function recovery after ablation or injury of the ipsilateral motor cortex, as shown by poor recovery of contralateral motor function after removal of both the motor cortex and basal ganglia.[96] Crossed cerebellar diaschisis, functional impairment at a remote site after injury to an anatomically connected area of brain, and loss of afferent input to the remote site (**Fig. 3**), is typically irreversible in adults.[97] However, it recovers with time in children. It also depends upon the timing of injury. Indeed, Kerrigan and colleagues[98] did not find evidence of crossed cerebellar diaschisis on FDG-PET scan in eight children with congenital hemiplegia. However, after examination of a larger group of subjects with unilateral brain injury, the same investigators found that crossed cerebellar diaschisis may occur in infants and children, if injury occurs postnatally.[99] They further observed the phenomenon of "paradoxic diaschisis" (paradoxically increased cerebellar glucose metabolism contralateral to cerebral injury) in several children

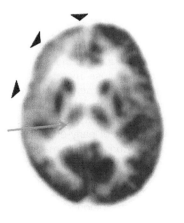
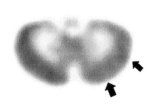

Fig. 3. FDG-PET scan in a child with a large epileptic focus in the right frontal-parietal-temporal cortex (*arrowheads*) associated with ipsilateral thalamic hypometabolism (*long green arrow*) and crossed cerebellar diaschisis (*black arrows*).

with congenital hemiplegia who had sustained their injury at or before 4 months of age.[99] Anatomic reorganization resulting in an "uncrossed" or "recrossed" corticopontocerebellar pathway may be responsible for the absence of crossed cerebellar diaschisis or presence of paradoxic diaschisis. Recent PET studies using C-11 flumazenil, a benzodiazepine antagonist, have also demonstrated that unlike adults, children with unilateral cortical damage show increased binding in both contralateral dentate nuclei and lateral cerebellar lobules, suggesting an age-dependent reorganization of GABA$_A$ receptors in cerebellum.[100]

Several studies on animal models have provided neuroanatomic support for increased plasticity during this period.[101,102] In human beings, studies evaluating the effects of early intervention on intellectual and academic achievement in disadvantaged children[103] and the effect of vocational activities on dendritic complexity[104,105] further strengthens this concept, though it is not clear why some domains (eg, language) show nearly complete recovery or sparing after early injury, yet others (eg, motor, visual) show only limited recovery. Furthermore, the neurobiologic rules that govern intrahemispheric versus interhemispheric reorganization of function are not well understood. However, it seems that LCMRglc changes not only indicate the location of various maturational processes going on in the brain, but also may indicate when brain plasticity is at a maximum. This may be of importance not only in understanding neurophysiology during normal growth or diseases, but also in planning of various clinical, social, and academic interventions, which can have far-reaching impacts.

PET evaluation of neuroreceptors, neurochemical mediators, and cerebral protein synthesis in brain development

Similar to blood flow, oxygen use, and glucose metabolism, there are also developmental changes in various neuroreceptors and neurotransmitters. Understanding their normal patterns of expression not only will help in understanding the functional aspects of regional brain maturation but also in understanding the pathophysiology of several neurologic disorders. Our understanding of the role played by neurotransmitter receptors in the developing brain has advanced in recent years. Although PET has been extensively used for neuroreceptor imaging and evaluation of neurotransmitters, very few studies are available that have evaluated their developmental and maturational aspects, particularly in human beings. Therefore, the discussion will be restricted to GABA$_A$ receptor binding, serotonin synthesis, and cerebral protein synthesis.

Postnatal maturation of human GABA receptor The major inhibitory neurotransmitter in the brain, GABA, acts to influence early developmental events, some of which occur before synapse formation; these include proliferation, migration, differentiation, or survival processes during neural development. To carry out these functions, different types of GABA$_A$ receptors need to be expressed both at the right time and at the right place. Several types of GABA$_A$ receptor transcripts and subunits have been described as components of functional GABA$_A$ receptors in rat neuroepithelial cells, neuroblasts, and glioblasts during spinal and cortical neurogenesis.[106–109]

It appears that activity-dependent synaptic plasticity in response to sensory experience in animals is related to developmental changes in GABA$_A$ neurotransmission.[110,111] There are significant changes in GABA$_A$ receptor subunit composition in the developing brain: for example, in the visual cortex,[112] somatosensory cortex,[113] and cerebellum.[114] The density of GABA$_A$ receptors in the rhesus monkey cortex increases after birth to peak (40% higher than adult value) at 2 to 4 months of age, and then gradually declines to adult values at 3 years of age.[115] There are also regional and laminar-specific developmental changes in the cortical and subcortical GABA$_A$ receptor subunits.[116–118]

Therefore, knowledge of GABA$_A$ receptor ontogeny in human beings is not only important for understanding brain maturation, but also to investigate how GABA function may play a role in the pathophysiology of a number of developmental disorders. C-11-flumazenil (FMZ), a ligand that binds to the α-subunit of the GABA$_A$ receptor, can be used to evaluate GABA$_A$ receptor complex in vivo with PET. Chugani and colleagues[119] measured age-related changes in the brain distribution of the GABA$_A$ receptor complex in vivo using FMZ-PET. They found that all brain regions showed the highest value for FMZ binding or FMZ VD (volume of distribution) at 2 years of age and then decreased exponentially with age until adult values were reached at around 20 years of age (**Fig. 4**).

Because not much data are available for children less than 2 years of age, it is difficult to say when FMZ binding is highest. It seems that high FMZ VD in early childhood may be related to a specific role of benzodiazepine-sensitive GABA$_A$ receptors in critical periods of synaptic plasticity during human brain development. The order of

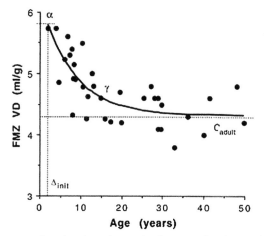

Fig. 4. Plot showing change in flumazenil volume of distribution (measure of its binding) with age. (*From* Chugani DC, Muzik O, Juhasz C, et al. Ann Neurol 2001;49:621; with permission.)

brain region (from highest to lowest FMZ binding) at 2 years of age is as follows: primary visual cortex, superior frontal cortex, medial temporal cortex, temporal lobe, prefrontal cortex, cerebellum, basal ganglia, and thalamus (**Fig. 5**). During development, medial temporal lobe structures, the primary visual cortex, and the thalamus show the largest decrease in FMZ VD (approximately 50% decreases), compared with the basal ganglia, cerebellum, and other cortical regions (25%–40% decreases). Subcortical brain regions reach adult values earlier (14–17.5 years) than cortical regions (18–22 years). Rank order of FMZ binding in various adult brain regions is given in the **Table 1**. Although their finding of earlier maturation of GABA$_A$ receptors in subcortical brain regions is consistent with results of previous studies of changes in glucose metabolism with

age,[56] investigators found that the time course of decline in synaptic density in visual cortex appears to more closely follow the time course of decrease in GABA$_A$ receptors than that of glucose metabolism.

Maturational changes in brain serotonin Serotonin (5-hydroxytryptamine or 5HT) is phylogenetically the oldest of the biogenic amine neurotransmitters and acts as a trophic or differentiating factor in addition to its role as a neurotransmitter. It has a regulatory role in neuronal proliferation, migration, and differentiation, and in preventing apoptotic cell death; indeed, change in its level during early stages of life is associated with altered brain development and maturation.

Stimulation of serotonin receptors in vitro accelerates cell division and increases DNA synthesis. In monkeys, high levels of serotonin expression have been reported in the proliferative zone of the occipital lobe during neurogenesis.[120] Cortical progenitors are also sensitive to serotonin levels and pharmacologic depletion of serotonin in the embryo induces microcephaly.[42] It seems that serotonin either plays a role in establishing the number of progenitors or their proliferation at the start of corticogenesis or is involved in modeling the length of the cell cycle. At early developmental stages, serotonin modulates the migration of several neural crest derivatives[121,122] and it has been postulated that serotonin influences the rate of migration by modulating the microtubule stability in specific neuronal populations. Serotonin depletion is associated with a delay in neurogenesis.[123] Decreased or increased brain serotonin during development has been shown to result in disruption of synaptic connectivity in sensory cortices.[124,125]

Developmental changes in brain serotonin content and serotonin receptor binding have

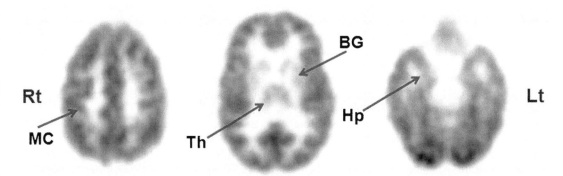

Fig. 5. FMZ-PET scan showing normal FMZ binding in a 2-year-old child (BG, basal ganglia; Hp, hippocampus; MC, motor cortex; Th, thalamus). Note the relatively low binding in the basal ganglia and thalamus, and the high degree of binding in hippocampus.

been demonstrated in nonhuman primates.[115,126] In the rhesus monkey, development of serotonin storage capacity and synthetic processes continues over a period of months and years and varies greatly in different cytoarchitectonic regions of the cerebral cortex.[126] There is a rise in serotonin content beginning before birth, reaching adult values between 2 and 5 months of age in most cortical regions. Changes in rates of synthesis of serotonin generally parallel developmental changes. A smaller but significant increase in serotonin metabolism takes place in the parietal and visual cortex between birth and 36 months. Serotonin receptors also show similar developmental changes in the rhesus monkey, reaching a maximum level between 2 and 4 months of age and then declining gradually to adult levels in all layers of sensory, motor, and association regions.[115]

Recent development of α[C-11] methyl-L-tryptophan (AMT) as a tracer for PET now allows a direct in vivo measurement of serotonin synthesis in human beings. AMT is an analog of tryptophan, the precursor for serotonin synthesis but, unlike tryptophan, AMT is not incorporated into protein in significant amounts. AMT is converted to alpha-methyl-serotonin (AM-5HT) by tryptophan hydroxylase, but because AM-5HT, unlike serotonin, is also not a substrate for the degradative enzyme monamine oxidase, it accumulates in neurons and nerve terminals along with the releasable pool of serotonin.[127,128] After intravenous injection, AMT accumulates in the brain for the first 20 minutes (less than 2% of the injected dose is present in the brain at peak values), after which a plateau is reached and maintained for up to 60 minutes, with no right-left asymmetry in normal adults.[129] Because AMT-PET does not allow the measurement of absolute rates of serotonin synthesis, the term "serotonin synthesis capacity" (an index of serotonin synthesis) has been applied. This measurement increases after birth, reaches twice the adult value by 3 years of age, remains at a plateau until 5 years of age, and then declines, reaching adult values by 14 years of age (**Fig. 6**).[130] Rank order of serotonin uptake values in various adult brain regions is given in the **Table 1** and the AMT uptake pattern in the brain is given in **Fig. 7**. Values in women are 10% to 20% higher throughout the brain and particularly higher in the transverse temporal gyrus, anterior cingulate cortex, and cerebellar vermis.[129]

There is evidence that abnormalities of serotonergic neurotransmission are associated with several neurologic and psychiatric disorders, including autism, migraine, sleep disorders, depression, various movement disorders, and epilepsy. Although there is evidence for the potential involvement of several other neurotransmitters in autism, the most consistent findings involve serotonin. While tryptophan depletion has been reported to result in an exacerbation of symptoms in autistic subjects,[131] administration of serotonin reuptake inhibitors appear to result in improvement of compulsive symptoms, repetitive movements, and social difficulties in autistic adults.[132] Chugani and colleagues[133] used AMT-PET scanning to study seizure-free children with autism (seven males, one female, 4–11 years of age) and their healthy nonautistic siblings (four males, one female, 8–14 years of age). Gross asymmetries of AMT standard uptake value in the frontal cortex, thalamus, and cerebellum were visualized in seven

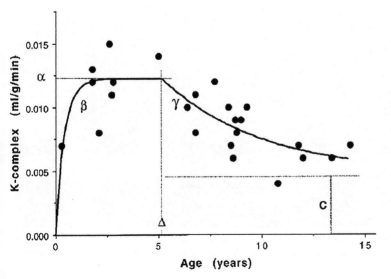

Fig. 6. Plot showing change in serotonin synthesis capacity (global brain values for K complex) with age. (*From* Chugani DC, Muzik O, Behen M, et al. Ann Neurol 1999;45:292; with permission.)

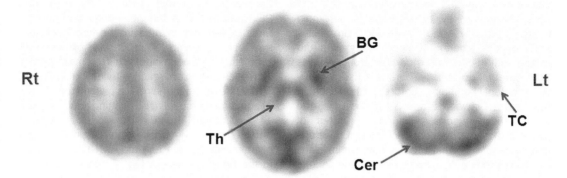

Fig. 7. AMT-PET scan showing normal AMT uptake in a 14 years old child (BG, basal ganglia; Cer, cerebellum; TC, temporal cortex; Th, thalamus). Note the very high activity in cerebellum.

autistic boys, but not in the one autistic girl studied nor in four of the five siblings. Decreased AMT accumulation was seen in the left frontal cortex and thalamus in five of seven autistic boys. This was accompanied by an elevated AMT accumulation in the right cerebellum, in the region of the dentate nucleus (**Fig. 8**). In the remaining two autistic boys, AMT accumulation was decreased in the right frontal cortex and thalamus and elevated in the left dentate nucleus. Subsequently, Chugani and colleagues[130] measured whole-brain serotonin synthesis capacity in 30 seizure free autistic children (24 males, 6 females, 2–15 years of age) and 8 of their healthy nonautistic siblings (6 males, 2 females, 2–14 years of age), and found that the trajectory of serotonin synthesis capacity in autistic children was abnormal, compared with normal children. The serotonin synthesis capacity in autistic children increased between the ages of 2 to 15 years to only 1.5 times of the adult

normal values, unlike normal siblings, in whom an increase of 2 times the adult value was found between 2 to 5 years of age.

Brain development and protein synthesis Virtually all aspects of brain development, such as neurogenesis, neuronal proliferation and migration, synaptogenesis and pruning, myelination, and most cognitive functions, such as learning, memory, and so forth are dependent upon protein synthesis. Therefore, it will be of large clinical significance to study brain protein synthesis during development and maturation. This can potentially enhance our understanding of normal brain development and various developmental disorders. PET with radio-labeled leucine can measure regional cerebral protein synthesis and presently is the only available noninvasive in vivo technique to allow such measurements. However, because of many technical, methodologic, and logistic

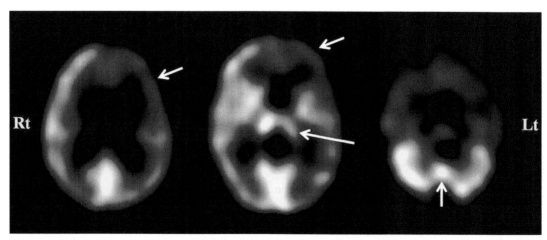

Fig. 8. AMT-PET scan in an autistic boy showing the typical pattern of decreased AMT uptake in the frontal cortex and thalamus (*left* side in this case), and increased uptake in the contralateral right cerebellum and dentate nucleus (*arrows*).

problems, it has not been used widely. Although no study on human brain development has been performed to date, several autoradiographic studies in animals have provided interesting insight.

Protein synthesis rates in most brain structures in cats at birth were found to be within the range of adult values (with some exceptions, such as the hippocampus and putamen).[134] Subsequently, most structures showed a transient developmental peak during which the rates became higher than that of adults. This peak often occurred at around postnatal day 60 (P60), but in some regions lasted from P30 to P90, indicating some regional heterogeneity in the maturation of brain protein synthesis. It seems that, like glucose metabolism, there is a transitory but generally significant increase in protein synthesis rate during early development that goes beyond stable, adult values. The majority of structures progressively reached peak values of leucine incorporation by P60, but thereafter a steady decline brought the values back down to P1/adult levels by the age of P120, a profile similar to that seen with glucose-use rates in kittens.[49] However, unlike glucose-use rate, no second peak was observed with the protein synthesis rate. The authors speculated that the developmental time course of protein synthesis was similar to and probably related to synaptogenesis.

Nehlig and colleagues[135] conducted protein synthesis studies in rats at P10 through P35 and in adult rats by measuring the incorporation of labeled methionine into brain proteins. They observed a pattern of maturation very similar to that described above for the cat, but with a different timing relative to birth. However, after making adjustments for the different time course of development in these two species, protein synthesis rates in cat and rat brains appeared to be similar. In another study also using rats, Sun and colleagues[136] measured local rates of leucine incorporation into cerebral protein (lCPSleu) from age P7 to P60. They found that in most brain regions the values were highest at P10 (except for white matter, with values peaking at P14–P20) and then gradually decreased with age. With the use of the quantitative autoradiographic L-[1-(14C] leucine method, Abrams and colleagues[137] measured lCPSleu in 35 regions of the central nervous system, pineal body, and whole brain of nine fetal sheep (118–139 days gestational age) and five newborn lambs (1–5 days of age). Regardless of age, lCPSleu was highest in the pineal body, brain stem, and hypothalamic nuclei and lowest in white matter, with lCPSleu correlating positively with prenatal age in sensorimotor cortex, corona radiata, pyramidal tracts, and whole brain.

These developmental data on cerebral protein synthesis add to our knowledge of normal brain development and how protein synthesis is important for the evolution of various neurologic functions. This information may provide us an insight into the pathogenesis of various developmental and neurologic disorders, particularly those related to neurogenesis, dendritic, and synaptic proliferation, and maturational processes such as myelination.

ROLE OF PET IN DEVELOPMENTAL DISORDERS

PET can play an extremely important role in the evaluation of various developmental disorders. It is beyond the scope of this article to provide an exhaustive review of all pediatric conditions where PET has been applied, but the following examples will illustrate the potential of PET in understanding various childhood neurologic disorders and altering management.

Childhood Epileptic Syndromes

Infantile spasms

Infantile spasms, also known as West syndrome, is an uncommon epileptic disorder of infancy that usually starts between 3 and 12 months of age. These seizures are characterized by sudden severe myoclonic contractions of the entire body, typically involving the neck flexor muscles, with the chin jerking toward the torso or the head drawing inward with simultaneous raising and bending of the arms, occurring in clusters. The infantile spasms are classified as symptomatic if an underlying cause is present or cryptogenic when an underlying neurologic disorder is suspected but cannot be diagnosed. Rarely, when no underlying cause is present and the spasms are physiologic, presumably because of immaturity of electrophysiologic systems, they are referred to as idiopathic. PET can play a very important role in cases of cryptogenic or idiopathic infantile spasms, in understanding the pathogenesis of the spasms, in prognostication of these cases, or in selecting children for surgical treatment. PET can also help in etiologic classification of infantile spasm, with many cryptogenic cases being reclassified as symptomatic, as 95 out of 97 cryptogenic cases were found to have one or more abnormalities on FDG-PET scan.[138]

FDG-PET in these infants usually shows focal areas of hypo- or hypermetabolism or multifocal abnormalities, which are usually associated with underlying cortical dysplasia (**Fig. 9**).[139–141] Symmetric, diffuse hypometabolism indicates

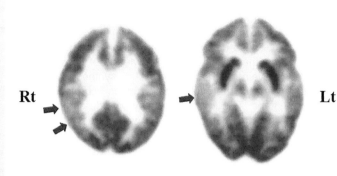

Rt   Lt

Fig. 9. FDG-PET scan in a 4-month-old child with infantile spasms showing hypometabolism in the right parietal and temporal cortex (*arrows*), and increased FDG uptake in bilateral basal ganglia.

neurometabolic or neurodegenerative disorders, rather than a lesional etiology.[142] FDG-PET also shows abnormalities in the primary sensorimotor area in asymmetric and asynchronous spasms.[143] Cortical hypometabolism may change with time, with persistence of hypometabolism indicating continuation of spasms and worse developmental prognosis.[144] Similarly, bitemporal hypometabolism on FDG-PET scan may indicate poor long-term outcome with autistic features in these children.[145]

Areas of PET abnormalities usually correspond well with the EEG localization of focal ictal or interictal abnormalities,[140,141] except when hypsarrhythmia is present, in which case focal electrographic abnormalities either preceding or following the presence of hypsarrhythmia correlate best with the PET abnormalities. Therefore, children with infantile spasms, particularly cryptogenic ones, should routinely undergo FDG-PET scan for further evaluation. In many cases it may be the only modality showing any brain abnormality and may help in surgical planning. As opposed to multifocal or diffuse bilateral PET abnormalities, children with unifocal lesion, consistent with electrophysiologic findings, may undergo surgical resection, which usually results in cessation of spasms (or improved spasms control) and improved long-term development.[140,141] PET may also help in intracranial electrode placements, to determine the area of resection, as leading spikes followed by fast-wave bursts have been shown to originate in and around glucose hypometabolic regions and whose resection is necessary for better surgical outcome.[146]

PET has been used to investigate the complex cortical-subcortical interactions believed to be important in the secondary generalization of focal cortical discharges resulting in spasms. PET studies have shown that, regardless of the type or extent of cortical abnormality, there is hypermetabolism in lenticular nuclei and brain stem in infants with spasms (see **Fig. 9**).[139] It seems that infantile spasms are initiated as cortical epileptic

discharges that, during a critical developmental period, may undergo secondary generalization in an age-dependent mechanism to emerge as spasms. The onset of spasms often coincides with the functional maturation of the cerebral cortex. The offending lesion may be a focal or diffuse cortical abnormality that, at a critical stage of maturation, causes abnormal functional interactions with brainstem raphe nuclei, which project widely throughout the brain. Raphe-cortical projections could mediate the hypsarrhythmic changes seen on EEG, and the prominent serotonergic raphe-striatal pathway and descending spinal pathways may be responsible for the secondary generalization of the cortical discharges resulting in the relatively symmetric spasms.[147,148] These pathogenic mechanisms can be further investigated using newer PET tracers, such as C-11 AMT (for serotonin synthesis; see above) and C-11 flumazenil (for GABA$_A$ receptor binding; see above).

Lennox-Gastaut syndrome

Lennox-Gastaut syndrome (LGS) is childhood-onset often-intractable epilepsy that usually starts between 2 and 6 years of age and is characterized by a slow spike-wave pattern (1 Hz–2.5 Hz) on the EEG, frequent seizures, and different seizure types, and is accompanied by mental retardation and developmental delay. The most common type of seizure is tonic, usually nocturnal, followed by myoclonic, atonic, atypical absence, complex partial, or tonic-clonic seizures. Status epilepticus is also common. Up to 20% children with infantile spasms may progress to LGS during the second year of life. Although there are many underlying pathologies, such as encephalopathy, tuberous sclerosis, hereditary metabolic diseases, inflammatory brain disease (such as encephalitis, meningitis, and toxoplasmosis), hypoxic-ischemic injury, and other birth injuries supposed to be involved in LGS, in up to one-third of cases it is cryptogenic or idiopathic. FDG-PET may show uni- or multifocal metabolic abnormalities (**Fig. 10**), which do not always correlate with anatomic or structural

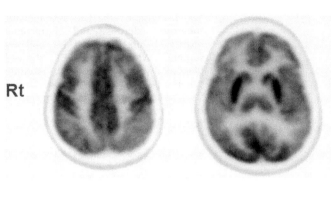

Fig. 10. FDG-PET scan showing multiple areas of severe cortical hypometabolism in a child with LGS and multiple seizure types. The motor cortex, occipital cortex, and basal ganglia appear relatively prominently.

Rt

Lt

abnormalities and thus can help in revealing the extent of pathology and understanding the pathomechanism of various functional expressions of this disorder.[149–155] FDG-PET has been used for metabolic classification of LGS into four predominant metabolic subtypes: unilateral focal hypometabolism, unilateral diffuse hypometabolism, bilateral diffuse hypometabolism, and normal glucose metabolism.[149] FDG-PET can play a particularly important role in cryptogenic cases by showing underlying abnormalities and in surgical management if there is a focal lesion.

Tuberous sclerosis

Tuberous sclerosis complex (TSC) is a neurocutaneous disorder, characterized by tumorous growths that involve multiple organs, including brain, retina, kidney, heart, and skin. Approximately 70% to 90% of patients with TSC have seizures, which are attributed to the presence of brain cortical malformations. Tubers typically show up as areas of cortical hypometabolism on interictal FDG-PET scan;[156,157] these hypometabolic areas are believed to be caused by the decreased number of neurons and simplified dendritic pattern in the tubers. Interictal FDG-PET can even detect small cortical tubers not visualized on T2 MR imaging. However, these hypometabolic areas often extend beyond the structural lesions visible on MR imaging[158] and it has been shown that the seizure activity often originates from the mildly hypometabolic regions adjacent to the cortical tubers. Furthermore, in the case of multiple tubers, FDG-PET is not able to identify which of the multiple tubers are epileptogenic and, therefore, is not useful to guide surgical resection in TSC patients with medically intractable seizures.

The PET tracer AMT can be used to differentiate epileptogenic from nonepileptogenic tubers, as it shows increased AMT uptake interictally in only epileptogenic tubers (**Fig. 11**). In epileptogenic tubers, there is increased uptake and subsequent intracellular accumulation of the AMT because of

activation of the kynurenine pathway,[129] which leads to the production of neurotoxic and convulsant metabolites, such as quinolinic acid.[159] AMT-PET can identify epileptogenic tubers in almost two-thirds of children with tuberous sclerosis and intractable epilepsy.[129,158,160] While the specificity of AMT-PET is very high, its sensitivity is suboptimal, and appears to be related to the underlying pathology as well as the method of image analysis. In patients with tuberous sclerosis and intractable epilepsy, MR imaging-based quantitative assessment almost doubles the sensitivity of AMT-PET to 79%, from 44.4%, with visual assessment.[161] This apparent discrepancy is because of the fact that nonepileptogenic tubers typically show decreased AMT uptake, and that some epileptogenic tubers showing relatively increased AMT uptake cannot be easily differentiated from adjacent normal cortex without quantitative analysis. The authors also found good correlation between resection of epileptogenic tubers suggested by AMT-PET and seizure outcome.[162] Tubers with at least 10% increase of AMT uptake were all found to be epileptogenic. A cutoff threshold of 1.02 for AMT uptake ratio provided 83% accuracy for detecting tubers that need to be resected to achieve a seizure-free outcome.[158,162]

The use of PET has also contributed to our understanding of the neurobehavioral phenotypes of TSC, which include autism, attention deficit hyperactivity disorder, aggression, and cognitive impairment. Application of PET, by combining FDG and AMT, has revealed the role of both cortical and subcortical dysfunction in the pathophysiology of autism in TSC.[163] Glucose hypometabolism in the bilateral, lateral temporal cortex has been found to be associated with the severity of communication disturbance, whereas hypermetabolism in the deep cerebellar nuclei and increased AMT uptake in the caudate nucleus has been found to be related to stereotyped behavior, impaired social interaction, and communication disturbance.[164] A recent PET study of

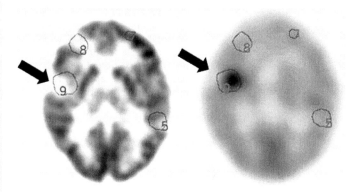

Fig. 11. Multiple tubers in a child with tuberous sclerosis and intractable seizures being evaluated for epilepsy surgery. Whereas FDG-PET showed glucose hypometabolism in multiple tubers (*left*), AMT-PET scan (*right*) showed intense uptake in a right frontal tuber (*arrow*) corresponding to the EEG focus.

cerebellar tubers has shown that right-sided cerebellar lesions were associated with higher social isolation and communicative and developmental disturbance compared with left-sided cerebellar lesions,[165] supporting an important role of the cerebellum in autism.

Sturge-Weber syndrome

Sturge-Weber syndrome (SWS) is a neurocutaneous syndrome characterized by facial capillary nevus (port-wine stain) in the distribution of one or more divisions of the fifth cranial nerve and ipsilateral leptomeningeal angiomatosis. Neurologic consequences include intracerebral calcification, epilepsy, hemiparesis, hemianopia, and glaucoma. In children with SWS, FDG-PET reveals hypometabolism ipsilateral to the facial nevus and usually identifies additional areas of abnormal cortex extending beyond the lesion visible on MR imaging.[43,166] However, some infants may show increased glucose metabolism interictally in the cortex underlying the leptomenigeal angioma, which with time becomes hypometabolic.[43] In some patients, serial FDG-PET scans show rapidly progressing hypometabolism in the affected area, probably because of rapid demise of the brain tissue associated with the angioma.[167] These patients usually show improvement in seizure status and cognitive function and therefore may not require surgical intervention (**Fig. 12**). Probably, early and rapid progression of unilateral disease, associated with destruction of underlying brain tissue, leads to early and more efficient reorganization in the contralateral cortex. Indeed, a recent FDG-PET study showed decreased glucose metabolism in the visual and parietal cortex on the side of the angioma but increased metabolism on the contralateral side.[168] In particular, glucose metabolism was found to be very high in contralateral visual cortex of children with SWS and visual field defect, indicating that early, severe unilateral cortical damage in SWS may induce increased glucose metabolism in the

contralateral visual cortex, probably reflecting reorganization.

On the other hand, persistent mild hypometabolism of the lesion may indicate ongoing functional deterioration and these patients may show persistent seizures and developmental delay.[167] These are the patients who require surgical intervention to control their seizures and to improve their cognitive development by allowing the brain to reorganize itself while brain plasticity is still at a maximum. In SWS, damaging metabolic changes occur before 3 years of age,[166] coinciding with a rapid increase in developmentally regulated cerebral metabolic demand.[56] Progressive hypometabolism is associated with high seizure frequency in these children. However, metabolic abnormalities may remain limited or even partially recover later in some children with well-controlled seizures. Metabolic recovery accompanied by neurologic improvement suggests a window for therapeutic intervention in children with unilateral SWS.[166] O-15 water PET studies have also been used to evaluate the functional activation of calcified hypoperfused brain areas during language and motor tasks.[169] It was found that hypoperfused areas may become activated during language and motor performance, and progressive calcification in SWS is associated with functional reorganization in the language and motor domains. Interhemispheric reorganization was found to be more pronounced for language than for motor functions.

Landau-Kleffner syndrome

Landau-Kleffner syndrome, also called "acquired epileptic aphasia" or "aphasia with convulsive disorder," is a rare childhood neurologic disorder occurring between 4 and 8 years of ages and is characterized by the sudden or gradual development of aphasia in an epileptic child, who had developed typically, including normal language, until that time. While many of the affected children have clinical seizures, some may have only

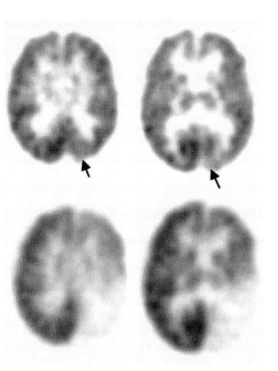

Fig. 12. In a child with SWS and meningeal hemangioma of the left posterior quadrant (*arrow*), serial FDG scans showed progression of the cortical hypometabolism, indicating degenerative changes in the brain tissue associated with the angioma. The child showed improvement in seizure status and cognitive function.

electrographic seizures, including electrographic status epilepticus of sleep. FDG-PET has shown bilateral temporal lobe involvement, particularly superior and medial.[170–172] FDG-PET has also revealed the possible involvement of temporal lobes in the generation of continuous spike waves during slow-wave sleep.[173,174] FDG-PET can be further used to monitor dynamic changes of glucose metabolism in the temporal lobe during episodes of aphasia and remission (**Fig. 13**).[175]

Hemimegalencephaly

Hemimegalencephaly is a developmental brain malformation characterized by congenital hypertrophy of one cerebral hemisphere with ipsilateral ventriculomegaly and is associated with epilepsy, hemianopsia, and varying degrees of developmental delay. The larger hemisphere is the more abnormal one and is highly epileptogenic, often requiring hemispherectomy for alleviation of the seizures. FDG-PET usually shows varying level of hypometabolism in the affected hemisphere.[176] However, the apparently normal hemisphere also may show metabolic abnormalities (**Fig. 14**), indicating dysfunction of the structurally normal

hemisphere, and which could be the reason for not as good a surgical outcome of hemispherectomy when compared with children undergoing the same operation for SWS, chronic focal encephalitis of Rasmussen, or hemiplegic cerebral palsy. Therefore, FDG-PET can be used for the presurgical evaluation of the functional integrity of the apparently normal hemisphere. In fact, the degree and pattern of the metabolic involvement of the apparently uninvolved hemisphere has been found to be correlated with surgical outcome and overall prognosis.[176]

Perinatal Hypoxic-ischemic Encephalopathy

FDG-PET can delineate the extent of brain damage and provide new perspective on the mechanisms of neonatal brain injury and prognostic information about subsequent functional sequelae. Cerebral perfusion PET studies in preterm infants with intraventricular and intracerebral hemorrhage have demonstrated large areas of hypoperfusion, involving the whole affected hemisphere.[177] Similarly, FDG-PET studies found areas of hypometabolism extending beyond the affected regions shown by CT scan.[178] In full-term neonates with perinatal asphyxia, PET usually shows relative hypoperfusion in the parasagittal regions.[179] Transient hypermetabolism in the basal ganglia at the time of birth, followed by severe hypometabolism in the lenticular nuclei and thalami, has been found in newborns who suffered perinatal hypoxic-ischemic encephalopathy (HIE) and developed dystonic cerebral palsy later (**Fig. 15**), suggesting that transient hypermetabolism in the basal ganglia following perinatal hypoxia may be related to excitotoxic damage, causing permanent neurologic symptoms in the form of dystonic cerebral palsy.[180] Similarly, total CMRglc has been found to be inversely correlated with the severity of HIE, with neonates having low CMRglc subsequently developing cerebral palsy.[181] Another FDG-PET study in children with suspected HIE found that those with abnormal development had persistently low cerebral glucose metabolism.[182] Therefore, it appears that FDG-PET can provide valuable information for the prediction of neurologic outcome in cases of HIE.

Cerebral Palsy

Cerebral palsy is a nonprogressive neurologic disorder which may, in some cases, be related to perinatal brain injury. Depending upon the motor impairments, which depends upon the area of the brain damaged, cerebral palsy has been classified into four major types: spastic (spastic

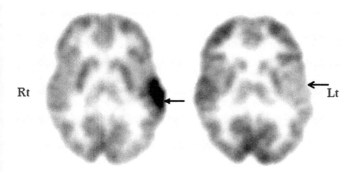

Rt   Lt

Fig. 13. FDG-PET images from a child with Landau-Kleffner syndrome showing marked hypermetabolism in the left temporal region (*arrow*) during the peak of his aphasic episode. EEG during the PET tracer uptake period showed frequent and repetitive spike-and-wave activities from this area. A repeat FDG-PET scan during his remission state showed hypometabolism in the same region (*arrow*).

hemiplegia, diplegia, or quadriplegia), athetoid/dyskinetic, ataxic, and mixed. PET can help in identifying the involvement of various cortical and subcortical structures and the extent of their damage in these various forms of cerebral palsy. FDG-PET studies have shown that the distribution of metabolic impairment almost invariably extends beyond the region of anatomic involvement. Whereas FDG-PET shows focal areas of cortical hypometabolism in the absence of apparent structural abnormality in spastic diplegic patients, a relatively normal pattern of cortical metabolism is seen in some children with choreoathetoid cerebral palsy, along with marked hypometabolism in the thalamus and lenticular nuclei and relative sparing of the caudate nucleus (see **Fig. 15**).[98] Relative sparing of the cerebral cortex is consistent with the clinical observation that many of these children have relative preservation of cognitive function compared with their severe motor impairment. Use of FMZ-PET has demonstrated increased GABA receptor binding in the bilateral motor and visual cortex and decreased binding in the brain stem, indicating the role of GABA receptors in poor motor control.[183]

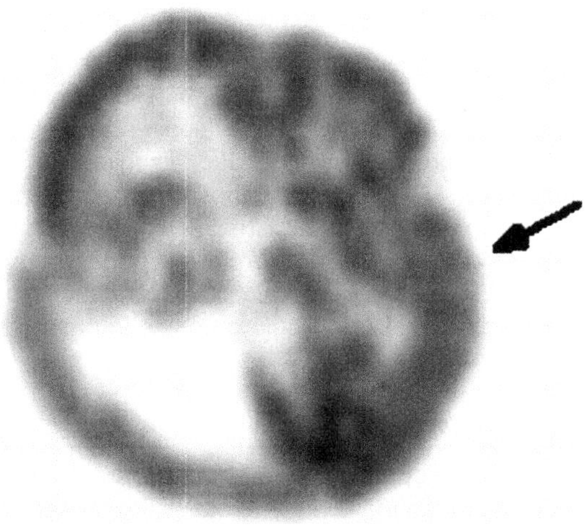

Developmental Dyslexia

Dyslexia is a specific learning disability that manifests primarily as a difficulty with written language, particularly with reading and spelling. Various PET studies have shown the involvement of bilateral posterior temporal and parietal cortices. PET studies using O-15 labeled water in dyslexic subjects showed a failure to activate the left temporoparietal cortex during a rhyme detection task, and reduced activation/unusual deactivation in mid- and posterior temporal cortex bilaterally, and also in the inferior parietal cortex, predominantly on the left side, during both pronunciation and decision making.[184,185] In contrast, dyslexic men demonstrated essentially normal activation of the left inferior frontal cortex during both phonologic and orthographic decision making. In another PET study, the dyslexic group showed less activation than the control group in the right superior temporal and right postcentral gyri, and also in the left cerebellum.[186] Other PET studies revealed lower activation in right cerebellar cortex and left cingulate gyrus,[187] and functional disconnection of the left angular gyrus from other parts of the reading network in adults with persistent developmental dyslexia.[188] A recent O-15 PET study of the learning of phoneme categorization found a different pattern of activation in dyslexic subjects compared with normal controls.[189] A strongly left-lateralized activation involving the superior temporal, inferior parietal, and inferior lateral frontal cortex was found during the speech mode in normal readers. Frontal and parietal subparts of these left-sided regions were found to be significantly more activated in the control group than in the dyslexic group. However, activations in the right frontal cortex were found to be larger in the dyslexic group than in the control group for both speech and acoustic modes compared with rest.

Fig. 14. FDG-PET scan in a child with right hemimegalencephaly showing an enlarged malformed right hemisphere and additional area of mild hypometabolism (*arrow*) in the opposite hemisphere.

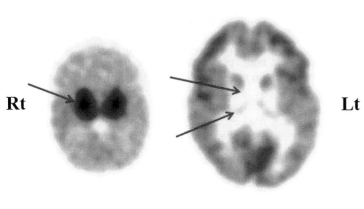

Fig. 15. FDG-PET scans of a child who suffered hypoxic ischemic encephalopathy at birth and later developed dystonic/choreoathetoid cerebral palsy. The left image from the newborn period showed intense hypermetabolism in the basal ganglia (*arrow*). The right image at 5 years showed severe hypometabolism in the lenticular nuclei and thalami (*arrows*). Note the relative preservation of metabolism in the cerebral cortex.

Dyslexic subjects also showed an unexpected large deactivation in the medial occipital cortex for the acoustic mode.

FDG-PET studies have shown less asymmetry in glucose uptake in prefrontal and lingual (inferior) regions of the occipital lobe during reading in dyslexic subjects, indicating that brain regions are activated differently in them.[190] Another FDG-PET study showed significantly higher absolute and relative brain metabolism along an anterior-posterior gradient, including medial temporal lobe, in dyslexic subjects compared with normal during auditory syllable discrimination task.[191] The authors have also found several patterns of abnormal glucose metabolism, including bilateral temporal and parietal hypometabolism, bilateral temporal hypometabolism, and unilateral left temporal hypometabolism in dyslexic subjects, which is in agreement with neuropsychologic data indicating heterogeneity in patients with developmental dyslexia (**Fig. 16**).

Tourette Syndrome

Tourette syndrome is an inherited neurologic disorder with onset in childhood and is characterized by the presence of multiple motor tics and at least one vocal tic for more than 1 year; these tics characteristically wax and wane. In the few children with Tourette syndrome who have been studied with FDG-PET, no consistent abnormalities have been found. These patients have been reported to have decreased normalized metabolic rates in paralimbic and ventral prefrontal cortices, particularly in orbitofrontal, inferior insular, and parahippocampal regions.[192] Similar decreases were observed in subcortical regions, including the ventral striatum (nucleus accumbens/ventromedial caudate) and in the midbrain. These changes were more robust and occurred with greater frequency in the left hemisphere and were associated with concomitant bilateral increases in metabolic activity of the supplementary motor, lateral premotor, and Rolandic cortices. Cerebral perfusion PET studies have been used for the investigation of neuronal circuits involved in tic generation in patients with Tourette syndrome. One O-15 PET study showed robust activation of cerebellum, insula, thalamus, and putamen during tic release.[193] Another O-15 PET study showed significant tics related activation in medial and lateral premotor cortices, anterior cingulate cortex, dorsolateral-rostral prefrontal cortex, inferior parietal cortex, putamen, and caudate, as well as primary motor cortex, Broca's area, superior temporal gyrus, insula, and

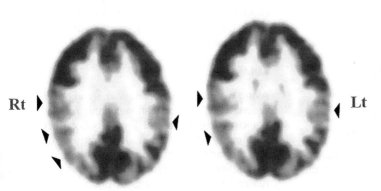

Fig. 16. FDG-PET scan of a child with developmental dyslexia and normal MR imaging showing bilateral parietal cortex hypometabolism (*arrowheads*).

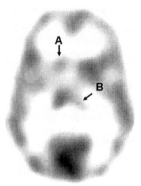

Right   Left

Fig. 17. AMT-PET scan in a child with Tourette syndrome showing decreased AMT uptake in the right basal ganglia (A) and the left thalamus (B).

claustrum.[194] Aberrant activity in the interrelated sensorimotor, language, executive, and paralimbic circuits identified in this study may account for the initiation and execution of diverse motor and vocal behaviors that characterize tics in Tourette syndrome, as well as for the urges that often accompany them.

Several studies evaluated various aspects of dopaminergic transmission, as it is believed that disturbances in the dopaminergic system contribute to the pathophysiology of Tourette syndrome. Such studies reported elevated striatal dopamine transporter levels,[195] abnormal presynaptic DOPA decarboxylase activity,[196] and significantly lower D2 receptor availability in the orbitofrontal cortex, primary motor cortex, anterior

cingulate gyrus, mediodorsal nucleus of thalamus, and hippocampus, areas important for motivation and reward, sensory gating, movement, and attention, in subjects with Tourette syndrome.[197] Another study also demonstrated increased dopamine release in the striatum, particularly putamen, of Tourette patients.[198,199] Imaging data using AMT-PET appear to support the role of abnormal serotonergic neurotransmission in the pathophysiology of Tourette syndrome and some of its comorbid conditions, such as attention deficit hyperactivity disorder and obsessive-compulsive disorder.[200] Increased serotonin receptor binding was found not only in regions closely related to subcortical regions in patients with Tourette syndrome, but also in most other brain regions.[201] Decreased AMT uptake in bilateral dorsolateral prefrontal cortical and bilaterally increased uptake in the thalamus with bilateral increased ratio of AMT uptake in subcortical structures to dorsolateral prefrontal cortex was reported in Tourette syndrome children.[200] However, thalamic and basal ganglia asymmetry in AMT uptake is also frequently found in these children (**Fig. 17**).

Neuronal Ceroid Lipofuscinoses or Spielmeyer-Vogt Disease

The neuronal ceroid lipofuscinoses are a group of autosomal recessive neurodegenerative disorders that are characterized, in general, by seizures, developmental regression, and progressive visual impairment. While children with the juvenile form (CLN-3) or Spielmeyer-Vogt (or Batten) disease show decreased glucose metabolism in the calcarine cortex early in the course of the disease (**Fig. 18**), children with late infantile neuronal ceroid lipofuscinosis (CLN-2; Jansky-Bielschowsky disease, with curvilinear inclusions) show rapid degeneration with generalized cortical and subcortical hypometabolism.[202–206] As the juvenile form of the disease progresses, a rostral spread of glucose hypometabolism to other cortical areas is observed.[206] Therefore, the rate of disease progression can be monitored with PET. PET Studies have also shown reduced striatal dopamine D1 receptors in juvenile neuronal ceroid lipofuscinosis.[207]

SUMMARY

Along with various molecular imaging agents in its arsenal, PET can play an invaluable role in understanding the structural and functional changes that occur during brain development and how these changes relate to behavioral and cognitive maturation in the infant and child. This article has reviewed various aspects of brain development,

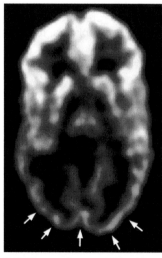

Fig. 18. FDG-PET image from a child with neuronal ceroid lipofuscinosis showing selective hypometabolism in the occipital cortex bilaterally (*arrows*).

such as the ontogeny of brain glucose metabolism, protein synthesis, and maturation and development of neurotransmitter systems, and has emphasized that a thorough understanding of normal maturational patterns seen on PET is a prelude to the application of this technology in understanding the pathogenesis and neurologic basis of various developmental and neurologic disorders. Application of PET methods may help in following disease evolution and progression, planning, and development of various social and therapeutic interventions, timing these interventions and monitoring their responses, as well as allowing for long-term prognostication.

REFERENCES

1. Rakic P. The neocortex: ontogeny and phylogeny. New York: Plenum Press; 1990.
2. Spreen O, Risser AT, Edgell D. Developmental neuropsychology. New York: Oxford Univ Press; 1995.
3. Lenroot RK, Giedd JN. Brain development in children and adolescents: insights from anatomical magnetic resonance imaging. Neurosci Biobehav Rev 2006;30:718–29.
4. Rakic P, Bourgeois JP, Eckenhoff MF, et al. Concurrent overproduction of synapses in diverse regions of the primate cerebral cortex. Science 1986;232:232–5.
5. Becker LE, Armstrong DL, Chan F, et al. Dendritic development in human occipital cortical neurons. Brain Res 1984;315:117–24.
6. Huttenlocher PR. Dendritic and synaptic development in human cerebral cortex: time course and critical periods. Dev Neuropsychol 1999;16:347–9.
7. Huttenlocher PR. Synaptic density in human frontal cortex—developmental changes and effects of aging. Brain Res 1979;163:195–205.
8. Huttenlocher PR, Dabholkar AS. Regional differences in synaptogenesis in human cerebral cortex. J Comp Neurol 1997;387:167–78.
9. Huttenlocher PR, de Courten C, Garey LJ, et al. Synaptogenesis in human visual cortex-evidence for synapse elimination during normal development. Neurosci Lett 1982;33:247–52.
10. Inder TE, Huppi PS. In vivo studies of brain development by magnetic resonance techniques. Ment Retard Dev Disabil Res Rev 2000;6:59–67.
11. Levitt P. Structural and functional maturation of the developing primate brain. J Pediatr 2003;143:S35–45.
12. Paus T, Collins DL, Evans AC, et al. Maturation of white matter in the human brain: a review of magnetic resonance studies. Brain Res Bull 2001;54:255–66.
13. Volpe JJ. Overview: normal and abnormal human brain development. Ment Retard Dev Disabil Res Rev 2000;6:1–5.
14. Levine D, Barnes PD. Cortical maturation in normal and abnormal fetuses as assessed with prenatal MR imaging. Radiology 1999;210:751–8.
15. Dekaban AS. Changes in brain weights during the span of human life: relation of brain weights to body heights and body weights. Ann Neurol 1978;4:345–56.
16. Giedd JN, Blumenthal J, Jeffries NO, et al. Brain development during childhood and adolescence: a longitudinal MRI study. Nat Neurosci 1999;2:861–3.
17. Pakkenberg B, Gundersen HJ. Neocortical neuron number in humans: effect of sex and age. J Comp Neurol 1997;384:312–20.
18. Scheff SW, Price DA, Sparks DL. Quantitative assessment of possible age-related change in synaptic numbers in the human frontal cortex. Neurobiol Aging 2001;22:355–65.
19. Marner L, Nyengaard JR, Tang Y, et al. Marked loss of myelinated nerve fibers in the human brain with age. J Comp Neurol 2003;462:144–52.
20. Clancy B, Darlington RB, Finlay BL. The course of human events: predicting the timing of primate neural development. Dev Sci 2000;3:57–66.
21. Finlay BL, Darlington RB. Linked regularities in the development and evolution of mammalian brains. Science 1995;268:1578–84.
22. Shaw P, Greenstein D, Lerch J, et al. Intellectual ability and cortical development in children and adolescents. Nature 2006;440:676–9.
23. Shaw P, Kabani NJ, Lerch JP, et al. Neurodevelopmental trajectories of the human cerebral cortex. J Neurosci 2008;28:3586–94.
24. Clark AS, MacLusky NJ, Goldman-Rakic PS. Androgen binding and metabolism in the cerebral cortex of the developing rhesus monkey. Endocrinology 1988;123:932–40.
25. Giedd JN, Vaituzis AC, Hamburger SD, et al. Quantitative MRI of the temporal lobe, amygdala, and hippocampus in normal human development: ages 4–18 years. J Comp Neurol 1996;366:223–30.
26. Morse JK, Scheff SW, DeKosky ST. Gonadal steroids influence axon sprouting in the hippocampal dentate gyrus: a sexually dimorphic response. Exp Neurol 1986;94:649–58.
27. Gogtay N, Giedd JN, Lusk L, et al. Dynamic mapping of human cortical development during childhood through early adulthood. Proc Natl Acad Sci U S A 2004;101:8174–9.
28. Marsh R, Gerber AJ, Peterson BS. Neuroimaging studies of normal brain development and their relevance for understanding childhood neuropsychiatric disorders. J Am Acad Child Adolesc Psychiatry 2008;47:1233–51.

29. Paus T, Zijdenbos A, Worsley K, et al. Structural maturation of neural pathways in children and adolescents: in vivo study. Science 1999;283:1908–11.

30. Lenroot RK, Gogtay N, Greenstein DK, et al. Sexual dimorphism of brain developmental trajectories during childhood and adolescence. Neuroimage 2007;36:1065–73.

31. Mesulam MM. From sensation to cognition. Brain 1998;121(Pt 6):1013–52.

32. Sowell ER, Peterson BS, Thompson PM, et al. Mapping cortical change across the human life span. Nat Neurosci 2003;6:309–15.

33. Sowell ER, Thompson PM, Leonard CM, et al. Longitudinal mapping of cortical thickness and brain growth in normal children. J Neurosci 2004; 24:8223–31.

34. Levitt P, Reinoso B, Jones L. The critical impact of early cellular environment on neuronal development. Prev Med 1998;27:180–3.

35. Johnson MH. Functional brain development in humans. Nat Rev Neurosci 2001;2:475–83.

36. Atkinson J. Human visual development over the first 6 months of life. A review and a hypothesis. Hum Neurobiol 1984;3:61–74.

37. Johnson MH. Cortical maturation and the development of visual attention in early infancy. J Cogn Neurosci 1990;2:81–95.

38. Diamond A, Goldman-Rakic PS. Comparison of human infants and rhesus monkeys on Piaget's AB task: evidence for dependence on dorsolateral prefrontal cortex. Exp Brain Res 1989;74:24–40.

39. Muller RA. The study of autism as a distributed disorder. Ment Retard Dev Disabil Res Rev 2007; 13:85–95.

40. Sokoloff L. Localization of functional activity in the central nervous system by measurement of glucose utilization with radioactive deoxyglucose. J Cereb Blood Flow Metab 1981;1:7–36.

41. Lujan R, Shigemoto R, Lopez-Bendito G. Glutamate and GABA receptor signalling in the developing brain. Neuroscience 2005;130:567–80.

42. Vitalis T, Parnavelas JG. The role of serotonin in early cortical development. Dev Neurosci 2003;25:245–56.

43. Chugani HT, Mazziotta JC, Phelps ME. Sturge-Weber syndrome: a study of cerebral glucose utilization with positron emission tomography. J Pediatr 1989;114:244–53.

44. Kennedy C, Sakurada O, Shinohara M, et al. Local cerebral glucose utilization in the newborn macaque monkey. Ann Neurol 1982;12:333–40.

45. Gregoire N, Pontier R, Salamon G. Local cerebral glucose utilization in the newborn brain. Eur Neurol 1981;20:162–8.

46. Duffy TE, Cavazzuti M, Cruz NF, et al. Local cerebral glucose metabolism in newborn dogs: effects of hypoxia and halothane anesthesia. Ann Neurol 1982;11:233–46.

47. Abrams RM, Ito M, Frisinger JE, et al. Local cerebral glucose utilization in fetal and neonatal sheep. Am J Physiol 1984;246:R608–18.

48. Nehlig A, de Vasconcelos AP, Boyet S. Quantitative autoradiographic measurement of local cerebral glucose utilization in freely moving rats during postnatal development. J Neurosci 1988;8: 2321–33.

49. Chugani HT, Hovda DA, Villablanca JR, et al. Metabolic maturation of the brain: a study of local cerebral glucose utilization in the developing cat. J Cereb Blood Flow Metab 1991;11:35–47.

50. Winfield DA. The postnatal development of synapses in the visual cortex of the cat and the effects of eyelid closure. Brain Res 1981;206:166–71.

51. Winfield DA. The postnatal development of synapses in the different laminae of the visual cortex in the normal kitten and in kittens with eyelid suture. Brain Res 1983;285:155–69.

52. Kennedy C, Sokoloff L. An adaptation of the nitrous oxide method to the study of the cerebral circulation in children; normal values for cerebral blood flow and cerebral metabolic rate in childhood. J Clin Invest 1957;36:1130–7.

53. Chiron C, Raynaud C, Maziere B, et al. Changes in regional cerebral blood flow during brain maturation in children and adolescents. J Nucl Med 1992;33:696–703.

54. Takahashi T, Shirane R, Sato S, et al. Developmental changes of cerebral blood flow and oxygen metabolism in children. AJNR Am J Neuroradiol 1999;20:917–22.

55. Chugani HT, Phelps ME. Maturational changes in cerebral function in infants determined by 18FDG positron emission tomography. Science 1986;231: 840–3.

56. Chugani HT, Phelps ME, Mazziotta JC. Positron emission tomography study of human brain functional development. Ann Neurol 1987;22:487–97.

57. Chugani HT. Metabolic imaging: a window on brain development and plasticity. Neuroscientist 1999;5: 29–40.

58. Kennedy C, Grave GD, Juhle JW, et al. Changes in blood flow in the component structures of the dog brain during postnatal maturation. J Neurochem 1972;19:2423–33.

59. Kinnala A, Suhonen-Polvi H, Aarimaa T, et al. Cerebral metabolic rate for glucose during the first six months of life: an FDG positron emission tomography study. Arch Dis Child Fetal Neonatal Ed 1996;74:F153–7.

60. Van Bogaert P, Wikler D, Damhaut P, et al. Regional changes in glucose metabolism during brain development from the age of 6 years. Neuroimage 1998; 8:62–8.

61. Rabinowicz T. The differential maturation of the human cerebral cortex. In: Falkner F, Tanner JM,

editors. Human growth, vol. 3. New York: Plenum; 1979. p. 97–123.

62. Andre-Thomas CY, Saint-Anne Dargassies S. The Neurological examination of the infant. London: Medical Advisory Committee of the National Spastic Society; 1960.

63. Bronson G. The postnatal growth of visual capacity. Child Dev 1974;45:873–90.

64. Parmelee AH, Sigman MD. Perinatal brain development and behavior. In: Haith M, Campos J, editors. Biology and infancy, vol. II. New York: Wiley; 1983. p. 95–155.

65. von Hofsten C, Fazel-Zandy S. Development of visually guided hand orientation in reaching. J Exp Child Psychol 1984;38:208–19.

66. Kellaway P. An orderly approach to visual analysis: parameters of the normal EEG in adults and children. In: Klass DW, Daly DD, editors. Current practice of clinical Electroencephalography. New York: Raven; 1979. p. 69–147.

67. Emde RN, Gaensbauer TJ, Harmon RJ. Emotional expression in infancy: a behavioral study. vol. 10. New York: Intl Univ Press; 1976.

68. Kagan J. Do infants think? Sci Am 1972;226:74–82.

69. Fuster JM. The prefrontal cortex. 3rd edition. Philadelphia: Lippincott-Raven; 1997.

70. Mata M, Fink DJ, Gainer H, et al. Activity-dependent energy metabolism in rat posterior pituitary primarily reflects sodium pump activity. J Neurochem 1980;34:213–5.

71. Morest DK. The growth of dendrites in the mammalian brain. Z Anat Entwicklungsgesch 1969;128: 290–317.

72. Hubel DH, Wiesel TN. The period of susceptibility to the physiological effects of unilateral eye closure in kittens. J Physiol 1970;206:419–36.

73. Timney B. The effects of early and late monocular deprivation on binocular depth perception in cats. Brain Res 1983;283:235–43.

74. Spinelli DN, Jensen FE, Viana Di Prisco G. Early experience effect on dendritic branching in normally reared kittens. Exp Neurol 1980;68: 1–11.

75. Curtiss S. Feral children, vol. XII. New York: Brunner/Mazel; 1981.

76. Elbert T, Pantev C, Wienbruch C, et al. Increased cortical representation of the fingers of the left hand in string players. Science 1995;270:305–7.

77. Schwartz TL, Linberg JB, Tillman W, et al. Monocular depth and vernier acuities: a comparison of binocular and uniocular subjects. Invest Ophthalmol Vis Sci 1987;28(Suppl):304 [abstract].

78. Veraart C, De Volder AG, Wanet-Defalque MC, et al. Glucose utilization in human visual cortex is abnormally elevated in blindness of early onset but decreased in blindness of late onset. Brain Res 1990;510:115–21.

79. De Volder AG, Bol A, Blin J, et al. Brain energy metabolism in early blind subjects: neural activity in the visual cortex. Brain Res 1997;750:235–44.

80. Wanet-Defalque MC, Veraart C, De Volder A, et al. High metabolic activity in the visual cortex of early blind human subjects. Brain Res 1988; 446:369–73.

81. Sadato N, Pascual-Leone A, Grafman J, et al. Activation of the primary visual cortex by Braille reading in blind subjects. Nature 1996;380:526–8.

82. Catalan-Ahumada M, Deggouj N, De Volder A, et al. High metabolic activity demonstrated by positron emission tomography in human auditory cortex in case of deafness of early onset. Brain Res 1993; 623:287–92.

83. Neville HJ. Intermodal competition and compensation in development. Evidence from studies of the visual system in congenitally deaf adults. Ann N Y Acad Sci 1990;608:71–87 [discussion: p. 91].

84. Wolff AB, Thatcher RW. Cortical reorganization in deaf children. J Clin Exp Neuropsychol 1990;12: 209–21.

85. Muller RA, Rothermel RD, Behen ME, et al. Brain organization of language after early unilateral lesion: a PET study. Brain Lang 1998;62:422–51.

86. Muller RA, Rothermel RD, Behen ME, et al. Plasticity of motor organization in children and adults. Neuroreport 1997;8:3103–8.

87. Molteni B, Oleari G, Fedrizzi E, et al. Relation between CT patterns, clinical findings and etiological factors in children born at term, affected by congenital hemiparesis. Neuropediatrics 1987;18: 75–80.

88. Trauner DA, Chase C, Walker P, et al. Neurologic profiles of infants and children after perinatal stroke. Pediatr Neurol 1993;9:383–6.

89. Ptito A, Lassonde M, Lepore F, et al. Visual discrimination in hemispherectomized patients. Neuropsychologia 1987;25:869–79.

90. Vargha-Khadem F, Isaacs EB, Papaleloudi H, et al. Development of language in six hemispherectomized patients. Brain 1991;114(Pt 1B):473–95.

91. Nass R, deCoudres Peterson H, Koch D. Differential effects of congenital left and right brain injury on intelligence. Brain Cogn 1989;9:258–66.

92. Chugani HT, Jacobs B. Metabolic recovery in caudate nucleus of children following cerebral hemispherectomy. Ann Neurol 1994;36:794–7.

93. Dauth GW, Gilman S, Frey KA, et al. Basal ganglia glucose utilization after recent precentral ablation in the monkey. Ann Neurol 1985;17:431–8.

94. Kling A, Tucker TJ. Effects of combined lesions of frontal granular cortex and caudate nucleus in the neonatal monkey. Brain Res 1967;6:428–39.

95. McGeorge AJ, Faull RL. The organization of the projection from the cerebral cortex to the striatum in the rat. Neuroscience 1989;29:503–37.

96. Olmstead CE, Villablanca JR. Effects of caudate nuclei or frontal cortical ablations in cats and kittens: paw usage. Exp Neurol 1979;63:559–72.

97. Pantano P, Baron JC, Samson Y, et al. Crossed cerebellar diaschisis. Further studies. Brain 1986; 109(Pt 4):677–94.

98. Kerrigan JF, Chugani HT, Phelps ME. Regional cerebral glucose metabolism in clinical subtypes of cerebral palsy. Pediatr Neurol 1991;7:415–25.

99. Shamoto H, Chugani HT. Glucose metabolism in the human cerebellum: an analysis of crossed cerebellar diaschisis in children with unilateral cerebral injury. J Child Neurol 1997;12:407–14.

100. Niimura K, Chugani DC, Muzik O, et al. Cerebellar reorganization following cortical injury in humans: effects of lesion size and age. Neurology 1999; 52:792–7.

101. Beaulieu C, Colonnier M. Number and size of neurons and synapses in the motor cortex of cats raised in different environmental complexities. J Comp Neurol 1989;289:178–81.

102. Sirevaag AM, Black JE, Shafron D, et al. Direct evidence that complex experience increases capillary branching and surface area in visual cortex of young rats. Brain Res 1988;471:299–304.

103. Ramey CT, Ramey SL. Prevention of intellectual disabilities: early interventions to improve cognitive development. Prev Med 1998;27:224–32.

104. Jacobs B, Batal HA, Lynch B, et al. Quantitative dendritic and spine analyses of speech cortices: a case study. Brain Lang 1993;44:239–53.

105. Jacobs B, Scheibel AB. A quantitative dendritic analysis of Wernicke's area in humans. I. Lifespan changes. J Comp Neurol 1993;327:83–96.

106. LoTurco JJ, Owens DF, Heath MJ, et al. GABA and glutamate depolarize cortical progenitor cells and inhibit DNA synthesis. Neuron 1995;15: 1287–98.

107. Ma W, Barker JL. Complementary expressions of transcripts encoding GAD67 and GABAA receptor alpha 4, beta 1, and gamma 1 subunits in the proliferative zone of the embryonic rat central nervous system. J Neurosci 1995;15:2547–60.

108. Ma W, Liu QY, Maric D, et al. Basic FGF-responsive telencephalic precursor cells express functional GABA(A) receptor/Cl-channels in vitro. J Neurobiol 1998;35:277–86.

109. Serafini R, Maric D, Maric I, et al. Dominant GABA(A) receptor/Cl- channel kinetics correlate with the relative expressions of alpha2, alpha3, alpha5 and beta3 subunits in embryonic rat neurones. Eur J Neurosci 1998;10:334–49.

110. Ramoa AS, Paradiso MA, Freeman RD. Blockade of intracortical inhibition in kitten striate cortex: effects on receptive field properties and associated loss of ocular dominance plasticity. Exp Brain Res 1988;73:285–96.

111. Wolf W, Hicks TP, Albus K. The contribution of GABA-mediated inhibitory mechanisms to visual response properties of neurons in the kitten's striate cortex. J Neurosci 1986;6:2779–95.

112. Huntsman MM, Isackson PJ, Jones EG. Lamina-specific expression and activity-dependent regulation of seven GABAA receptor subunit mRNAs in monkey visual cortex. J Neurosci 1994;14:2236–59.

113. Golshani P, Truong H, Jones EG. Developmental expression of GABA(A) receptor subunit and GAD genes in mouse somatosensory barrel cortex. J Comp Neurol 1997;383:199–219.

114. Carlson BX, Elster L, Schousboe A. Pharmacological and functional implications of developmentally-regulated changes in GABA(A) receptor subunit expression in the cerebellum. Eur J Pharmacol 1998;352:1–14.

115. Lidow MS, Goldman-Rakic PS, Rakic P. Synchronized overproduction of neurotransmitter receptors in diverse regions of the primate cerebral cortex. Proc Natl Acad Sci U S A 1991;88:10218–21.

116. Hornung JP, Fritschy JM. Developmental profile of GABAA-receptors in the marmoset monkey: expression of distinct subtypes in pre- and postnatal brain. J Comp Neurol 1996;367:413–30.

117. Huntsman MM, Munoz A, Jones EG. Temporal modulation of GABA(A) receptor subunit gene expression in developing monkey cerebral cortex. Neuroscience 1999;91:1223–45.

118. Kultas-Ilinsky K, Leontiev V, Whiting PJ. Expression of 10 GABA(A) receptor subunit messenger RNAs in the motor-related thalamic nuclei and basal ganglia of Macaca mulatta studied with in situ hybridization histochemistry. Neuroscience 1998; 85:179–204.

119. Chugani DC, Muzik O, Juhasz C, et al. Postnatal maturation of human GABAA receptors measured with positron emission tomography. Ann Neurol 2001;49:618–26.

120. Lidow MS, Rakic P. Neurotransmitter receptors in the proliferative zones of the developing primate occipital lobe. J Comp Neurol 1995;360:393–402.

121. Lauder JM. Neurotransmitters as morphogens. Prog Brain Res 1988;73:365–87.

122. Lauder JM, Zimmerman EF. Sites of serotonin uptake in epithelia of the developing mouse palate, oral cavity, and face: possible role in morphogenesis. J Craniofac Genet Dev Biol 1988;8:265–76.

123. Lauder JM. Neurotransmitters as growth regulatory signals: role of receptors and second messengers. Trends Neurosci 1993;16:233–40.

124. Bennett-Clarke CA, Leslie MJ, Lane RD, et al. Effect of serotonin depletion on vibrissa-related patterns of thalamic afferents in the rat's somatosensory cortex. J Neurosci 1994;14:7594–607.

125. Cases O, Vitalis T, Seif I, et al. Lack of barrels in the somatosensory cortex of monoamine oxidase

A-deficient mice: role of a serotonin excess during the critical period. Neuron 1996;16:297–307.

126. Goldman-Rakic PS, Brown RM. Postnatal development of monoamine content and synthesis in the cerebral cortex of rhesus monkeys. Brain Res 1982;256:339–49.

127. Diksic M, Nagahiro S, Sourkes TL, et al. A new method to measure brain serotonin synthesis in vivo. I. Theory and basic data for a biological model. J Cereb Blood Flow Metab 1990;10:1–12.

128. Madras BK, Sourkes TL. Metabolism of alpha-methyltryptophan. Biochem Pharmacol 1965;14:1499–506.

129. Chugani DC, Muzik O, Chakraborty P, et al. Human brain serotonin synthesis capacity measured in vivo with alpha-[C-11]methyl-L-tryptophan. Synapse 1998;28:33–43.

130. Chugani DC, Muzik O, Behen M, et al. Developmental changes in brain serotonin synthesis capacity in autistic and nonautistic children. Ann Neurol 1999;45:287–95.

131. McDougle CJ, Naylor ST, Cohen DJ, et al. Effects of tryptophan depletion in drug-free adults with autistic disorder. Arch Gen Psychiatry 1996;53:993–1000.

132. Cook EH Jr, Rowlett R, Jaselskis C, et al. Fluoxetine treatment of children and adults with autistic disorder and mental retardation. J Am Acad Child Adolesc Psychiatry 1992;31:739–45.

133. Chugani DC, Muzik O, Rothermel R, et al. Altered serotonin synthesis in the dentatothalamocortical pathway in autistic boys. Ann Neurol 1997;42:666–9.

134. Hovda DA, Villablanca JR, Chugani HT, et al. Metabolic maturation of the brain: a study of local cerebral protein synthesis in the developing cat. Brain Res 2006;1113:54–63.

135. Nehlig A, Daval JL, Vasconcelos PD, et al. Postnatal maturation of regional levels of cerebral protein synthesis in the rat. Circ Métab Cerveau 1991;8:175–6 [in French].

136. Sun Y, Deibler GE, Jehle J, et al. Rates of local cerebral protein synthesis in the rat during normal postnatal development. Am J Physiol 1995;268:R549–61.

137. Abrams RM, Burchfield DJ, Sun Y, et al. Rates of local cerebral protein synthesis in fetal and neonatal sheep. Am J Physiol 1997;272:R1235–44.

138. Chugani HT, Conti JR. Etiologic classification of infantile spasms in 140 cases: role of positron emission tomography. J Child Neurol 1996;11:44–8.

139. Chugani HT, Shewmon DA, Sankar R, et al. Infantile spasms: II. Lenticular nuclei and brain stem activation on positron emission tomography. Ann Neurol 1992;31:212–9.

140. Chugani HT, Shewmon DA, Shields WD, et al. Surgery for intractable infantile spasms: neuroimaging perspectives. Epilepsia 1993;34:764–71.

141. Chugani HT, Shields WD, Shewmon DA, et al. Infantile spasms: I. PET identifies focal cortical dysgenesis in cryptogenic cases for surgical treatment. Ann Neurol 1990;27:406–13.

142. Asano E, Chugani DC, Juhasz C, et al. Surgical treatment of West syndrome. Brain Dev 2001;23:668–76.

143. Gaily EK, Shewmon DA, Chugani HT, et al. Asymmetric and asynchronous infantile spasms. Epilepsia 1995;36:873–82.

144. Maeda N, Watanabe K, Negoro T, et al. Evolutional changes of cortical hypometabolism in West's syndrome. Lancet 1994;343:1620–3.

145. Chugani HT, Da Silva E, Chugani DC. Infantile spasms: III. Prognostic implications of bitemporal hypometabolism on positron emission tomography. Ann Neurol 1996;39:643–9.

146. Asano E, Juhasz C, Shah A, et al. Origin and propagation of epileptic spasms delineated on electrocorticography. Epilepsia 2005;46:1086–97.

147. Chugani HT, Chugani DC. Basic mechanisms of childhood epilepsies: studies with positron emission tomography. Adv Neurol 1999;79:883–91.

148. Juhasz C, Chugani HT, Muzik O, et al. Neuroradiological assessment of brain structure and function and its implication in the pathogenesis of West syndrome. Brain Dev 2001;23:488–95.

149. Chugani HT, Mazziotta JC, Engel J Jr, et al. The Lennox-Gastaut syndrome: metabolic subtypes determined by 2-deoxy-2[18F]fluoro-D-glucose positron emission tomography. Ann Neurol 1987;21:4–13.

150. Ferrie CD, Maisey M, Cox T, et al. Focal abnormalities detected by 18FDG PET in epileptic encephalopathies. Arch Dis Child 1996;75:102–7.

151. Gur RC, Sussman NM, Alavi A, et al. Positron emission tomography in two cases of childhood epileptic encephalopathy (Lennox-Gastaut syndrome). Neurology 1982;32:1191–4.

152. Iinuma K, Yanai K, Yanagisawa T, et al. Cerebral glucose metabolism in five patients with Lennox-Gastaut syndrome. Pediatr Neurol 1987;3:12–8.

153. Miyauchi T, Nomura Y, Ohno S, et al. Positron emission tomography in three cases of Lennox-Gastaut syndrome. Jpn J Psychiatry Neurol 1988;42:795–804.

154. Theodore WH, Rose D, Patronas N, et al. Cerebral glucose metabolism in the Lennox-Gastaut syndrome. Ann Neurol 1987;21:14–21.

155. Yanai K, Iinuma K, Matsuzawa T, et al. Cerebral glucose utilization in pediatric neurological disorders determined by positron emission tomography. Eur J Nucl Med 1987;13:292–6.

156. Rintahaka PJ, Chugani HT. Clinical role of positron emission tomography in children with tuberous sclerosis complex. J Child Neurol 1997;12:42–52.

157. Szelies B, Herholz K, Heiss WD, et al. Hypometabolic cortical lesions in tuberous sclerosis with epilepsy: demonstration by positron emission tomography. J Comput Assist Tomogr 1983;7:946–53.

158. Asano E, Chugani DC, Muzik O, et al. Multimodality imaging for improved detection of epileptogenic foci in tuberous sclerosis complex. Neurology 2000;54:1976–84.

159. Stone TW. Kynurenines in the CNS: from endogenous obscurity to therapeutic importance. Prog Neurobiol 2001;64:185–218.

160. Fedi M, Reutens DC, Andermann F, et al. alpha-[11C]-Methyl-L-tryptophan PET identifies the epileptogenic tuber and correlates with interictal spike frequency. Epilepsy Res 2003;52:203–13.

161. Juhász C, Chugani DC, Asano E, et al. Alpha[11C]-methyl-L-tryptophan positron emission tomography scanning in 176 patients with intractable epilepsy. Ann Neurol 2002;53:S118 [abstract].

162. Kagawa K, Chugani DC, Asano E, et al. Epilepsy surgery outcome in children with tuberous sclerosis complex evaluated with alpha-[11C]methyl-L-tryptophan positron emission tomography (PET). J Child Neurol 2005;20:429–38.

163. Asano E, Chugani DC, Muzik O, et al. Autism in tuberous sclerosis complex is related to both cortical and subcortical dysfunction. Neurology 2001;57:1269–77.

164. Luat AF, Makki M, Chugani HT. Neuroimaging in tuberous sclerosis complex. Curr Opin Neurol 2007;20:142–50.

165. Eluvathingal TJ, Behen ME, Chugani HT, et al. Cerebellar lesions in tuberous sclerosis complex: neurobehavioral and neuroimaging correlates. J Child Neurol 2006;21:846–51.

166. Juhasz C, Batista CE, Chugani DC, et al. Evolution of cortical metabolic abnormalities and their clinical correlates in Sturge-Weber syndrome. Eur J Paediatr Neurol 2007;11:277–84.

167. Lee JS, Asano E, Muzik O, et al. Sturge-Weber syndrome: correlation between clinical course and FDG PET findings. Neurology 2001;57:189–95.

168. Batista CE, Juhasz C, Muzik O, et al. Increased visual cortex glucose metabolism contralateral to angioma in children with Sturge-Weber syndrome. Dev Med Child Neurol 2007;49:567–73.

169. Muller RA, Chugani HT, Muzik O, et al. Language and motor functions activate calcified hemisphere in patients with Sturge-Weber syndrome: a positron emission tomography study. J Child Neurol 1997;12:431–7.

170. da Silva EA, Chugani DC, Muzik O, et al. Landau-Kleffner syndrome: metabolic abnormalities in temporal lobe are a common feature. J Child Neurol 1997;12:489–95.

171. Honbolygo F, Csepe V, Fekeshazy A, et al. Converging evidences on language impairment in Landau-Kleffner Syndrome revealed by behavioral and brain activity measures: a case study. Clin Neurophysiol 2006;117:295–305.

172. Shiraishi H, Takano K, Shiga T, et al. Possible involvement of the tip of temporal lobe in Landau-Kleffner syndrome. Brain Dev 2007;29:529–33.

173. Maquet P, Hirsch E, Dive D, et al. Cerebral glucose utilization during sleep in Landau-Kleffner syndrome: a PET study. Epilepsia 1990;31:778–83.

174. Rintahaka PJ, Chugani HT, Sankar R. Landau-Kleffner syndrome with continuous spikes and waves during slow-wave sleep. J Child Neurol 1995;10:127–33.

175. Luat AF, Chugani HT, Asano E, et al. Episodic receptive aphasia in a child with Landau-Kleffner syndrome: PET correlates. Brain Dev 2006;28:592–6.

176. Rintahaka PJ, Chugani HT, Messa C, et al. Hemimegalencephaly: evaluation with positron emission tomography. Pediatr Neurol 1993;9:21–8.

177. Volpe JJ, Herscovitch P, Perlman JM, et al. Positron emission tomography in the newborn: extensive impairment of regional cerebral blood flow with intraventricular hemorrhage and hemorrhagic intracerebral involvement. Pediatrics 1983;72:589–601.

178. Doyle LW, Nahmias C, Firnau G, et al. Regional cerebral glucose metabolism of newborn infants measured by positron emission tomography. Dev Med Child Neurol 1983;25:143–51.

179. Volpe JJ, Herscovitch P, Perlman JM, et al. Positron emission tomography in the asphyxiated term newborn: parasagittal impairment of cerebral blood flow. Ann Neurol 1985;17:287–96.

180. Batista CE, Chugani HT, Juhasz C, et al. Transient hypermetabolism of the basal ganglia following perinatal hypoxia. Pediatr Neurol 2007;36:330–3.

181. Thorngren-Jerneck K, Ohlsson T, Sandell A, et al. Cerebral glucose metabolism measured by positron emission tomography in term newborn infants with hypoxic ischemic encephalopathy. Pediatr Res 2001;49:495–501.

182. Suhonen-Polvi H, Kero P, Korvenranta H, et al. Repeated fluorodeoxyglucose positron emission tomography of the brain in infants with suspected hypoxic-ischaemic brain injury. Eur J Nucl Med 1993;20:759–65.

183. Lee JD, Park HJ, Park ES, et al. Assessment of regional GABA(A) receptor binding using 18F-fluoroflumazenil positron emission tomography in spastic type cerebral palsy. Neuroimage 2007;34:19–25.

184. Rumsey JM, Andreason P, Zametkin AJ, et al. Failure to activate the left temporoparietal cortex in dyslexia. An oxygen 15 positron emission tomographic study. Arch Neurol 1992;49:527–34.

185. Rumsey JM, Nace K, Donohue B, et al. A positron emission tomographic study of impaired word recognition and phonological processing in dyslexic men. Arch Neurol 1997;54:562–73.

186. McCrory E, Frith U, Brunswick N, et al. Abnormal functional activation during a simple word repetition task: a PET study of adult dyslexics. J Cogn Neurosci 2000;12:753–62.

187. Nicolson RI, Fawcett AJ, Berry EL, et al. Association of abnormal cerebellar activation with motor learning difficulties in dyslexic adults. Lancet 1999;353:1662–7.

188. Horwitz B, Rumsey JM, Donohue BC. Functional connectivity of the angular gyrus in normal reading and dyslexia. Proc Natl Acad Sci U S A 1998;95:8939–44.

189. Dufor O, Serniclaes W, Sprenger-Charolles L, et al. Top-down processes during auditory phoneme categorization in dyslexia: a PET study. Neuroimage 2007;34:1692–707.

190. Gross-Glenn K, Duara R, Barker WW, et al. Positron emission tomographic studies during serial word-reading by normal and dyslexic adults. J Clin Exp Neuropsychol 1991;13:531–44.

191. Hagman JO, Wood F, Buchsbaum MS, et al. Cerebral brain metabolism in adult dyslexic subjects assessed with positron emission tomography during performance of an auditory task. Arch Neurol 1992;49:734–9.

192. Braun AR, Stoetter B, Randolph C, et al. The functional neuroanatomy of Tourette's syndrome: an FDG-PET study. I. Regional changes in cerebral glucose metabolism differentiating patients and controls. Neuropsychopharmacology 1993;9:277–91.

193. Lerner A, Bagic A, Boudreau EA, et al. Neuroimaging of neuronal circuits involved in tic generation in patients with Tourette syndrome. Neurology 2007;68:1979–87.

194. Stern E, Silbersweig DA, Chee KY, et al. A functional neuroanatomy of tics in Tourette syndrome. Arch Gen Psychiatry 2000;57:741–8.

195. Krause KH, Dresel S, Krause J, et al. Elevated striatal dopamine transporter in a drug naive patient with Tourette syndrome and attention deficit/hyperactivity disorder: positive effect of methylphenidate. J Neurol 2002;249:1116–8.

196. Ernst M, Zametkin AJ, Jons PH, et al. High presynaptic dopaminergic activity in children with Tourette's disorder. J Am Acad Child Adolesc Psychiatry 1999;38:86–94.

197. Gilbert DL, Christian BT, Gelfand MJ, et al. Altered mesolimbocortical and thalamic dopamine in Tourette syndrome. Neurology 2006;67:1695–7.

198. Singer HS, Szymanski S, Giuliano J, et al. Elevated intrasynaptic dopamine release in Tourette's syndrome measured by PET. Am J Psychiatry 2002;159:1329–36.

199. Wong DF, Brasic JR, Singer HS, et al. Mechanisms of dopaminergic and serotonergic neurotransmission in Tourette syndrome: clues from an in vivo neurochemistry study with PET. Neuropsychopharmacology 2008;33:1239–51.

200. Behen M, Chugani HT, Juhasz C, et al. Abnormal brain tryptophan metabolism and clinical correlates in Tourette syndrome. Mov Disord 2007;22:2256–62.

201. Haugbol S, Pinborg LH, Regeur L, et al. Cerebral 5-HT2A receptor binding is increased in patients with Tourette's syndrome. Int J Neuropsychopharmacol 2007;10:245–52.

202. De Volder AG, Cirelli S, de Barsy T, et al. Neuronal ceroid-lipofuscinosis: preferential metabolic alterations in thalamus and posterior association cortex demonstrated by PET. J Neurol Neurosurg Psychiatr 1990;53:1063–7.

203. Iannetti P, Messa C, Spalice A, et al. Positron emission tomography in neuronal ceroid lipofuscinosis (Jansky-Bielschowsky disease): a case report. Brain Dev 1994;16:459–62.

204. Philippart M, Chugani B. Neuronal ceroid-lipofuscinosis: late infantile form or juvenile form? Brain Dev 1995;17:225.

205. Philippart M, da Silva E, Chugani HT. The value of positron emission tomography in the diagnosis and monitoring of late infantile and juvenile lipopigment storage disorders (so-called Batten or neuronal ceroid lipofuscinoses). Neuropediatrics 1997;28:74–6.

206. Philippart M, Messa C, Chugani HT. Spielmeyer-Vogt (Batten, Spielmeyer-Sjogren) disease. Distinctive patterns of cerebral glucose utilization. Brain 1994;117(Pt 5):1085–92.

207. Rinne JO, Ruottinen HM, Nagren K, et al. Positron emission tomography shows reduced striatal dopamine D1 but not D2 receptors in juvenile neuronal ceroid lipofuscinosis. Neuropediatrics 2002;33:138–41.

208. Pfund Z, Chugani DC, Muzik O, et al. Alpha[11C] methyl-L-typtophan positron emission tomography in patients with alternating hemiplegia of childhood. J Child Neurol 2002;17:253–60.

Clinical Application of PET in Pediatric Brain Tumors

Wei Chen, MD, PhD[a,b,*]

KEYWORDS

• Brain tumors • Pediatric • PET • Diagnosis • Treatment

While rare in adults, central nervous system (CNS) tumor is the most common solid tumor in childhood, accounting for 21.2% of all cancers, and is the leading cause of cancer death in children.[1] Childhood brain tumors are different from those in adults in epidemiology, histologic features, and responses to treatment.[2] Although the outcome for children with brain tumors is poor, survival rates are better than in adults with similar tumors.[2] Five-year survival for children with CNS tumors is reported as high as 74%.[1]

Gliomas make up over one-half of all childhood brain tumors.[2] According to the World Health Organization (WHO) classification, there are three main types of gliomas based on their histologic features: astrocytomas, oligodendrogliomas, and mixed oligoastrocytomas.[3] These tumors are typically heterogeneous in nature in that different levels of malignant degeneration can occur in different regions within the same tumor. Analysis of the most malignant region of the tumors establishes grading: low-grade or WHO grades I and II, and high-grade or WHO grades III (anaplastic tumor) and IV (glioblastoma). In children, low-grade (grade I and grade II tumors) tumor is the most common type of glioma.[4] In particular, grade I pilocytic astrocytoma, which is rare in adults, accounts for 24% of total childhood gliomas. Grade I pilocytic astrocytoma typically is considered curable surgically. Clinical course and treatment for grade II to IV gliomas in children are similar to those in adults, although less developed.[5] Grade II gliomas are more indolent than their high-grade counterparts, but they are associated with significant neurologic disability. In children, grade II tumors have a better prognosis than those in adults in that surgical resection may result in cure, and spontaneous regression has been reported.[6] However, tumor cells can acquire genetic defects, which result in anaplastic transformation to a high-grade lesion.[7] They may also progress without anaplastic transformation. The clinical course of glioblastoma is usually rapid and fatal, with the median survival of 1 year. Median survival for anaplastic tumors is 2 to 3 years. After the initial treatment, these tumors invariably recur. Patients are treated with a variety of chemotherapeutic agents, although response to conventional cytotoxic chemotherapy agents and radiation therapy is often poor, and therapy-related morbidity is a significant problem in children.[8] A recent study demonstrated that pediatric glioblastomas may have distinct genetic alterations different from adult glioblastomas.[9] Targeted therapy is an area of active research.

Metastasis from systemic tumors to the brain through hematogenous spread is uncommon in childhood. A review of the literature showed a 4.08% incidence of cerebral metastasis in 2,035 pediatric patients.[10] The top three most common childhood cancers that metastasize to the brain were melanoma (13.6%), germ cell tumors (13.5%), and osteosarcoma (6.5%).

This work was supported by grants P50 CA086306 from the National Institutes of Health – National Cancer Institute, and U.S Department of Energy Contract DE-FC03-87-ER60615.

[a] Department of Molecular and Medical Pharmacology, David Geffen School of Medicine, University of California Los Angeles, 200 Medical Plaza, Suite B114-61, Los Angeles, CA 90095, USA

[b] Department of Radiology, Kaiser Permanente Woodland Hills Medical Center, 5601 De Soto Ave, Woodland Hills, CA 91367, USA

* Department of Molecular and Medical Pharmacology, David Geffen School of Medicine, University of California Los Angeles, 200 Medical Plaza, Suite B114-61, Los Angeles, CA 90095.

E-mail address: weichen@mednet.ucla.edu

PET Clin 3 (2009) 517–529
doi:10.1016/j.cpet.2009.03.005
1556-8598/09/$ – see front matter © 2009 Elsevier Inc. All rights reserved.

Patients are followed clinically for neurologic symptoms and by neuroimaging with MR imaging, the current clinical gold standard. However, imaging the extent of contrast enhancement in malignant gliomas is limited by the difficulty in distinguishing between tumor extent and treatment-induced changes, such as radiation necrosis.[11] Proton MR spectroscopic imaging is being developed in pediatric patients to better characterizing tumor activity.[12] Metabolic imaging with PET plays a significant role in evaluation of these tumors, and exciting progresses have been made in recent years. PET applications and advances in evaluation of brain tumors in adults have been reviewed recently.[13,14] However, PET studies in childhood brain tumors are relatively limited when compared with those in adults.[15] This article emphasizes PET applications in childhood brain tumors, focusing on mainly gliomas with regard to tumor-grading and prognosis, distinguishing tumor recurrence from radiation necrosis, and PET-guided diagnosis and treatment.

PET FOR TUMOR GRADING AND PROGNOSIS

The clinical gold-standard imaging procedure, MR imaging, provides excellent anatomic details. Standard T1- and T2-weighted MR images detect brain tumors with high sensitivity with regard to size and localization, as well as mass effect, edema, hemorrhage, necrosis, and signs of increased intracranial pressure. A high-grade glioma usually presents as an irregular, hypodense lesion on T1-weighted MR imaging, with various degrees of contrast enhancement and edema. Ring-like enhancement surrounding irregularly shaped foci of presumed necrosis is suggestive of glioblastoma. However, anaplastic tumors can often present as nonenhancing tumors and even glioblastoma may present initially as a nonenhancing lesion. Likewise, some low-grade-appearing tumors may contain areas of anaplastic tumor. Early and adequate tissue sampling is important, given the potential for nonenhancing tumors to be anaplastic gliomas rather than low-grade gliomas. Grading of tumors by noninvasive imaging is especially important when tissue biopsy is difficult to obtain because of tumor location.

PET uptake with 18F-Fluorodeoxyglucose (FDG) is generally high in high-grade tumors. It is well established that FDG uptake has prognostic value in that high-FDG uptake in a previously known low-grade tumor establishes the diagnosis of anaplastic transformation.[16,17] Coregistration of FDG-PET images with MR imaging greatly improves the performance of FDG-PET.[18] Tumor grading by FDG-PET image fusion with MR

imaging was prospectively studied in 19 pediatric patients with primary CNS tumors.[19] Before the start of treatment, FDG-PET was obtained in all 19 patients. Sixteen patients were also studied with $H_2{}^{15}O$-PET. The semiquantitative determination of the FDG scan consisted of a 10-mm diameter circular region-of-interest (ROI) after coregistration and image fusion to MR imaging to localize the tumor. Same-diameter reference ROIs were selected in the temporal cortex and white matter contralateral to the tumor. Tumors were graded using references to the gray- and white-matter uptakes. FDG uptake was positively correlated with malignancy grading, whereas $H_2{}^{15}O$-PET uptake showed no correlation with malignancy (**Fig. 1**). Digitally performed PET/MR imaging coregistration increased information on tumor characterization in 90% of cases.

Amino acid and amino acid analog-PET tracers constitute another class of tumor imaging agents.[20,21] They are particularly attractive for imaging brain tumors because of the high uptake in tumor tissue and low uptake in normal brain tissue, thus higher tumor-to-normal tissue contrast. The best studied amino acid tracer is ^{11}C-methionine.[22,23] Because of the short half-life of ^{11}C ($t_{1/2} = 20$ min), ^{18}F-labeled aromatic amino acid analogs have been developed for tumor imaging.[24] Tumor uptake of O-2- [^{18}F]fluoroethyl-L-tyrosine (FET) and 3,4-dihydroxy-6- [^{18}F]-fluoro-L-phenylalanine (FDOPA) have been reported to be similar to L-[methyl-^{11}C] methionine (MET).[25,26] FDOPA metabolite 3-O-methyl-6-[^{18}F]fluoro-L-DOPA has also been investigated for brain tumor imaging with PET.[27] Superior diagnostic accuracy of FDOPA to FDG in evaluating recurrent low-grade and high-grade gliomas was reported.[28,29]

FDOPA as an amino acid analog was shown to be taken up at the blood-brain barrier in normal brains by the neutral amino acid transporter. In the most detailed and comprehensive study published of FDOPA in brain tumors, FDOPA was compared with FDG in 30 patients with brain tumors and the diagnostic accuracy of FDOPA was evaluated in a subsequently expanded study to additional 51 patients.[28] FDOPA demonstrated excellent visualization of high- and low-grade tumors (**Fig. 2**). However, no significant differences between FDOPA standard uptake values (SUVs) or tumor-to-normal brain ratio could be found between low-grade and high-grade tumors. No FDOPA study in pediatric brain tumors has been reported.

MET-PET is perhaps the best studied amino acid tracer and also the best studied amino acid tracer in pediatric brain tumors. MET-PET was

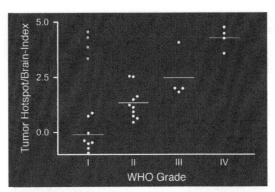

Fig. 1. The tumor hotspot/brain index is significantly positively correlated with the WHO malignancy grading, although the benign hypermetabolic tumors confound the correlation (marked with *green*, not included in mean for WHO grade 1 tumors). (*Adapted from* Borgwardt L, Hojgaard L, Carstensen H, et al. Increased Fluorine-18 2-Fluoro-2-Deoxy-D-Glucose (FDG) uptake in childhood CNS tumors is correlated with malignancy grade: A study with FDG positron emission tomography/magnetic resonance imaging coregistration and image fusion. J Clin Oncol 2005;23:3030–7; with permission).

compared with FDG-PET in 27 pediatric patients with previously untreated primary CNS tumors.[30] Metabolic characteristics as assessed with FDG and MET SUV and SUV-to-normal brain ratio were compared with pathologic markers, such as proliferation index (Ki-67), vascular, apoptotic, and cell-density indices. Investigators found that both FDG and MET uptakes were significantly higher in high-grade than in low-grade tumors, but there were significant overlaps (**Fig. 3**). Thus, no clear limits of SUVs or SUV-to-normal brain ratios can be set between low-grade and high-grade tumors. In univariate analysis, FDG-PET, MET-PET, and apoptotic index were independent predictors of event-free survival.

In a larger study, MET-PET uptake was determined in 52 pediatric patients with CNS tumors: 26 newly diagnosed, 26 recurrent diseases.[31] The study evaluated the relationship between the MET uptake and histopathologic grading, as well as the prognostic value. ROIs were defined manually with knowledge of the clinical and MR imaging data. The MET-uptake index was established using the ratio of tumor ROI and MET uptake in the contralateral gray matter. Although there was significant difference in MET uptake between the higher-grade tumors and those of grade I tumors (pilocytic astrocytoma, $n = 3$) and benign lesions ($n = 8$), no significant differences in the MET-uptake index between tumor grades for either

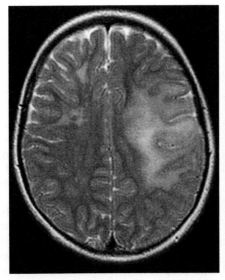
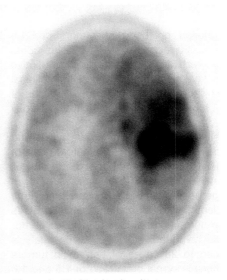

Fig. 2. MR imaging and FDOPA-PET in a 12-year-old boy with grade III oligodendroglioma.

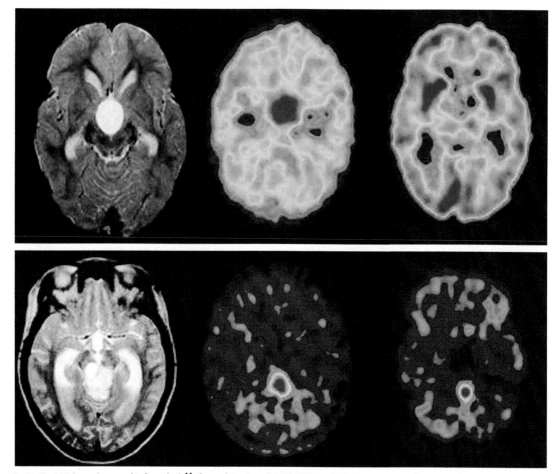

Fig. 3. T$_2$-MR imaging and L-[methyl-^{11}C] methionine (MET)-PET and FDG-PET scans of two pediatric patients with optic tract pilocytic astrocytoma (*upper*) and anaplastic astrocytoma (*lower*). Both tumors exhibited high MET accumulation, whereas only anaplastic astrocytoma exhibited high FDG accumulation. (*Adapted from* Utriainen M, Metahonkala L, Salmi TT, et al. Metabolic characterization of childhood brain tumors: comparison of ^{18}F-fluorodeoxyglucose and ^{11}C-methionine positron emission tomography. Cancer 2002;95:1376–86; with permission).

newly diagnosed or recurrent tumors can be demonstrated. Furthermore, no thresholds could be found at which MET uptake could be predictive of survival. Investigators concluded that clinical use of MET should be focused on evaluations of recurrence, tumor volume delineation, and biopsy guidance.

It is possible that correlations between PET and tumor grade may be different for different types of tumors. MET-PET uptake and tumor grade, as well as proliferative index Ki-67, was studied in a mixed-age population of 67 pediatric and adult glioma patients.[32] No correlations between SUVs or tumor-to-normal brain ratios to Ki-67 or tumor grade could be found. However, when analysis was confined to 28 cases of astrocytic tumors only, a tumor-to-normal brain ratio of 1.5 and 1.6 was found to distinguish between low-grade and

high-grade tumor, and a correlation was also found between MET-PET uptake and Ki-67.

RADIATION NECROSIS VERSUS RECURRENT TUMOR
Radiation Necrosis

Necrosis of the brain tissue after radiation is a known complication and potential synergistic effects of high-dose chemotherapy, and radiation therapy is being investigated.[33] Clinical and radiographic data were assessed in 49 pediatric patients with brain tumors treated with high-dose chemotherapy and autologous hematopoietic stem cell rescue, preceded or followed by radiation.[33] Multiple enhancing cerebral lesions were frequently seen on MR imaging scans soon after high-dose chemotherapy and radiation. Of the

49 children, 18 had abnormal MR imaging findings occurring at a median of 8 months after radiation and beginning to regress at a median of 13 months after onset. Such findings pose a major diagnostic challenge in differential diagnosis.

Radiosurgery is another approach in the treatment of brain tumors. Stereotactic radiosurgery has the potential to ablate small tumors that are not surgically respectable, while reducing the damage to the brain tissue associated with delivering a high-radiation dose to the developing brain. Outcome of stereotactic radiosurgery was investigated in 90 children with brain tumors.[34] Nineteen patients suspected to have radiation necrosis underwent reoperation after an interval of 0.6 to 62 months. Pathology revealed necrosis with no evidence of tumor in nine patients, whereas a mix of radiation necrosis and tumor was seen in the rest of the patients.

Various treatment-related changes can be seen on MR imaging. After resection of brain tumors, late transient treatment-induced lesions in 11 pediatric patients were evaluated.[35] Seventeen foci of abnormality located outside of the tumor bed, which occurred after radiation or chemotherapy, were detected. The median lesion diameter was 1 cm or smaller, without mass effect, and occurred 10 months after radiation therapy, 11 months after chemotherapy, and resolved by 3 months.

FDG-PET

Diagnostic limitations of FDG-PET have been demonstrated.[36,37] Because of the high physiologic glucose metabolic rate of normal brain tissue, the detectability of tumors with only modest increases in glucose metabolism, such as low-grade tumors and in some cases recurrent high-grade tumors, can be difficult. There can be significant variability in FDG uptake in that high-grade tumors may actually have uptake that is only similar to or slightly above the white matter uptake, especially for high-grade tumors after treatment.[36]

In general, methods to define a cut-off FDG-SUV value is not reliable, as relative use of glucose and FDG varied widely for brain tumors and was different from that for the normal brain.[38] Attempts to use lesion to contralateal normal white-matter or gray-matter tissue yielded poor results.[37] This is because of the fact that the treated brain area has a wide range of background metabolic activity and is usually lower than the metabolic activity of the normal untreated brain. As recurring tumors may have FDG uptakes equal to or lower than the normal cortex, reference with MR imaging delineates the area of interest. In the area of interest, any FDG uptake higher than the expected background, based on references to the adjacent brain, should be considered a recurrent tumor if that corresponds to abnormalities on MR imaging, even though the uptake may be equal or less than the uptake of a normal cortex.

Thus, when interpreting FDG-PET in a treated brain to distinguish recurrent tumor from radiation necrosis, it is (a) critical to evaluate lesion activity not by the absolute uptake value, not by the ratio to untreated normal brain tissue, but by whether it is above the expected background activity based on referencing to the uptake in the adjacent brain; and (b) to have the MR imaging structural information available for correlation. In a series of 44 lesions treated with stereotactic radiosurgery, FDG-PET alone had a sensitivity of 65% in subjects with metastases, but reached 86% when MR imaging and PET images were coregistered.[39] Any area of FDG uptake higher than the uptake of expected background activity using the adjacent brain as a reference should be considered suspicious, as was any FDG uptake in a region showing contrast enhancement on the coregistered MR images. In a series of 117 patients after radiotherapy when such criteria was used, a sensitivity of 96% and specificity of 77% in evaluating recurrent tumor versus radiation necrosis were demonstrated.[40]

Sensitivity of FDG-PET can be increased by imaging at delayed intervals of 3 to 8 hours after injection, improving distinction between tumor and normal gray matter.[41] The investigators hypothesized that there would be increased excretion of glucose from the cells at extended intervals between FDG administration and PET data acquisition, and this excretion is greater in normal brain tissue than in tumor. Therefore, imaging at delayed intervals may improve the delineation of tumor from normal gray matter (**Fig. 4**). In 19 patients with gliomas imaged from 0 to 90 minutes, and once or twice later at 180 to 480 minutes after injection, SUV was greater in the tumors than in normal gray or white matter at delayed times.[41] Investigators used kinetic modeling to demonstrate that the rate constant of FDG-6-phosphate degradation k_4 values were not significantly different between tumor and normal brain tissue in early imaging times, but were lower in tumor than normal brain tissue in extended-time data, suggesting that higher FDG-6-phosphate degradation at delayed times may be responsible for higher excretion of FDG from normal tissue than tumor. A potentially useful approach is to use dual-phase imaging to evaluate radiation necrosis. An attractive hypothesis would be that, similar to normal brain tissue, FDG excretion from necrotic tissue would also be greater than tumor at delayed times. Further studies are

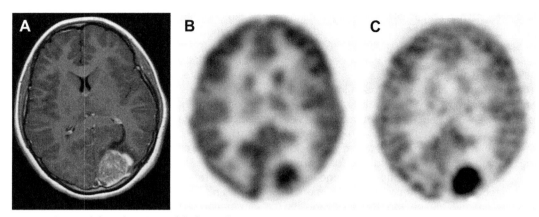

Fig. 4. MR image (A) and FDG-PET (B) showed a metastatic osteogenic sarcoma in a 15-year-old girl. Delayed FDG-PET at 4 hours after injection (C) showed much higher tumor-to-background ratio.

needed to evaluate whether this approach could increase the diagnostic accuracy to distinguish radiation necrosis from recurrent tumor.

Amino acid-PET

As amino acid tracers appear more sensitive to visualize tumor; they have the potential to have better diagnostic performance than FDG-PET in evaluating radiation necrosis. However, amino acid uptake in radiation necrosis lesions is not well known. Uptakes of FET, FDG, and ^{18}F-Choloine (FCH) were compared in acute cerebral-radiation injury lesions (inflammatory cells) as well as acute cryolesions (disruption of blood-brain barrier) in rat.[42] Both FDG and FCH were accumulated in macrophages, a common inflammatory mediator in radiation necrosis, but FET uptake was absent in macrophages. Moreover, FET-uptake ratio in radiation necrosis versus normal cortex was much lower than that of FDG and FCH, suggesting that FET is promising for differentiating radiation necrosis from tumor recurrence. Although these results appear promising, larger systematic studies are needed to evaluate the diagnostic accuracies of these amino acid tracers in differentiating radiation necrosis from recurrent tumor.

A promising role of MET-PET for differentiation of recurrent tumors from radiation necrosis was found in a study of 77 patients who had been previously treated with radiotherapy for metastatic brain tumor ($n = 51$) or glioma ($n = 26$).[43] A definitive diagnosis was made on the basis of pathologic examination or clinical course. Lesions that showed spontaneous shrinkage or remained stable in size on MR imaging for more than 6 months were assumed to be radiation necrosis. Uptakes of MET-PET tended to be higher for tumor recurrence than for radiation necrosis (Fig. 5). Receiver operating characteristic analysis

demonstrated that a tumor-to-normal mean SUV of 1.41 provided best sensitivity and specificity for metastatic brain tumor (79% and 75%, respectively), and a tumor-to-normal mean SUV of greater than 1.58 provided the best sensitivity and specificity for glioma (75% and 75%, respectively). Thus, quantitative analysis of MET-PET may be useful in distinguishing between recurrent tumor and radiation necrosis.

Recurrent Tumor

FDG-PET

High FDG uptake in a previously diagnosed low-grade glioma with low FDG uptake is diagnostic of anaplastic transformation. This high-FDG uptake is strongly prognostic.[16] FDG-PET performs generally well in identifying growing high-grade glioma. In lesions that are equivocal on MR imaging, FDG-PET may have limited sensitivity.[28] FDG-PET also is generally not sensitive in identifying recurrent low-grade tumors without anaplastic transformation.

Amino acid-PET

In contrast to FDG, amino acid uptake has been shown to be increased relative to normal brain tissue in most low- and high-grade tumors and radio-labeled amino acid might therefore be preferable for evaluating recurrent tumors. Usefulness of MET-PET in 45 brain lesions that did not show increased uptake on FDG-PET was evaluated.[44] MET demonstrated increased uptake in 31 out of 35 tumors, with 89% sensitivity. For 24 gliomas, MET demonstrated a positive uptake in 22 tumors, with 92% sensitivity. All 10 benign brain lesions (cysticerosis, radiation necrosis, tuberculous granuloma, hamanigoma, organized infarction, and benign cyst) showed normal or decreased MET uptake (100% specificity). MET was false-negative in cases of intermediate oligodendroglioma, metastatic tumor, chordoma, and cyctic ganglioma. In

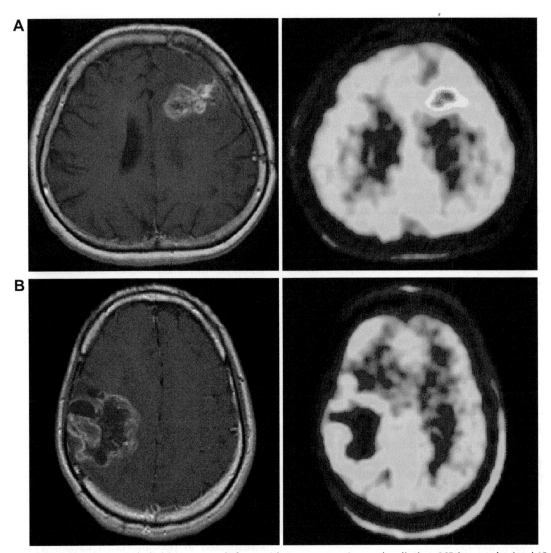

Fig. 5. (A) Previously treated glioblastoma multiform with tumor resection and radiation. MR image obtained 13 months after initial surgery, showing contrast-enhanced lesion in left frontal lobe. MET-PET image showing obvious accumulation of tracer corresponding to abnormality on MR image. Lesion-to-normal ratio was 1.70. Recurrent tumor was pathologically confirmed by second surgery. (B) Previously treated anaplastic astrocytoma with tumor resection and radiation. MR image obtained 21 months after initial surgery, showing ringlike enhancement of lesion in right frontoparietal area. MET-PET image showing slight accumulation of tracer corresponding to abnormality on MR image. Lesion-to-normal ratio was 1.44. Gliosis without tumor was pathologically demonstrated by second surgery. (Adapted from Terakawa Y, Tsuyuguchi N, Iwai Y, et al. Diagnostic accuracy of ^{11}C-Methionine PET for differentiation of recurrent brain tumors from radiation necrosis after radiotherapy. J Nucl Med 2008;49:694–9; with permission).

pediatric patients, MET-PET was found helpful to identify tumor recurrence when performed in 11 patients with suspicion of disease.[45]

The diagnostic value of FET-PET was evaluated in 53 patients with clinically suspected recurrent glioma.[46] All patients had gliomas (43 high grade and 10 low grade) and initially underwent surgery and various additional treatment modalities. All 42 patients with confirmed recurrent tumors had

focally increased FET uptake, whereas only low homogeneous FET uptakes were seen at the margins of the resection cavity in 11 patients without recurrence. Thus, focal- and high-FET uptake was considered suspicious for tumor recurrence, whereas low and homogenous uptake around the resection cavity was considered benign, after treatment changes from disrupted blood-brain barrier. Using a threshold value of

2.0 for the maximum SUV-to-background ratio, or a threshold of 2.2 for the absolute maximum SUV, FET was able to distinguish reliably between recurrent tumor and therapy-induced benign changes with 100% accuracy.

In another study, diagnostic accuracies of FET-PET and MR imaging were compared in 45 patients with 34 high-grade and 11 low-grade gliomas.[47] FET-PET and MR imaging demonstrated a correct diagnosis in 44 and 36 patients, respectively. Using a threshold of 2.2 for the maximum SUV, the specificity of FET-PET was 92.9% and sensitivity was 100%. Sensitivity of MR imaging was 93.5% and specificity was 50%. FET-PET was concordant with MR imaging in 37 patients and discordant in 8 patients. The investigators suggested MR imaging be used for the screening test first, as it has high sensitivity but poor specificity. In the event of suspected tumor recurrence, additional FET-PET investigation seems to differentiate between after-treatment changes and tumor recurrence and to avoid both under- and over-treatment.

The higher tumor-to-normal tissue ratio in FDO-PA-PET proved useful in detecting low-grade as well as recurrent tumors. Standard visual analysis of FDOPA-PET seemed adequate in that it provides a high sensitivity in identifying tumor.[28] The specificity of FDOPA brain-tumor imaging could be greatly increased by using thresholds of tumor-to-striatum ratio (T/S) of 0.75 or 1.0, tumor-to-normal hemispheric brain ratio (T/N) of 1.3, or tumor-to-normal white matter ratio (T/W) of 1.6. It may prove particularly valuable for examining recurrent low-grade gliomas.

PET TO GUIDE DIAGNOSIS

Accurate grading and diagnosis are important to direct therapeutic approach and provide prognosis, and it is especially important in patients with nonresectable tumors. As amino acid tracers have shown higher sensitivity in imaging tumors that are either hypo- or iso-metabolic to normal cortex with FDG, combining FDG and amino acid tracer to guide biopsy has been investigated.

FDG and MET to guide stereotactic biopsy were studied in 32 patients with unresectable gliomas.[48] The double-tracer approach was proposed for these patients because they presented with a tumor considered unresectable and located in the cortical or subcortical gray matter, hence were likely to have lower sensitivity with FDG. PET images were coregistered with MR imaging and were analyzed to determine which tracer offered the best information for target definition. FDG was used for target selection when its uptake was higher in tumor than the gray matter (14 patients). MET was used for target selection when FDG uptake was less than or equal to the gray matter (18 patients). Sixty-one of the 70 stereotactic trajectories were based on PET-defined targets and had abnormal MET uptake. All 61 MET-positive trajectories yielded a diagnosis of tumor. All of the remaining nine MET negative trajectories were nondiagnostic. The investigators concluded from the study that because MET provides a more sensitive signal, it is the tracer of choice for single-tracer PET-guided neurosurgical procedures in gliomas.

Added value of FET-PET was investigated in 31 patients with suspected gliomas.[49] PET and MR imaging were coregistered and 52 neuronavigated tissue biopsies were taken from lesions with both abnormal MR image signal and increased FET uptake (match), as well as from areas with abnormal MR image signal but normal FET or vice versa (mismatch). FET was negative in three patients with ischemic infarct and demyelinating disease, and these three patients were excluded from the study. In the remaining 28 patients, tumor was diagnosed in 23 and the other 5 patients had reactive changes. Diagnostic performances with MR imaging alone or MR imaging combined with FET were compared. MR imaging yielded a sensitivity of 96% for the detection of tumor tissue but a specificity of 53%. Combined use of MR imaging and FET-PET yielded a sensitivity of 93% and a specificity of 94%. The investigators concluded that combined use of MR imaging and FET-PET significantly improves the identification of tumor tissue.

Amino acid-PET to guide biopsy has also been investigated in pediatric brain tumors (**Fig. 6**). FET-PET was used to enhance diagnostic yield in diffuse glial tumors with bithalamic involvement.[50] In one case, FET-PET revealed an unexpected lesion in the left cerebellar hemisphere and biopsy showed anaplastic astrocytoma. MET-PET was used with MR imaging to guide stereotactic biopsy in nine children.[51] The lesion was either so ill-defined and showed such diffuse infiltration of the surrounding structures that no relevant-representative target could be selected, or it was located in critical areas so that multiple sampling could severely increase operative morbidity. PET-guided stereotactic biopsy based on selecting hypermetabolic areas provided accurate histologic diagnosis in all patients and allowed a reduction of the number of trajectories in lesions located in functional areas. Moreover, it offered additional prognostic information, allowing better understanding of the outcome in some children and led to decision making of performing secondary surgery.

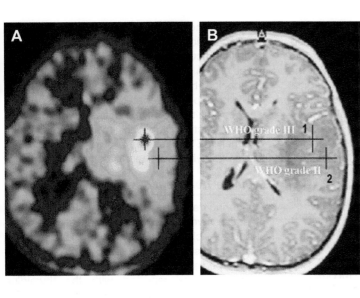

Fig. 6. Infiltrative anaplastic astrocytoma (WHO grade III) in a 9-year-old boy. The biopsy sampling of the trajectory guided by the increased MET uptake yielded the anaplastic diagnosis, while the second trajectory guided outside the area of increased MET uptake yielded a low-grade diagnosis. (*Adapted from* Pirotte B, Acerbi F, Lubansu A, et al. PET Imaging in the surgical management of pediatric brain tumors. Childs Nerv Syst 2007;23:739–51; with permission).

PET TO GUIDE TREATMENT
Planning Resection

The localization and identification of functional cortical areas in pediatric brain tumor patients provide the neurosurgeon with the ability to achieve aggressive resections with preservation of neurologic function (**Fig. 7**). Five children with hemispheric brain tumors adjacent to the eloquent cortex were studied with PET for preoperative neurosurgical planning.[52] PET imaging with FDG, MET, or a combination of the two was performed to grade the tumors, and a [^{15}O] H$_2$O uptake study was used to characterize the anatomic relationships of the tumors to functional cortex. The cortical activation maps were obtained during control periods and during behavioral tasks and were used to document motor, visual, speech, and language organizational areas. The investigators found the combination of PET measurements

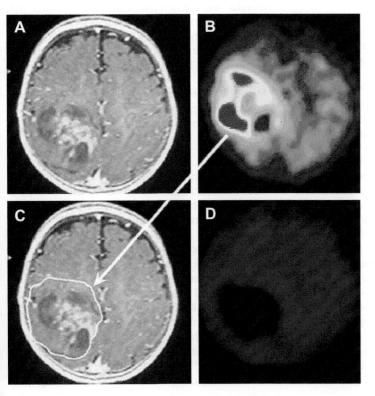

Fig. 7. Parietal ganglioglioma (WHO grade I) in a 10-month-old boy. Tumor boundaries were ill defined on MR images (*A*). MET-PET showed a sharply delineation (*B*) that was subsequently projected on stereotactic MR images (*C*). Combination of MET-PET and MR tumor contours showed in this case that PET-defined contour was more extended than the contour on MR, allowing a complete tumor resection, as confirmed by postoperative MET-PET (*D*). (*Adapted from* Pirotte B, Acerbi F, Lubansu A, et al. PET imaging in the surgical management of pediatric brain tumors. Childs Nerv Syst 2007;23:739–51; with permission).

were useful in characterizing and grading tumors and instrumental in achieving effective neurosurgical planning. Postoperative results suggest that preoperative functional brain mapping has the potential to improve outcome by defining a surgical plan to maximize resection and minimize the risk of neurologic sequelae. PET-guided surgical planning may also be useful in infiltrative low-grade tumors. In 22 children with infiltrative low-grade tumors, MET-PET was combined with MR imaging in planning of a navigation procedure.[53] These children presented with low-grade tumors located close to functional areas with tumor boundaries ill-defined on MR imaging and could not be clearly identified for allowing a complete, or at least large, image-guided resection. The level and extent of MET uptake were analyzed to define the PET contour, subsequently projected onto MR imaging scans to define a final-target contour for volumetric resection. Investigators found that in 20 of 22 children, PET improved tumor delineation and contributed to define a final-target contour different from that obtained with MR imaging alone. MET-PET guidance allowed a total resection of MET uptake in 17 cases, as the operative margin contained nontumor tissue. Because the quality of resection represents a key factor for increasing the child's survival in low-grade brain tumors, investigators suggest that the technique could improve the prognosis of children harboring ill-defined brain tumors.

After the surgery, when postoperative MR imaging presented signals that raised the question of residual tumor, PET could be used to evaluate the metabolic uptake of the signals. MET-PET and FDG-PET, used in 20 children operated on for total resection, presented a signal on postoperative MR, raising the question of a possible tumor residue.[54] An increased uptake found in 14 children led to reoperation on 11 of them, confirming the tumor histologically. Absence of PET uptake led to conservative management in six children in whom MR imaging follow-up showed no tumor progression. The investigators conclude that early postoperative PET appears to be a valid basis for complementary therapeutic decisions, especially second-look surgery, as a radical resection is a key factor for prognosis.

In a large series of 400 pediatric brain tumor patients, MET-PET or FDG-PET were integrated in the diagnostic work-up of 126 selected cases.[55] These 126 cases were selected when MR imaging showed limitations for (a) assessing the evolving nature of an incidental lesion (n = 54), (b) selection targets for contributive and accurate biopsy (n = 32), and (c) delineating tumor tissue for maximal resection (n = 40). Investigators found

that assessing functional data with PET improved the diagnostic, surgical, and postoperative steps. It was particularly helpful when the newly diagnosed lesion was an incidental finding, so that the choice between surgery and conservative MR follow-up was debated, and when the lesion was so infiltrative or ill-defined on MR that biopsy/resection target selection was difficult. Whether PET-guidance improves outcome in terms of survival will need to be assessed.

Evaluate Treatment Response

Monitoring treatment response with PET is an area of active investigation. However, little is known about the clinical value of PET in assessing treatment response in pediatric oncology, especially in pediatric brain tumors.[56] In adults, promising data was reported with the thymidine analog 3'-deoxy-3'- [^{18}F]-fluorothymidine (FLT)-PET.[57] FLT-PET was developed as a noninvasive method to evaluate tumor cell proliferation.[58] Uptakes of FLT correlates with thymidine kinase-1 (TK1) activity, an enzyme expressed during the DNA synthesis phase of the cell cycle.[59] Phosphorylation of FLT intracellularly by TK1 results in trapping of the negatively charged FLT monophosphate.[60,61] FLT uptake has been investigated in brain tumors [62–67] and correlations with proliferation index Ki-67 have been observed.[62–64] Thus, FLT as a prognostic marker has the potential to monitor treatment response. This potential was investigated in 19 patients with malignant gliomas treated with the antiangiogenesis inhibitor bevacizumab and irinotecan.[57] A more than 25% reduction in tumor FLT uptake as measured by SUV was found to be a predictive metabolic response. Metabolic responders (9 out of 19) lived three times as long as nonresponders (10.8 months versus 3.4 months).

SUMMARY

Clinical application of PET imaging in brain tumors has demonstrated that it is helpful in tumor grading, establishing prognosis, defining targets for biopsy, and planning resection. PET imaging may also be an effective method to distinguish recurrent tumor from treatment-induced changes. In addition to FDG-PET, amino acid-PET seems particularly suited for imaging brain tumors. Although PET studies in pediatric brain tumors are relatively limited when compared with adults, an active collaborative research network has been established to the study of correlative tumor biology and new therapies for primary CNS tumors of childhood.[68] The future will see significant progress in integrating functional neuroimaging, such as PET, into the clinical management of pediatric patients with brain tumors, as well as in our understanding of tumor biology through imaging various aspects of tumor metabolism, and ultimately in improving the patient outcome.

REFERENCES

1. American Cancer Society. Cancer facts and figures. Surveillance research. 2008. Available at: www.cancer.org/downloads/STT/CAFF2008AAacspdf2008.pdf. Accessed October 26, 2008.
2. Packer R. Brain tumors in children. Arch Neurol 1999;56:421–5.
3. Kleihurs P, Cavenee WK, editors. World Health Organization Classification of Tumors: pathology and genetics of tumors of the nervous system. New York: Oxford University Press; 2000. p. 15–75.
4. Central brain tumor registry of the United States, 2005–2006. Available at: http://www.cbtrus.org. Accessed October 15, 2008.
5. Burzynski S. Treatments for astrocytic tumors in children. Paediatr Drugs 2006;8:167–78.
6. Schmandt S, Packer R, Vezina L, et al. Spontaneous regression of low-grade astrocytomas in childhood. Pediatr Neurosurg 2000;32:132–6.
7. Olson JD, Riedel E, DeAngelis LM. Long-term outcome of low-grade oligodendroglioma and mixed glioma. Neurology 2000;54:1442–8.
8. Pytel P. Spectrum of pediatric gliomas: implications for the development of future therapies. Expert Rev Anticancer Ther 2007;7:S51–60.
9. Sarkar C, Suri V, Das P, et al. Pediatric glioblastomas: a histopathological and molecular genetic study. Neuro Oncol 2008 [Epub ahead of print].
10. Curless R, Toledano S, Ragheb J, et al. Hematogenous brain metastasis in children. Pediatr Neurol 2002;26:219–21.
11. Levivier M, Becerra A, De Witte O, et al. Radiation necrosis or recurrence. J Neurosurg 1996;84:148–9.
12. Tzika A. Proton magnetic resonance spectroscopic imaging as a cancer biomarker for pediatric brain tumors. Int J Oncol 2008;32:517–26.
13. Chen W. Clinical applications of PET in brain tumors. J Nucl Med 2007;48:1468–81.
14. Chen W, Silverman DHS. Advances in evaluation of primary brain tumors. Semin Nucl Med 2008;38:240–50.
15. Jadvar H, Connolly L, Fahey F, et al. PET and PET/CT in pediatric oncology. Semin Nucl Med 2007;37:316–31.
16. Padoma MV, Said S, Jacobs M, et al. Prediction of pathology and survival by FDG PET in gliomas. J Neurooncol 2003;64:227–37.
17. De Witte O, Levivier M, Violon P, et al. Prognostic value of positron emission tomography with [18F]Fluoro-2-D-glucose in the low-grade glioma. J Neurosurg 1996;39:470–7.
18. Wong TZ, Turkington TG, Hawk TC, et al. PET and brain tumor image fusion. Cancer J 2004;10:234–42.
19. Borgwardt L, Hojgaard L, Carstensen H, et al. Increased fluorine-18 2-fluoro-2-deoxy-D-glucose (FDG) uptake in childhood CNS tumors is correlated with malignancy grade: a study with FDG positron emission tomography/magnetic resonance imaging coregistration and image fusion. J Clin Oncol 2005;23:3030–7.
20. Ishiwata K, Kutota K, Murakami M, et al. Re-evaluation of amino acid PET studies: can the protein synthesis rates in brain and tumor tissues be measured in vivo? J Nucl Med 1993;34:1936–43.
21. Jager PL, Vaalburg W, Pruim J, et al. Radiolabeled amino acids: basic aspects and clinical applications in oncology. J Nucl Med 1993;42:432–45.
22. Herholz K, Holzer T, Bauer B, et al. 11C-methionine PET for differential diagnosis of low-grade gliomas. Neurology 1998;50:1316–22.
23. Coope DJ, Cizek J, Eggers C, et al. Evaluation of primary brain tumors using 11C-methionine PET with reference to a normal methionine uptake map. J Nucl Med 2007;48:1971–80.
24. Laverman P, Boerman OC, Corstens FHM, et al. Fluorinated amino acids for tumour imaging with positron emission tomography. Eur J Nucl Med Mol Imaging 2002;29:681–90.
25. Weber WA, Wester HJ, Grosu AL, et al. O-(2-[18F]fluoroethyl)-L-tyrosine and L-[methyl-11C]methionine uptake in brain tumours: initial results of a comparative study. Eur J Nucl Med Mol Imaging 2000;27:542–9.
26. Becherer A, Karanikas G, Szabo M, et al. Brain tumour imaging with PET: a comparison between [18F]fluorodopa and [11C]methionine. Eur J Nucl Med Mol Imaging 2003;30:1561–7.
27. Bethien-Baumann B, Bredow J, Burchert W, et al. 3-O-Methyl-6-[18F]fluoro-L-DOPA and its evaluation in brain tumor imaging. Eur J Nucl Med Mol Imaging 2003;30:1004–8.
28. Chen W, Silverman DHS, Delaloye S, et al. 18F-FDOPA PET imaging of brain tumors: comparison study with 18F-FDG PET and evaluation of diagnostic accuracy. J Nucl Med 2006;47:904–11.
29. Schiepers C, Chen W, Cloughesy T, et al. 18F-FDOPA kinetics in brain tumors. J Nucl Med 2007;48:1651–61.
30. Utriainen M, Metahonkala L, Salmi TT, et al. Metabolic characterization of childhood brain tumors: comparison of 18F-fluorodeoxyglucose and 11C-methionine positron emission tomography. Cancer 2002;95:1376–86.
31. Ceyssens S, Van Laere K, Groot T, et al. [11C]methionine PET, histopathology, and survival in primary brain tumors and recurrence. Am J Neuroradiol 2006;27:1432–7.

32. Torii K, Tsuyuguchi N, Kawabe J, et al. Correlation of amino-acid uptake using methionine PET and histological classifications in various gliomas. Ann Nucl Med 2005;19:677–83.

33. Spreafico F, Gandola L, Marchiano A, et al. Brain magnetic resonance imaging after high-dose chemotherapy and radiotherapy for childhood brain tumors. Int J Radiat Oncol Biol Phys 2008;70:1011–9.

34. Hodgson D, Goumnerova L, Loeffler J, et al. Radiosurgery in the management of pediatric brain tumors. Int J Radiat Oncol Biol Phys 2001;50:929–35.

35. Helton J, Edwards M, Steen R, et al. Neuroimaging-detected late transient treatment-induced lesions in pediatric patients with brain tumors. J Neurosurg 2005;102:S179–86.

36. Olivero WC, Dulebohn SC, Lister JR. The use of PET in evaluating patients with primary brain tumors: is it useful? J Neurol Neurosurg Psychiatr 1995;58:250–2.

37. Ricci PE, Karis JP, Heiserman JE, et al. Differentiating recurrent tumor from radiation necrosis: time for re-evaluation of positron emission tomography? Am J Neuroradiol 1998;19:407–13.

38. Hustinx R, Smith RJ, Benard F, et al. Can the standardized uptake value characterize primary brain tumors on FDG-PET? Eur J Nucl Med Mol Imaging 1999;26:1501–9.

39. Chao ST, Suh JH, Raja S, et al. The sensitivity and specificity of FDG PET in distinguishing recurrent brain tumors from radionecrosis in patients treated with stereotactic radiosurgery. Int J Cancer 2001;96:191–7.

40. Wang SX, Boethius J, Ericson K. FDG-PET on irradiated brain tumor: ten years' summary. Acta Radiol 2006;47:85–90.

41. Spence AM, Muzi M, Mankoff DA, et al. [18F]-FDG PET of gliomas at delayed intervals: improved distinction between tumor and normal gray matter. J Nucl Med 2004;45:1653–9.

42. Spaeth N, Wyss MT, Weber B, et al. Uptake of [18F]-fluorocholine, [18F]-fluoroethtyl-L-tyrosine, and [18F]-FDG in acute cerebral radiation injury in the rat: implications for separation of radiation necrosis from tumor recurrence. J Nucl Med 2004;45:1931–8.

43. Terakawa Y, Tsuyuguchi N, Iwai Y, et al. Diagnostic accuracy of [11C]-methionine PET for differentiation of recurrent brain tumors from radiation necrosis after radiotherapy. J Nucl Med 2008;49:694–9.

44. Chung JK, Kim YK, Kim SK, et al. Usefulness of [11C]-methionine PET in the evaluation of brain lesions that are hypo- or isometabolic on [18F]-FDG PET. Eur J Nucl Med Mol Imaging 2002;29:176–82.

45. Sorensen J, Savitcheva I, Engler H, et al. Utility of PET and 11C-methionine in the pediatric brain tumors. Clin Positron Imaging 2000;3:157–8.

46. Popperl G, Gotz C, Rachinger W, et al. Value of O-(2-[18F]fluoroethyl)-L-tyrosine PET for the diagnosis of recurrent glioma. Eur J Nucl Med Mol Imaging 2004;31:1464–70.

47. Rachinger W, Goetz C, Popperl G, et al. Positron emission tomography with O-(2-[18F]fluoroehtyl)-L-tyrosine versus magnetic resonance imaging in the diagnosis of recurrent gliomas. Neurosurgery 2005;57:505–11.

48. Pirotte B, Goldman S, Massager N, et al. Comparison of 18F-FDG and 11C-methionine for PET-guided stereotactic brain biopsy of gliomas. J Nucl Med 2004;45:1293–8.

49. Pauleit D, Floeth F, Hamacher K, et al. O-(2-[18F]fluoroethyl)-L-tyrosine PET combined with MRI improves the diagnostic assessment of cerebral gliomas. Brain 2005;128:678–87.

50. Messing-Junger A, Floeth F, Pauleit D, et al. Multimodal target point assessment for stereotactic biopsy in children with diffuse bithalamic astrocytomas. Childs Nerv Syst 2002;18:445–9.

51. Pirotte B, Goldman S, Salzberg S, et al. Combined positron emission tomography and magnetic resonance imaging for the planning of stereotactic brain biopsies in children: experience in 9 cases. Pediatr Neurosurg 2003;38:146–55.

52. Kaplan A, Bandy D, Manwaring K, et al. Functional brain mapping using positron emission tomography scanning in preoperative neurosurgical planning for pediatric brain tumors. J Neurosurg 1999;91:797–803.

53. Pirotte B, Goldman S, Bogaert P, et al. Integration of [11C]methionine-postitron emission tomographic and magnetic resonance imaging for image-guided surgical resection of infiltrative low-grade brain tumors in children. Neurosurgery 2005;57:128–39.

54. Pirotte B, Levivier M, Morelli D, et al. Positron emission tomography for the early postsurgical evaluation of pediatric brain tumors. Childs Nerv Syst 2005;21:294–300.

55. Pirotte B, Acerbi F, Lubansu A, et al. PET Imaging in the surgical management of pediatric brain tumors. Childs Nerv Syst 2007;23:739–51.

56. Franzius C, Schober O. Assessment of therapy response by FDG PET in pediatric patients. Q J Nucl Med 2003;47:41–5.

57. Chen W, Delaloye S, Silverman DH, et al. Predicting treatment response of malignant gliomas to bevacizumab and irinotecan by imaging proliferation with [18F] fluorothymidine positron emission tomography: a pilot study. J Clin Oncol 2007;25:4714–21.

58. Shields A, Grierson J, Dohmen B, et al. Imaging proliferation in vivo with F-18 FLT and positron emission tomography. Nat Med 1998;4:1334–6.

59. Rasey IS, Grierson JR, Wierns LW, et al. Validation of FLT uptake as a measure of thymidine kinase-1 activity in A549 carcinoma cells. J Nucl Med 2002;43:1210–7.

60. Toyohara J, Waki A, Takamatsu S, et al. Basis of FLT as a cell proliferation marker: comparative uptake studies with [^{3}H]thymidine and [^{3}H]arabinothymidine, and cell-analysis in 22 asynchronously growing tumor cell lines. Nucl Med Biol 2002;29:281–7.

61. Schwartz JL, Grierson JR, Rasey JS, et al. Rates of accumulation and retention of 3′-deoxy-3′-fluorothymidine (FLT) in different cell lines. J Nucl Med 2001; 42:283–90.

62. Chen W, Cloughesy T, Kamdar N, et al. Imaging proliferation in brain tumors with 18F-FLT PET: comparison with FDG. J Nucl Med 2005;46: 945–52.

63. Jacobs AH, Thomas A, Kracht LW, et al. ^{18}F-Fluoro-L-thyumidine and [11]C 65 methymethione as markers of increased transport and proliferation in brain tumors. J Nucl Med 2005;46:1948–58.

64. Choi SJ, Kim JS, Kim JH, et al [^{18}F]3′-deoxy-3′-fluorothymidine PET for the diagnosis and grading of brain tumors. Eur J Nucl Med Mol Imaging 2005; 32:653–9.

65. Yamamoto Y, Wong TZ, Turkington TC, et al. 3′-Deoxy-3′-[F-^{18}]fluorothymidine positron emission tomography in patients with recurrent glioblastoma multiforme: comparison with Gd-DTPA enhanced magnetic resonance imaging. Mol Imaging Biol 2006;8:340–7.

66. Saga T, Kawashima H, Araki N, et al. Evaluation of primary brain tumors with FLT-PET: usefulness and limitations. Clin Nucl Med 2006;31:774–80.

67. Schiepers C, Chen W, Dahlbom M, et al. ^{18}F–fluorothymidine kinetics of malignant brain tumors. Eur J Nucl Med Mol Imaging 2007;34:1003–11.

68. Poussaint T, Phillips P, Vajapeyam S, et al. The neuroimaging center of the pediatric brain tumor consortium-collaborative neuroimaging in pediatric brain tumor research: a work in progress. Am J Neuroradiol 2007;28:603–7.

The Use of PET in the Evaluation of Tumors in Children with Neurofibromatosis Type 1

Michael J. Fisher, MD[a,b,]*

KEYWORDS

- Neurofibromatosis type 1
- Positron emission tomography
- Plexiform neurofibroma
- Malignant peripheral nerve sheath tumor
- Optic pathway glioma • Low-grade glioma

Neurofibromatosis type 1 (NF1) is one of the most common genetic disorders with an incidence of 1/2500–1/3000.[1,2] Although it is an autosomal dominant disease, up to half of cases are believed to be sporadic.[3] The diagnosis is based on the presence of two or more clinical criteria (**Table 1**).[4] The gene has been localized to the long arm of chromosome 17 (17q11.2).[5–7] The complications of NF1 are varied and include bony abnormalities, hypertension, congenital heart disease, cerebrovascular disease, seizures, macrocephaly, neurocognitive deficits, and both benign and malignant tumors.

The *nf1* gene protein product, neurofibromin, acts as a tumor suppressor by negative regulation of the oncogene *ras*.[8] Activating mutations of *ras* have been noted in over 10% of human cancers.[9] Malignancies are four to six times more common in patients with NF1 than the general population.[10,11] The most common NF1-associated malignancies in children are optic pathway gliomas, other central nervous system gliomas, and malignant peripheral nerve sheath tumors (MPNST). Less common malignancies include juvenile myelomonocytic leukemia[10,12,13] and rhabdomyosarcoma.[10] In adults with NF1, pheochromocytomas,[14] gastrointestinal stromal tumor,[15] and breast cancer[16] are also noted. The most common benign tumor in NF1 is the neurofibroma.

Computed tomography (CT) and magnetic resonance (MR) imaging are the primary imaging modalities used for the evaluation of solid tumors. Although these anatomic imaging techniques are useful for tumor detection, delineating tumor extent and diagnosing distant metastases, they provide minimal information to help with differentiating benign from malignant lesions, grading of tumors, distinguishing residual/relapsed tumor from postoperative edema or radiation injury, and predicting tumor behavior. In contrast, positron emission tomography (PET) provides functional information on a variety of metabolic processes including glucose utilization, protein synthesis, DNA synthesis, membrane biosynthesis, cerebral blood flow, and hypoxia. The role of PET for

a Department of Pediatrics, University of Pennsylvania School of Medicine, Philadelphia, PA, USA
b Division of Oncology, Children's Hospital of Philadelphia, 34th Street and Civic Center Boulevard, Philadelphia, PA 19104, USA
* Corresponding author. Division of Oncology, Children's Hospital of Philadelphia, 34th Street and Civic Center Boulevard, Philadelphia, PA 19104.
E-mail address: fisherm@email.chop.edu

PET Clin 3 (2009) 531–549
doi:10.1016/j.cpet.2009.04.005

Table 1
NIH consensus diagnostic criteria for neurofibromatosis type 1

The Patient must at least Two of the Following

- 6 or more café-au-lait macules
  - ≥5 mm in prepubertal individuals
  - ≥15 mm in postpubertal individuals
- Axillary or inguinal freckling
- 2 or more neurofibromas of any type or 1 plexiform neurofibroma
- 2 or more Lisch nodules (iris hamartomas)
- Optic pathway glioma
- A distinctive bony lesion, such as
  - sphenoid wing dysplasia
  - dysplasa/thinning of long bone cortex
- First degree relative with NF-1

Data from Neurofibromatosis. Conference statement. National Institutes of Health Consensus Development Conference. Arch Neurol 1988;45(5):575–8.

distinguishing tumor from nonmalignant processes, detecting and grading tumors, evaluating tumor margins, predicting prognosis, directing biopsy, planning treatment, and evaluating response to therapy has been established for a wide variety of benign and malignant tumors. Combining this functional imaging technique with anatomic localization using CT only further enhances the power of this imaging tool.

Although the utility of PET has been established in adult oncology and is gaining acceptance in pediatric oncology, there is less information available on its value in the management of tumors associated with NF1. This article reviews the literature regarding the use of PET in NF1 patients. The focus is on the more common NF1-associated tumors of childhood including MPNST, plexiform neurofibromas (PN), and optic pathway and other central nervous system gliomas. Although there is a growing literature on the use of PET for pheochromocytoma,[17–19] gastrointestinal stromal tumor[20–22] and breast cancer,[23–25] these tumors are rarely seen in children with NF1, and therefore are beyond the scope of this review.

MALIGNANT PERIPHERAL NERVE SHEATH TUMOR

MPNSTs (also called neurofibrosarcoma, neurogenic sarcoma, and malignant schwannoma) are soft tissue sarcomas. They account for 10% of all soft tissue sarcomas and approximately half occur in patients with NF1.[26,27] Although the incidence in the general population is 0.001%,[27]

patients with NF1 have a lifetime risk of 8%–13%.[28] In the latter group, most arise from the malignant degeneration of a plexiform neurofibroma (PN).[27,29] They are more likely to occur at a younger age in the setting of NF1[26,27,29] and they are the main cause of mortality in children with NF1.[30]

MPNST are aggressive, likely to metastasize (40%–82%),[31] and associated with a poor prognosis. Five-year overall survival is 42%–53% for sporadic MPNST but only 16%–32% in NF1.[27,31,32] Tumor size, extent of resection, and presence of metastases at diagnosis are poor prognostic factors.[27,32] Therefore, early detection is crucial for long-term survival.

Unfortunately, MPNST are difficult to diagnose in patients with NF1. "Bumps" (neurofibromas) are common in patients with NF1, and the symptoms accepted to be indicative of MPNST (rapid growth, persistent pain, change in texture, new neurologic deficit),[27,33] are not specific and frequently associated with the benign PN as well. Given the stark prognosis of MPNST, one might advocate for the resection of all concerning lesions. However, PN are extensive and often locally infiltrate or surround crucial structures such as large blood vessels, solid organs, and major nerves, which makes resection of suspicious lesions challenging and usually unfeasible. In addition, the heterogeneous nature of transforming lesions limits the ability to target a biopsy to the malignant portion of a tumor, thus risking a false negative biopsy result due to sampling error. Although MR imaging is useful for defining tumor site and extent, it is not reliable for differentiating benign PN from MPNST.

PET using [18F]fluorodeoxyglucose (FDG) is able to detect levels of glucose metabolism throughout the body.[34–36] Like glucose, FDG uptake is proportional to the metabolic rate of the cell. FDG PET plays an important role in staging various malignancies and its role in the diagnosis of cancer is expanding. It is particularly useful in distinguishing benign processes from malignant tumors[37] and in predicting grade in various tumor types.[38–42]

Studies of the utility of FDG PET in musculoskeletal tumors have shown a high correlation between tumor grade and uptake of FDG.[43–49] In aggregate, these studies included 325 patients, of which 35 had peripheral nerve sheath tumors. Most of these studies measured FDG uptake using a semiquantitative approach called standardized uptake value (SUV),[43,45,47,49] which normalizes the uptake for the dose given and the patient's weight, and revealed that mean SUV is higher for malignant than benign musculoskeletal tumors. Because many of the prior studies were small or used varied methods to evaluate FDG uptake, Ioannidis and colleagues[50] performed a meta-analysis to evaluate the utility of FDG for the diagnosis and grading soft tissue sarcoma. They examined 15 studies with a total of 441 soft tissue lesions, including 57 peripheral nerve sheath tumors, and concluded that FDG PET is "very good" at distinguishing benign from malignant soft tissue lesions but inadequate for differentiating low-grade tumors from benign lesions. It is not clear whether "low-grade tumors" refers to low-grade malignancy or includes benign tumors such as PN.

Lodge and colleagues[47] reported that there is a significant difference in the "time-activity response of benign and high-grade tumors." They showed that soft tissue sarcoma peak FDG uptake occurs at approximately 4 hours, while benign lesions have peak uptake within 30 minutes, resulting in increased separation between benign and malignant lesions at the later time-point (eg, comparison of mean SUV for benign versus high-grade malignant lesions was 2.00 versus 7.98 at 60 minutes, but 1.84 versus 11.43 at 255 minutes). Others have also shown that malignant tumors do not reach maximal FDG uptake until 4–5 hours post injection.[51]

Other groups have used amino acid PET imaging instead of FDG. The higher proliferative rate of malignant cells requires an increase in protein synthesis with a consequently increased need for amino acids. Therefore, labeled amino acids may be taken up to a greater extent into malignant cells.[52] Watanabe and colleagues[49] compared L-[3-^{18}F]-a-methyltyrosine (FMT) with FDG in 75 patients with musculoskeletal tumors (only 12 had peripheral nerve sheath tumors). There was a significant correlation between FMT and FDG uptake for all lesions. Of note, the accuracy for distinguishing benign from malignant lesions was higher with FMT (81.3%) than FDG (68%).

Wegner and colleagues[53] examined the impact of PET on clinical decision-making in 165 pediatric cancer patients (19 with sarcoma). This retrospective study relied on questionnaire results sent to the treating physicians. Thirty-three PET scans were performed in the sarcoma group for the diagnosis of a suspicious lesion or suspected recurrence, staging, monitoring of therapy, or the assessment of disease status following treatment. PET results led to a change in management in 13% of the 30 evaluable sarcoma cases (change in surgical approach from planned surgery to no treatment or to more aggressive resection). However, PET was proven wrong in 13% of cases (two false negative and two false positive scans).

Overall, PET was noted to be helpful in 80% of cases (changed management, helped locate the best site for biopsy, or reassured the clinician in the management plan).

There have been several case reports of the use of FDG PET in NF1 patients with MPNST.[54–57] FDG PET was used to help differentiate benign from malignant tissue,[57] for treatment planning and follow-up,[55,57] for identifying metastases,[54,56] and for evaluation of recurrence/residual disease.[55,57] Four series used FDG PET to differentiate benign PN from MPNST.[58–61] Ferner and colleagues[61] evaluated 23 PN (in 18 NF1 patients) suspicious for malignant change on the basis of symptomatology (pain, rapid increased size, new/unexplained neurologic deficit). Seven MPNST and 15 benign PN were identified. One tumor had clinical features of malignancy, but the histology was inconclusive. Qualitative PET assessment classified 13 of the tumors as benign and ten as malignant. No malignant tumors were misclassified, but two benign tumors were classified as malignant. SUVs were calculated for twenty tumors and were significantly higher in the malignant tumors (mean 5.4) than in the benign tumors (mean 1.54), although there was a range of SUV values (2.7–3.3) in which there was overlap between benign and malignant tumors. They noted improved differentiation between benign and malignant if SUV was calculated on imaging performed 200 minutes after FDG injection.

Cardona and colleagues[59] examined 25 neurogenic soft tissue tumors suspicious for malignancy in 13 patients (five with NF1) and found a significantly higher median SUV for MPNST (2.9, range 1.8–12.3) than benign PN (1.1, range 0.5–1.8). Of note, SUV was calculated on images taken 55–60 minutes after FDG injection. By qualitative assessment, no malignant tumors were thought to be benign, but three benign tumors were classified as malignant. They proposed a cut-off value of SUV 1.8, which differentiated MPNST from benign neurogenic tumors with 100% sensitivity and 83% specificity. In four of the patients, the information provided by PET influenced the treatment plan either by directing resection to only those lesions with high FDG uptake or by identifying recurrent or second primary tumors.

Recently, Ferner and colleagues[60] expanded their initial series to 105 NF1 patients (ages 5–71 years) with 116 PN concerning for malignant transformation. Delayed imaging was performed at 240 minutes based on their initial data showing increased separation of SUV values between benign and malignant lesions with later imaging. Surgical excision or biopsy was performed on 59 lesions that were either "positive" on FDG PET or because of clinical indications. PET was used to direct biopsies to the site of highest SUV. Twenty-nine MPNST, 23 PN, five "atypical neurofibroma" ("hypercellularity and nuclear atypia without mitosis or necrosis"), and two other cancers were identified histologically. The other 57 tumors were classified as benign based on lack of "clinical evidence of malignant disease" on follow-up (greater than 2 years for all patients and greater than 5 years for most). Mean SUV_{max} for the 29 MPNST (5.7, 95% CI 3.9–7.7) was significantly higher than in the 80 PN (1.5, 95% CI 1.3–1.8). There were no MPNST with SUV < 2.5, but three PN with SUV > 3.5 (4.1, 4.8, 6.4). Thirteen tumors (seven PN, six MPNST) had an SUV between 2.5 and 3.5. They noted that FDG PET and PET/CT were also useful for identifying subclinical metastases and second primaries. They recommend resection of all symptomatic neurofibromas with $SUV_{max} \geq 3.5$ and close observation for those lesions with SUV_{max} of 2.5–3.5.

Brenner and colleagues[62] evaluated SUV as a prognostic factor in 16 patients with NF1 and MPNST (age 16–57 years) who underwent FDG PET before wide resection of the tumor. Of these, only two underwent adjuvant treatment (radiotherapy). The mean SUV for the entire group was 5.7 (range 2.1–11.6), consistent with that found by Ferner and colleagues,[60] despite the fact that SUV was calculated on images acquired 45 minutes post FDG injection. There was no significant difference in survival between patients with grade II and grade III lesions. However, there was a significant difference in SUV between those alive after 3 years (SUV 2.5, range 2.1–2.8, n = 3) and those who had died (SUV 6.3, range 3.2–11.6, n = 12). When SUV of 3 is used as a cut-off, the mean survival of those with SUV > 3 was 13 months and those with SUV < 3 was 52 months. When compared with tumor grade, the accuracy of SUV < 3 for predicting survival was superior (94% versus 69%). Although promising, it is important to note that the sample size is quite low, especially of the low SUV group (n = 3). Larger studies will be needed to corroborate this finding.

One group added [^{11}C]methionine (MET), a common amino acid tracer, to their evaluation of lesions suspected of being MPNST (by clinical symptoms or new necrosis or hemorrhage detected by MR imaging) in patients with NF1.[58] Fifty lesions were identified in 45 patients using FDG PET. FDG had an accuracy of 82% in detecting MPNST (there were eight false positive and one false negative FDG PET scan). In addition, subclinical lesions were discovered by FDG PET in five patients and thereby contributed to the treatment

planning. Ten patients underwent MET PET imaging because of either equivocal FDG uptake or a discrepancy between uptake and clinical findings. Initial FDG uptake was increased in nine of these patients, of which six had no abnormal MET uptake and biopsy or clinical follow-up was negative for malignancy. Of the three patients with increased FDG and MET uptake, two patients had MPNST and one patient had a benign peripheral nerve sheath tumor on histology. One patient had no FDG or MET uptake and was negative for malignancy by clinical follow-up. The addition of MET PET improved the specificity of PET from 72% to 91% by decreasing the number of false positives from eight to two. Although FDG uptake was assessed by SUV calculated on images taken 45 to 60 minutes after tracer injection, it does not appear that delayed imaging would have improved the accuracy of FDG PET in this study, given that delayed imaging is more likely to reduce the false negative than the false positive rate.

In a retrospective evaluation of the impact of FDG PET in the management of 16 PN suspected of malignant transformation, the PET results led to a change in management in 56%.[53] In most cases, a planned biopsy or resection was deferred and the patient observed instead. Other management changes based on the PET results included a change from planned biopsy to extensive resection and radiotherapy and a change in the selection of lesion for resection. In addition, PET was noted to be helpful in 69% of cases. In contrast, PET was thought to be unhelpful in four cases (25%), three of whom would have undergone surgery anyway and one false positive PET scan.

Extrapolation from the soft tissue sarcoma literature—as well as the more limited literature focused on NF1 patients—supports the use of FDG PET in the evaluation of PN suspected of malignant change. Although the series suffer from verification bias (ie, many of the lesions designated as PN were not biopsied), the follow-up period for the largest studies was at a minimum one[58] or 2 years[60] and certainly sufficient to clinically differentiate a PN from an MPNST. Clearly, FDG PET is useful in differentiating benign from malignant peripheral nerve sheath tumors and in deciding which lesions should be biopsied or resected (**Fig. 1**). Suspicious lesions should be evaluated with PET, and the degree of FDG uptake should be used in conjunction with the clinical scenario to direct management. For lesions that are undergoing biopsy only, trajectories should be targeted to the area of highest FDG uptake. PET/CT is clearly useful for anatomic localization of highest tracer uptake in this setting. If FDG uptake is equivocal, the lesion should be

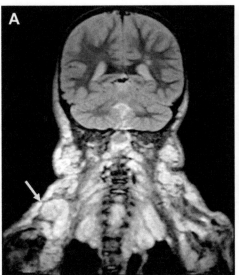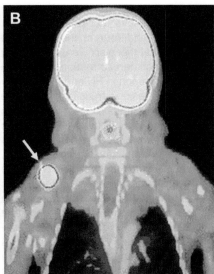

Fig. 1. MR (*A*) and FDG PET (*B*) images of a child with NF1 and extensive plexiform neurofibromas of the neck and chest. Over 8 months, a right supraclavicular lesion (*arrow*) progressed to a significant extent without associated symptoms. FDG PET scan revealed the lesion to have an SUV of 7.6. The lesion was resected with good margins and the histology confirmed to be a low-grade MPNST. There were no other FDG avid lesions concerning for metastases.

monitored closely. Perhaps MET PET may improve the accuracy of PET in this scenario, however, further study is needed before the use of MET PET can be advocated. In addition to differentiating benign from malignant, preoperative FDG PET may improve tumor staging by detecting metastases or second primary malignant lesions, and therefore may significantly alter clinical management. Last, FDG PET appears promising for predicting survival within a group of MPNST. If this is validated in larger studies, perhaps degree of FDG uptake may help stratify MPNST patients into different treatment arms.

PLEXIFORM NEUROFIBROMA

Plexiform neurofibromas (PN) occur in 16.8% to 39% of NF1 patients.[63–65] They are benign tumors composed of axons, Schwann cells, fibroblasts, perineural cells, mast cells, collagen fibrils, and extracellular matrix. They form along branches of nerves, nerve plexus, or spinal nerve roots, and often involve multiple fascicles of a nerve.[66] Although malignant transformation is the most worrisome complication, fortunately it is rare. In contrast, benign PN are a major cause of morbidity in NF1 by causing pain and disfigurement and impairing normal function when located in the extremities or orbit. In addition, they may be life-threatening if they compress vital structures such as the great vessels, trachea, or spinal cord.[65,67] PN growth is often unpredictable, with periods of rapid growth for some lesions and periods of

slow growth, inconsistent growth or relative quiescence for others.[66]

FDG PET is certainly useful in identifying PN[58–61,68,69] as well as cutaneous and subcutaneous neurofibromas,[70] but the gold standard for detecting and defining PN extent is MR imaging using short T1 inversion recovery (STIR) or T2-weighted sequences.[71] MR imaging is also used to detect changes in PN volume over time, and this is more sensitively assessed using volumetric analysis.[72] However, individual MR imaging studies are not able to predict which PN are likely to progress. The ability to predict which tumors are likely to progress is inherently valuable, allowing for the initiation of appropriate therapies before a tumor has grown larger and caused problematic complications. Because anatomic imaging techniques have limited prognostic value in predicting progression, using a functional imaging modality, such as PET, is attractive in this setting.

Schulte and colleagues[48] reported on the utility of FDG PET for the evaluation of 102 soft tissue tumors (29 benign, of which four were peripheral nerve sheath tumors). Not only was there a significant difference in FDG uptake between malignant and benign tumors, but also FDG uptake was significantly higher in "aggressive" versus "active" or "latent" benign lesions.

A case report evaluated twenty neurofibromas (ranging in size from 1–8 cm) in an NF1 patient with FDG PET before surgical resection.[70] Most of the lesions were cutaneous or subcutaneous and well circumscribed. Only six were PN. FDG uptake was evaluated 60 minutes after tracer injection using a qualitative four-point scale. Six lesions were painful and four of these showed growth. They imply that these six were concerning clinically for malignant transformation, but these same features are common in PN and it is unlikely to have six separate lesions transforming in one individual at the same time. Nine of the lesions had moderate to high FDG uptake. On histologic examination, all 20 were benign neurofibromas without evidence of malignant transformation. There was no association between FDG uptake and type of neurofibroma. However, there was a statistically significant association between FDG uptake and tumor growth, implying that FDG uptake may predict which PN are progressing. Unfortunately, no semiquantitative analysis was performed, eliminating the ability to compare FDG uptake with PN in other studies as well as between PN that were growing versus those that were stable in this study.

Only one study has assessed the ability of FDG PET to predict PN tumor growth.[73] Eighteen NF1 patients (age 6–27 years, only two older than 17 years) with stable PN by MRI (but who were considered "high-risk" for progression because of the likelihood of significant impairment of function, pain, or disfigurement if the tumor progressed) were studied with FDG PET with the intent of correlating FDG uptake with changes in quantitative MR imaging over the ensuing year. None of these lesions were concerning for malignant change. Nineteen lesions in 13 patients were evaluable for PN volume change. The SUV_{max} of these lesions ranged from 0.9 to 4 (mean 1.67, median 1.5), which is consistent with the FDG uptake values for PN noted in other series.[58–61] There was a significant difference in the percent increase in PN volume in the following year for lesions that had an SUV > 2 compared with those with lower values ($P = .016$).

Although the data is limited, these studies support the hypothesis FDG PET is useful to predict PN growth rate. Most current clinical trials for PN require MR imaging evidence of increased tumor volume over a time period of less than 12 months for enrollment. The ability to predict progression before actual tumor growth would enable intervention before a PN causes morbidity. If validated in larger series, FDG PET may be used to assist clinicians in deciding which PN to treat and/or which are candidates for clinical trials.

In addition, FDG PET may also be valuable for assessing the response of PN to therapy. Because the growth rate of individual PN may vary over time, determining if growth arrest is caused by a particular therapeutic intervention or has occurred spontaneously as a natural course of the disease can be difficult. In contrast to malignant tumors, benign lesions do not always shrink following therapy and persistent tumor may not herald inevitable tumor progression; therefore, anatomic imaging may be limited in the evaluation of response. Functional imaging with PET may provide a surrogate marker of treatment response. FDG PET has been used to evaluate treatment response in a variety of solid tumors, including esophageal, gastric, colorectal, breast, and lung cancer. Tumor FDG uptake has been shown to decrease before a decrease in tumor size, and reductions in FDG uptake are predictive of prolonged disease remission.[23,74,75] The use of FDG PET for predicting treatment response is also promising for musculoskeletal tumors. In three of four patients with osteo- or undifferentiated sarcoma in whom FDG PET scans were performed pretherapy and after one cycle of neoadjuvant chemotherapy, change in FDG predicted tumor response.[76] Two patients had a decline in peak SUV and greater that 90% "tumor cell kill" at resection. One patient had an increase in SUV and developed metastases during treatment. FDG uptake in the fourth patient was unchanged despite greater than 90% tumor kill. In another study, change in FDG uptake from pre-treatment to after neoadjuvant chemotherapy correlated with tumor response in 27 osteosarcoma patients.[77] It is possible that FDG PET may demonstrate similar efficacy in predicting early response to treatment for PN.

LOW-GRADE GLIOMA

Brain tumors are the second most common tumor seen in patients with NF1. The relative risk is greater than 100 times that of the normal population,[78] with an increased risk at all ages[30,78] but highest among children. Tumors reported include medulloblastoma, ependymoma, oligodendroglioma, ganglioglioma, and high-grade glioma,[10,63,78–82] the latter seen more commonly in adults,[78] but the overwhelming majority of CNS tumors in NF1 are low-grade astrocytomas. They can occur anywhere in the brain but are principally located in the optic pathway, brainstem, or cerebellum in children. Adults have an increased frequency of cortical lesions.[78]

Optic pathway gliomas are low-grade astrocytomas that can arise anywhere in the optic pathway (including the optic nerves, chiasm, tracts, and radiations) and can result in decreased visual acuity and frank blindness. Their incidence in children with NF1 is 15%–20%, but fortunately they become symptomatic in no more than half of patients.[83–86] The majority are diagnosed before the age of five years. On histologic evaluation most optic pathway gliomas are pilocytic astrocytomas, but fibrillary astrocytomas are seen as well.[87–89] In contrast to sporadic optic pathway gliomas, NF1-related tumors are less likely be associated with visual impairment at diagnosis and more likely to stay stable over time.[84,90–93]

The incidence of non-optic pathway gliomas in NF1 has been reported to be as high as 5%,[94] although more often noted to be 2%–3%.[63,79,95,96] In one study of 88 children and 16 adults with NF1, approximately one-third of all CNS tumors noted were outside of the optic pathway; almost half of these tumors were in the brainstem.[81] As with tumors of the optic pathway, non-optic pathway gliomas in NF1 behave in a more indolent fashion than sporadic gliomas in similar locations. This is demonstrated most dramatically for brainstem gliomas, which tend to be highly aggressive and associated with poor survival in the general population. In contrast, brainstem gliomas in NF1 are less likely to progress, require treatment, or be life-threatening.[97–99]

PET is established as a valuable tool in the evaluation of adult brain tumors.[40] FDG is the most common tracer used, but amino acid imaging is increasing in frequency. Although there are comparatively fewer studies specifically focused on pediatric brain tumors, they suggest that the metabolism of low-grade gliomas (LGG) in children is comparable to that of adults.[40] In addition, several large studies have established the impact of PET on clinical decision making for pediatric brain tumors.[53,100] PET was deemed helpful in 77% of cases and resulted in a direct management change in 15%.[53] In particular, PET distinguished tumor from non-neoplastic tissue, defined tumor extent, and helped with tumor grading and evaluation of response to therapy and recurrence. In addition, PET is useful in the surgical management of patients, particularly when the choice is between resection versus observation for an incidental brain lesion and when deciding the surgical approach for a tumor that is ill-defined on MRI or infiltrates eloquent areas of the brain.[100] Specifically, PET improved the selection of targets for biopsy, limited the number of biopsy trajectories required in functional brain regions, and helped delineate tumor margins to enable maximal resection.

There is a dearth of literature specifically focused on optic pathway gliomas and brain tumors in NF1; however, the literature regarding the utility of PET in the evaluation of LGG is extensive. Most of the discussion here focuses on LGG in general, but there is no reason to expect that the metabolism of low-grade astrocytomas in the optic pathway is unique. Despite the proven value of PET for differentiating tumor recurrence from radiation injury with excellent sensitivity and specificity[101–105] and the potential promise of PET for radiation treatment planning (to help define the optimal target volume as well as to identify regions for dose escalation),[106–109] the utility of PET for these purposes is less relevant for brain tumors in NF1, as radiation should be avoided in this population if possible because of the profound risk of secondary tumors[110,111] and cerebrovascular complications.[112,113] The most promising uses of PET in NF1-associated brain tumors is for the differentiation of low-grade astrocytomas from non-neoplastic lesions and for predicting tumor progression. Other potential or less common uses include: tumor grading, guidance for biopsy, treatment planning, and evaluating treatment response.

Detection

One of the most promising uses of PET for gliomas in NF1 is for differentiating LGG from nonmalignant lesions seen on MR imaging scan. There is likely little added value of PET imaging for the detection of optic nerve or chiasm gliomas given their distinctive appearance on MR imaging. However, PET may help in the detection of tumors of the optic radiations and other non-optic pathway gliomas in NF1. This potential use of PET is important given the high incidence (up to 90%) of focal areas of high signal intensity on T2-weighted or FLAIR (fluid attenuated inversion recovery sequence) MR imaging sequences in NF1.[114,115] These non-neoplastic lesions, formerly referred to as unidentified bright objects (UBOs), occur commonly in the basal ganglia, cerebellum, brainstem, thalamus, and subcortical white matter (**Fig. 2**). They arise usually in late childhood and disappear in adulthood.[116] Histologically, these lesions are characterized by spongiotic or vacuolar change in the myelin.[117] They do not enhance with gadolinium, exert mass effect on surrounding structures, or enlarge to a significant extent.[98] At times, particularly in the brainstem, these T2 hyperintensities may be atypical in appearance or increase in size.[116] Given that only approximately one-third of low-grade astrocytomas in the brainstem in NF1 enhance with gadolinium,[97] distinguishing non-neoplastic T2 hyperintensities from low-grade astrocytomas can be difficult.

Two studies have evaluated FDG uptake into areas of T2 hyperintensity in a total of 14 NF1 patients (aged 9 to 20 years).[118,119] T2 hyperintensities were found to have either normal glucose

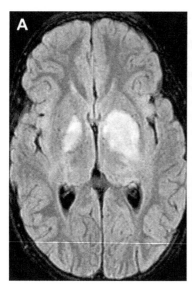
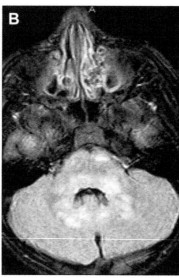

Fig. 2. FLAIR hyperintense lesions seen in the basal ganglia (*A*) and cerebellum (*B*) of a child with NF1. These lesions were nonenhancing on post-gadolinium imaging.

metabolism or low metabolism compared with adjacent areas of normal brain within the same structure. Small lesions (less than 0.5 cm) were not detected by FDG PET, either because they had normal glucose metabolism or because of volume averaging with adjacent tissue. In contrast, both FDG and MET are helpful in detecting gliomas and differentiating them from non-neoplastic lesions,[120–127] and therefore may be useful in differentiating low-grade astrocytomas from non-neoplastic T2 hyperintensities seen in NF1. However, FDG is more useful for evaluating higher-grade lesions. Given the high background uptake of FDG into normal brain tissue, especially gray matter,[36] differentiating low-grade lesions with minimal FDG uptake from normal brain tissue can sometimes be challenging. In contrast, because of its relatively minimal background uptake into normal brain,[36] MET appears to be more sensitive for detecting LGGs and delineating their margins than FDG.[128–132]

Prognosis

Although it is unclear whether FDG uptake is independent of tumor grade as a risk factor for glioma prognosis, it does appear to be prognostic within a given glioma grade. There is an extensive literature reporting an inverse correlation between FDG uptake and survival for high-grade gliomas.[133–137] Given the indolent nature of low-grade astrocytomas in NF1, predicting the likelihood of tumor progression is extremely important, so as to prevent unnecessary treatment of quiescent tumors. There are few reports evaluating FDG as a predictor of low-grade glioma progression in the absence of malignant transformation. In

a study of 28 patients, LGG with higher FDG uptake were more likely to progress and result in mortality that those without high uptake.[138] Other groups have reported a correlation between MET uptake and Mib-1 labeling index, a marker of tumor proliferative activity, for astrocytic tumors of all grades[139,140] and specifically for grade II astrocytomas,[141] implying that those tumors with higher MET uptake may behave more aggressively. The utility of MET uptake in separating grade II gliomas that will progress from those with stable disease has been confirmed in several studies.[108,121,142] In one study, an SUV threshold of 3.5 differentiated aggressive from stable lesions.[108] Ribom and colleagues[143,144] report an increase in MET uptake between baseline imaging and the time of low-grade glioma progression and an inverse correlation between change in MET uptake and time to progression. In contrast to FDG, MET does appear to be an independent risk factor for prognosis in gliomas,[139] and perhaps the "most important prognostic factor" for grade II astrocytomas.[145]

Grading

Although most gliomas in NF1 are low-grade, malignant transformation does occur at times. The utility of FDG PET for grading of brain tumors, including gliomas, was noted in one of the earliest reports of PET scanning[123] and has been established repeatedly in both adults and children.[120,122,126,127,146] In that early report, DiChiro and colleagues[123] showed that mean glucose metabolic rate was nearly twice as much for high-grade than LGG. Others have defined cut-off values of FDG uptake that differentiate high-grade from low-grade brain tumors with 94% sensitivity and 77% specificity.[122] Several studies of LGG suggest that an increase in FDG uptake in the tumor precedes or coincides with malignant change.[138,147] However, there is an overlap of signals between low-grade and high-grade lesions, which prevents complete segregation of the groups. In addition, although FDG PET may be useful for distinguishing grade II from higher-grade astrocytomas, more than half of LGG in NF1 patients (particularly the optic pathway gliomas) are pilocytic astrocytomas. The latter, although grade I and benign in behavior, have repeatedly been shown to have higher FDG uptake more similar to anaplastic astrocytomas,[130,148-150] and therefore limit the utility of FDG PET for differentiating them from high-grade gliomas. It is hypothesized that the vascular nature of pilocytic astrocytomas[148] or their increased expression of glucose transporters contributes to their unexpectedly high FDG uptake.[150,151]

MET PET has also been studied for the grading of gliomas, but its utility in this setting is less clear. Several studies have found a statistically significant relationship between MET uptake and tumor grade for grade II-IV gliomas.[121,152] Ribom and colleagues[143] showed that not only did MET uptake increase in LGG from baseline to the time of progression, but the degree of uptake was higher in those tumors that developed anaplasia than those whose histology remained the same.

Studies comparing MET and FDG PET for glioma grading are conflicting; some showing MET to be better[132] and others indicating that FDG is superior.[130] A recent study noted a significant difference in MET uptake between grade I and higher-grade gliomas but could not differentiate between individual grades. Given the weak relationship between MET uptake and glioma grade on static imaging, dynamic amino acid imaging is being studied. Popperl and colleagues[153] constructed time-activity curves of [18F]fluoroethyltyrosine (FET) uptake from five to sixty minutes following injection. They found improved separation between grade II and high-grade gliomas using this kind of evaluation, as the LGG exhibited slight but steady increase in FET uptake over time, while the high-grade gliomas had an earlier FET peak followed by a decrease. In contrast, dynamic MET PET imaging was not useful for glioma grading.[154]

Guidance for Biopsy

Because of the heterogeneous nature of brain tumors, especially gliomas,[155] it is crucial when biopsying a lesion suspected of transformation that the biopsy be targeted to the most malignant portion of the tumor, so as not to "under-grade" the tumor. Selecting biopsy targets solely on the basis of contrast-enhanced CT or MR imaging is unreliable;[156] in contrast, PET imaging is enormously helpful for this purpose. Given the utility of FDG for predicting tumor grade, targeting biopsy to the area of highest FDG uptake is likely to yield the most reliable results. Pirotte, Levivier and colleagues[107,157,158] have developed a technique to coregister stereotactically obtained PET images with either CT or MR images, and have shown that FDG PET is more accurate than contrast-enhanced CT or MR imaging for biopsy targeting of brain tumors.

Although FDG is probably more useful for detecting malignant transformation, the increased sensitivity of MET for detection of low-grade tumors (more reliable uptake into low-grade tumors and minimal background uptake into normal brain) is likely to provide an advantage over FDG for guiding biopsy trajectories to differentiate LGG from non-neoplastic tissue. The superiority of MET over FDG in differentiating tumor from surrounding brain has been shown for brain tumors,[159] and in particular gliomas,[160] in which FDG uptake was low or the lesion was adjacent to gray matter (which has an intrinsically high FDG uptake). FDG and MET were integrated with CT or MR imaging for stereotactic biopsy in 45 patients with brain lesions.[159] MET was the only useable tracer for targeting in 21 of 39 tumors. All 39 tumors had an area of abnormal MET uptake, and all trajectories (N = 73) in MET-positive areas yielded tumor tissue. In contrast, all six nontumorous lesions were MET-negative, and all trajectories in MET-negative areas yielded non-neoplastic tissue. When evaluating MET and FDG specifically for biopsy of gliomas (N = 32), all tumors had abnormal MET uptake, whereas only 27 had abnormal FDG uptake, and half of these had FDG uptake equal to that of adjacent gray matter.[160] In particular, biopsy trajectories in MET-positive regions yielded tumor in 100% of cases (N = 61), while all nine biopsies in MET-negative areas yielded nontumorous tissue. In nine of the ten LGG, MET was the superior tracer to guide biopsy. Of note, in all gliomas with increased uptake of MET and FDG, the focus of maximum tracer uptake was the same for both tracers, so the likelihood of missing malignant transformation using MET PET guidance instead of FDG is low.

Because the shorter half-life of MET (20 minutes) limits its use to institutions with their own cyclotron, other groups have looked at [18F]-labelled amino acid tracers (half-life 110 minutes) to direct biopsy. Pauleit and colleagues[161] studied [^{18}F]fluoroethyltyrosine (FET) for directing biopsy in 31 suspected gliomas (nine low-grade astrocytomas). Biopsies were performed into brain regions that were abnormal on MR images and had either increased or normal FET uptake. Biopsies from T2 hyperintense areas yielded tumor in only half of cases, whereas biopsies from regions that had increased FET uptake yielded tumor 86% of the time.

Surgical Planning

The frequent occurrence of non-neoplastic T2 hyperintensities in NF1 along with the fact that the borders of a low-grade astrocytoma may be ill defined (especially when part or all of the tumor is nonenhancing) make it challenging to delineate the margins of the tumor in NF1. PET guidance, particularly with MET, can help define the margins of a tumor that may be poorly defined by MR imaging scan and potentially help with surgical planning.[107,162] Pirotte and colleagues[163,164] have used MET PET to guide resections of LGG in both adults and children, with the goal of removing the entire area of MET uptake or the region of maximal MET uptake if the tumor was located in a brain area of functional importance. MET PET contributed to the final target resection volume in over 80% of cases and was more likely to extend the resection volume than focus it.[163] It is unclear if the patients gained a benefit in long-term survival using this technique.

In addition to delineating tumor margins, complete tumor resection is often limited by tumor location adjacent to functional brain regions. Techniques to define these eloquent brain regions, including Wada testing and intraoperative electrical stimulation or cortical somatosensory evoked potentials, may be unreliable and can cause complications.[165] PET imaging with radiolabeled water ([^{15}O] H_2O), which measures tissue perfusion and presumably is increased in activated brain regions, may assist in surgical planning by noninvasively identifying functionally important brain regions to avoid. Activation of cortical regions can be measured during motor, visual, articulation, and receptive language tasks, and the PET images coregistered with MR images. Duncan and colleagues[165] used this approach to localize areas of functional brain in 15 children with seizures (seven with tumors) and facilitate maximal resection of the seizure focus without significant neurologic sequelae. In a follow-up study, this approach altered the surgical plan to avoid critical speech/language or motor regions of brain in four of five children with tumors adjacent

to functionally important brain regions; aggressive resection was achieved without significant neurologic morbidity.[166] Combining [^{15}O] H_2O PET with FDG or MET may ultimately improve surgical outcomes by defining tumor margins and important functional brain regions for the neurosurgeon.

Treatment Response

For patients who undergo tumor resection, PET may be helpful in the postsurgical evaluation of residual disease. For low-grade astrocytomas that require treatment, complete surgical resection is the optimal therapy as long as the tumor is accessible for complete resection without significant risk of functional impairment.[167–169] In this clinical scenario, if there is residual tumor after initial surgery, many neurosurgeons consider reoperating to effect a gross total resection.[170,171] Unfortunately, it can often be difficult to distinguish residual tumor from postoperative changes on early postoperative MR imaging scans. Frequently, there may be residual linear enhancement around the tumor cavity or larger areas of T2 hyperintensity that may represent residual tumor or post-operative edema. FDG PET is unlikely to be useful in this regard, given its inconsistent uptake into low-grade tumors but high uptake by inflammatory cells, which are likely to infiltrate the resection cavity walls in the postoperative period.[172] In contrast, MET uptake is not as influenced by inflammation and is sensitive for the detection of LGG. Early postoperative PET scanning (2 to 7 days after surgery) in 20 children (18 with low-grade tumors) revealed increased MET uptake in 14.[173] Of these, three children had MR imaging scans with obvious residual tumor and 11 had MR imaging scans inconclusive for recurrence leading to re-operation, which confirmed residual tumor. Of the six MET-negative patients, three had clear MR imaging scans and three were inconclusive. Although the latter patients did not go back to the operating room, none of the MR imaging scans showed evidence of tumor progression during follow-up (4, 22, 40 months).

Another potential use for PET imaging for low-grade astrocytomas is in evaluating treatment response. Similar to other low-grade tumors, LGG do not always decrease in size with therapy. Therefore, it is difficult to know the clinical relevance of stable or persistent tumor after treatment. If the tumor cells have died, one would expect a drop in glucose metabolism and protein synthesis in the tumor. Similarly, an early decline in FDG or MET uptake may herald a good outcome. To date, the utility of PET for evaluating brain tumor response to therapy is unproven. The studies are mostly retrospective with limited outcome data and wide variability in timing of PET assessment. Surprisingly, PET imaging with FDG performed early after initiation of radiation or chemotherapy showed a correlation between increased glucose metabolism and better outcome.[137,174,175] Others suggest that this early increase in FDG uptake is transient and perhaps secondary to inflammation or a transient increase in glucose transport associated with cellular injury.[176,177] In contrast, in a study of chemotherapy for recurrent high-grade glioma, a decrease in FDG uptake from pretherapy to 2 weeks after treatment was correlated with response at 8 weeks.[178] Studies of MET PET in LGG show a decline in MET uptake following radiotherapy, but there was either no attempt to correlate this change with survival[108,179] or there was no link between MET decline and outcome.[144]

Optic Pathway Gliomas and Other NF1-Associated Low-Grade Astrocytomas

Although several of the studies on PET for brain tumors include a few subjects with optic pathway gliomas, extracting the data about these patients is difficult. There are anecdotal examples of FDG uptake in optic pathway gliomas (**Fig. 3**); however, the literature on the use of PET specifically for optic pathway gliomas or brain tumors in NF1 is sparse. One case report revealed high FDG uptake in an optic nerve/chiasm glioma with normal uptake in the other "unaffected" optic nerve in a 51-year-old man.[180] They report that the histology of the lesion was grade III; this is puzzling given the patient had symptoms for 7 years before surgery. Peng and colleagues[181] used [11C]methyltryptophan (AMT) to monitor a 16-year-old with an optic chiasm/hypothalamic glioma. They had previously reported increased AMT uptake in grade II astrocytic tumors.[182] In this patient, there was a decrease in AMT uptake into the tumor from pretreatment baseline to the completion of chemotherapy (greater than 1 year of treatment). Six months after treatment, new symptoms with associated decline in visual acuity were noted. Despite a stable MR imaging scan at the time, a new focus of AMT uptake was seen. They conclude that AMT may be useful for monitoring optic glioma progression and response to treatment.

A larger study retrospectively evaluated FDG PET as a prognostic factor in 24 patients with NF1 and optic pathway gliomas (N = 15) or low-grade astrocytomas of the brainstem or thalamus.[183] FDG uptake was qualitatively assessed. Ten tumors required treatment, because of clinical (all 10) and radiographic (nine of 10) disease progression. 70% of this group had increased FDG uptake. In contrast, only one (7%) of the 14 patients that did not need treatment had elevated FDG uptake. When evaluating clinical outcome, seven of eight patients with elevated FDG uptake had progressive disease, whereas all of the patients with FDG uptake that was not elevated had stable disease. In sum, FDG uptake appeared

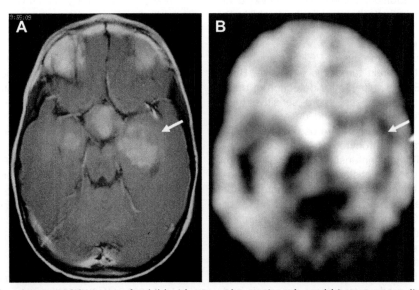

Fig. 3. MR (*A*) and FDG PET (*B*) images of a child with NF1 and an optic pathway (chiasm, tracts, radiations) glioma at the time of progression. FDG PET images indicate high uptake in the affected areas consistent with an actively progressing tumor.

to correlate with clinical outcome in 96% (23 of 24) of the patients. Prospective studies evaluating PET for predicting prognosis of low-grade astrocytomas are needed to validate this finding, perhaps with MET given its increased sensitivity for detecting LGG and probable increased utility in predicting tumor progression.

SUMMARY

Tumors are one of the most common and concerning complications in NF1. Fortunately, most of the tumors that arise in children with NF1 are low-grade; however, they can still be problematic by causing pain, functional deficits (including vision loss in optic pathway gliomas), and cosmetic disfigurement. In addition, these "benign" tumors can be life-threatening by exerting mass effect on surrounding structures or via malignant transformation. Functional imaging using PET has the ability to complement anatomic imaging with CT and MR imaging scan to improve the evaluation of NF1-related tumors. In particular, the utility of FDG PET imaging for detecting, grading, and evaluating malignant transformation of peripheral nerve sheath tumors is established. It is also useful for preoperative staging and to direct biopsy trajectories in these tumors. Last, it appears promising prognostically for both prediction of survival within a group of MPNST and for prediction of likelihood of PN growth. Future prospective studies may validate the use of FDG PET for peripheral nerve sheath tumor prognosis as well as evaluate its utility in predicting treatment response. In addition, evaluation of amino acid imaging may indicate its superiority or ability to complement these functions of PET imaging for PN sheath tumors.

The literature on the use of PET imaging in the management of brain tumors is extensive. Both FDG and MET are valuable for detection of brain tumors, but MET appears more sensitive than FDG for detection of LGG and delineating their margins. MET PET is therefore useful to differentiate low-grade astrocytomas from the nonneoplastic T2 hyperintensities associated with NF1, as well as to direct stereotactic biopsy trajectories and to help define tumor margins for improved resection. Multitracer PET (FDG or MET with $[^{15}O]H_2O$) appears valuable for planning tumor resection with minimal morbidity. Although malignant transformation of low-grade astrocytomas is infrequent in NF1, the role of FDG for assessing this is clear. To date the utility of PET for predicting low-grade astrocytoma prognosis and evaluating response to therapy is unproven. Future studies on the role of PET for low-grade astrocytomas in NF1, particularly focused on optic pathway gliomas, are needed and are likely to establish PET imaging as a valuable tool in the management of these patients. Although FDG and MET are still the most common tracers, amino acid agents with a longer half-life as well as newer tracers that measure DNA or cell membrane synthesis should be assessed.

ACKNOWLEDGMENTS

The author would like to thank Abass Alavi, MD for supplying **Fig. 3** and for helpful discussions.

REFERENCES

1. Huson SM, Compston DA, Harper PS. A genetic study of von Recklinghausen neurofibromatosis in south east Wales. II. Guidelines for genetic counselling. J Med Genet 1989;26(11):712–21.
2. Lammert M, Friedman JM, Kluwe L, et al. Prevalence of neurofibromatosis 1 in German children at elementary school enrollment. Arch Dermatol 2005;141(1):71–4.
3. Shen MH, Harper PS, Upadhyaya M. Molecular genetics of neurofibromatosis type 1 (NF1). J Med Genet 1996;33(1):2–17.
4. Neurofibromatosis. Conference statement. National Institutes of Health Consensus Development Conference. Arch Neurol 1988;45(5):575–8.
5. Barker D, Wright E, Nguyen K, et al. Gene for von Recklinghausen neurofibromatosis is in the pericentromeric region of chromosome 17. Science 1987;236(4805):1100–2.
6. Viskochil D, Buchberg AM, Xu G, et al. Deletions and a translocation interrupt a cloned gene at the neurofibromatosis type 1 locus. Cell 1990;62(1):187–92.
7. Wallace MR, Marchuk DA, Andersen LB, et al. Type 1 neurofibromatosis gene: identification of a large transcript disrupted in three NF1 patients. Science 1990;249(4965):181–6.
8. Feldkamp MM, Gutmann DH, Guha A. Neurofibromatosis type 1: piecing the puzzle together. Can J Neurol Sci 1998;25(3):181–91.
9. Walker K, Olson MF. Targeting Ras and Rho GTPases as opportunities for cancer therapeutics. Curr Opin Genet Dev 2005;15(1):62–8.
10. Matsui I, Tanimura M, Kobayashi N, et al. Neurofibromatosis type 1 and childhood cancer. Cancer 1993;72(9):2746–54.
11. Sorensen SA, Mulvihill JJ, Nielsen A. Long-term follow-up of von Recklinghausen neurofibromatosis. Survival and malignant neoplasms. N Engl J Med 1986;314(16):1010–5.
12. Shannon KM, O'Connell P, Martin GA, et al. Loss of the normal NF1 allele from the bone marrow of

children with type 1 neurofibromatosis and malignant myeloid disorders. N Engl J Med 1994; 330(9):597–601.

13. Stiller CA, Chessells JM, Fitchett M. Neurofibromatosis and childhood leukaemia/lymphoma: a population-based UKCCSG study. Br J Cancer 1994; 70(5):969–72.

14. Bryant J, Farmer J, Kessler LJ, et al. Pheochromocytoma: the expanding genetic differential diagnosis. J Natl Cancer Inst 2003;95(16): 1196–204.

15. Miettinen M, Fetsch JF, Sobin LH, et al. Gastrointestinal stromal tumors in patients with neurofibromatosis 1: a clinicopathologic and molecular genetic study of 45 cases. Am J Surg Pathol 2006;30(1):90–6.

16. Sharif S, Moran A, Huson SM, et al. Women with neurofibromatosis 1 are at a moderately increased risk of developing breast cancer and should be considered for early screening. J Med Genet 2007;44(8):481–4.

17. Ilias I, Chen CC, Carrasquillo JA, et al. Comparison of 6-18F-fluorodopamine PET with 123I-metaiodobenzylguanidine and 111in-pentetreotide scintigraphy in localization of nonmetastatic and metastatic pheochromocytoma. J Nucl Med 2008; 49(10):1613–9.

18. Mackenzie IS, Gurnell M, Balan KK, et al. The use of 18-fluoro-dihydroxyphenylalanine and 18-fluoro-deoxyglucose positron emission tomography scanning in the assessment of metaiodobenzylguanidine-negative phaeochromocytoma. Eur J Endocrinol 2007;157(4):533–7.

19. Shulkin BL, Thompson NW, Shapiro B, et al. Pheochromocytomas: imaging with 2-[fluorine-18]fluoro-2-deoxy-D-glucose PET. Radiology 1999;212(1): 35–41.

20. Antoch G, Kanja J, Bauer S, et al. Comparison of PET, CT, and dual-modality PET/CT imaging for monitoring of imatinib (STI571) therapy in patients with gastrointestinal stromal tumors. J Nucl Med 2004;45(3):357–65.

21. Kamiyama Y, Aihara R, Nakabayashi T, et al. 18F-fluorodeoxyglucose positron emission tomography: useful technique for predicting malignant potential of gastrointestinal stromal tumors. World J Surg 2005;29(11):1429–35.

22. Van den Abbeele AD. The lessons of GIST–PET and PET/CT: a new paradigm for imaging. Oncologist 2008;13(Suppl 2):8–13.

23. Kostakoglu L, Goldsmith SJ. 18F-FDG PET evaluation of the response to therapy for lymphoma and for breast, lung, and colorectal carcinoma. J Nucl Med 2003;44(2):224–39.

24. Lim HS, Yoon W, Chung TW, et al. FDG PET/CT for the detection and evaluation of breast diseases: usefulness and limitations. Radiographics 2007; 27(Suppl 1):S197–213.

25. Rosen EL, Eubank WB, Mankoff DA. FDG PET, PET/CT, and breast cancer imaging. Radiographics 2007;27(Suppl 1):S215–29.

26. Doorn PF, Molenaar WM, Buter J, et al. Malignant peripheral nerve sheath tumors in patients with and without neurofibromatosis. Eur J Surg Oncol 1995;21(1):78–82.

27. Ducatman BS, Scheithauer BW, Piepgras DG, et al. Malignant peripheral nerve sheath tumors. A clinicopathologic study of 120 cases. Cancer 1986; 57(10):2006–21.

28. Evans DG, Baser ME, McGaughran J, et al. Malignant peripheral nerve sheath tumours in neurofibromatosis 1. J Med Genet 2002;39(5):311–4.

29. King AA, Debaun MR, Riccardi VM, et al. Malignant peripheral nerve sheath tumors in neurofibromatosis 1. Am J Med Genet 2000;93(5):388–92.

30. Rasmussen SA, Yang Q, Friedman JM. Mortality in neurofibromatosis 1: an analysis using U.S. death certificates. Am J Hum Genet 2001;68(5):1110–8.

31. Stark AM, Buhl R, Hugo HH, et al. Malignant peripheral nerve sheath tumours–report of 8 cases and review of the literature. Acta Neurochir (Wien) 2001;143(4):357–63 [discussion: 63–4].

32. Carli M, Ferrari A, Mattke A, et al. Pediatric malignant peripheral nerve sheath tumor: the Italian and German soft tissue sarcoma cooperative group. J Clin Oncol 2005;23(33):8422–30.

33. Ferner RE, Gutmann DH. International consensus statement on malignant peripheral nerve sheath tumors in neurofibromatosis. Cancer Res 2002; 62(5):1573–7.

34. Hoh CK, Hawkins RA, Glaspy JA, et al. Cancer detection with whole-body PET using 2-[18F]fluoro-2-deoxy-D-glucose. J Comput Assist Tomogr 1993; 17(4):582–9.

35. Moog F, Bangerter M, Diederichs CG, et al. Lymphoma: role of whole-body 2-deoxy-2-[F-18]fluoro-D-glucose (FDG) PET in nodal staging. Radiology 1997;203(3):795–800.

36. Wong TZ, van der Westhuizen GJ, Coleman RE. Positron emission tomography imaging of brain tumors. Neuroimaging Clin N Am 2002;12(4): 615–26.

37. Zhuang H, Pourdehnad M, Lambright ES, et al. Dual time point 18F-FDG PET imaging for differentiating malignant from inflammatory processes. J Nucl Med 2001;42(9):1412–7.

38. Bastiaannet E, Groen H, Jager PL, et al. The value of FDG-PET in the detection, grading and response to therapy of soft tissue and bone sarcomas; a systematic review and meta-analysis. Cancer Treat Rev 2004;30(1):83–101.

39. Bombardieri E, Crippa F. PET imaging in breast cancer. Q J Nucl Med 2001;45(3):245–56.

40. Fisher MJ, Phillips PC. PET imaging of brain tumors. In: Charron M, editor. Practical pediatric

PET imaging. New York: Springer Science+Business Media, Inc.; 2006. p. 175–219.

41. Higashi K, Matsunari I, Ueda Y, et al. Value of whole-body FDG PET in management of lung cancer. Ann Nucl Med 2003;17(1):1–14.

42. Reske SN, Kotzerke J. FDG-PET for clinical use. Results of the 3rd German Interdisciplinary Consensus Conference, "Onko-PET III", 21 July and 19 September 2000. Eur J Nucl Med 2001; 28(11):1707–23.

43. Adler LP, Blair HF, Makley JT, et al. Noninvasive grading of musculoskeletal tumors using PET. J Nucl Med 1991;32(8):1508–12.

44. Eary JF, Conrad EU, Bruckner JD, et al. Quantitative [F-18]fluorodeoxyglucose positron emission tomography in pretreatment and grading of sarcoma. Clin Cancer Res 1998;4(5):1215–20.

45. Griffeth LK, Dehdashti F, McGuire AH, et al. PET evaluation of soft-tissue masses with fluorine-18 fluoro-2-deoxy-D-glucose. Radiology 1992;182(1): 185–94.

46. Kern KA, Brunetti A, Norton JA, et al. Metabolic imaging of human extremity musculoskeletal tumors by PET. J Nucl Med 1988;29(2):181–6.

47. Lodge MA, Lucas JD, Marsden PK, et al. A PET study of 18FDG uptake in soft tissue masses. Eur J Nucl Med 1999;26(1):22–30.

48. Schulte M, Brecht-Krauss D, Heymer B, et al. Fluorodeoxyglucose positron emission tomography of soft tissue tumours: is a non-invasive determination of biological activity possible? Eur J Nucl Med 1999;26(6):599–605.

49. Watanabe H, Inoue T, Shinozaki T, et al. PET imaging of musculoskeletal tumours with fluorine-18 alpha-methyltyrosine: comparison with fluorine-18 fluorodeoxyglucose PET. Eur J Nucl Med 2000; 27(10):1509–17.

50. Ioannidis JP, Lau J. 18F-FDG PET for the diagnosis and grading of soft-tissue sarcoma: a meta-analysis. J Nucl Med 2003;44(5):717–24.

51. Hamberg LM, Hunter GJ, Alpert NM, et al. The dose uptake ratio as an index of glucose metabolism: useful parameter or oversimplification? J Nucl Med 1994;35(8):1308–12.

52. Jager PL, Vaalburg W, Pruim J, et al. Radiolabeled amino acids: basic aspects and clinical applications in oncology. J Nucl Med 2001;42(3):432–45.

53. Wegner EA, Barrington SF, Kingston JE, et al. The impact of PET scanning on management of paediatric oncology patients. Eur J Nucl Med Mol Imaging 2005;32(1):23–30.

54. Basu S, Nair N. Potential clinical role of FDG-PET in detecting sarcomatous transformation in von Recklinghausen's disease: a case study and review of the literature. J Neurooncol 2006;80(1):91–5.

55. Chander S, Westphal SM, Zak IT, et al. Retroperitoneal malignant peripheral nerve sheath tumor:

evaluation with serial FDG-PET. Clin Nucl Med 2004;29(7):415–8.

56. Otsuka H, Graham MM, Kubo A, et al. FDG-PET/CT findings of sarcomatous transformation in neurofibromatosis: a case report. Ann Nucl Med 2005; 19(1):55–8.

57. Solomon SB, Semih Dogan A, Nicol TL, et al. Positron emission tomography in the detection and management of sarcomatous transformation in neurofibromatosis. Clin Nucl Med 2001;26(6):525–8.

58. Bredella MA, Torriani M, Hornicek F, et al. Value of PET in the assessment of patients with neurofibromatosis type 1. AJR Am J Roentgenol 2007; 189(4):928–35.

59. Cardona S, Schwarzbach M, Hinz U, et al. Evaluation of F18-deoxyglucose positron emission tomography (FDG-PET) to assess the nature of neurogenic tumours. Eur J Surg Oncol 2003; 29(6):536–41.

60. Ferner RE, Golding JF, Smith M, et al. [18F]2-fluoro-2-deoxy-D-glucose positron emission tomography (FDG PET) as a diagnostic tool for neurofibromatosis 1 (NF1) associated malignant peripheral nerve sheath tumours (MPNSTs): a long-term clinical study. Ann Oncol 2008;19(2):390–4.

61. Ferner RE, Lucas JD, O'Doherty MJ, et al. Evaluation of (18)fluorodeoxyglucose positron emission tomography ((18)FDG PET) in the detection of malignant peripheral nerve sheath tumours arising from within plexiform neurofibromas in neurofibromatosis 1. J Neurol Neurosurg Psychiatr 2000; 68(3):353–7.

62. Brenner W, Friedrich RE, Gawad KA, et al. Prognostic relevance of FDG PET in patients with neurofibromatosis type-1 and malignant peripheral nerve sheath tumours. Eur J Nucl Med Mol Imaging 2006; 33(4):428–32.

63. Huson SM, Harper PS, Compston DA. Von Recklinghausen neurofibromatosis. A clinical and population study in south-east Wales. Brain 1988;111(Pt 6):1355–81.

64. Tonsgard JH, Kwak SM, Short MP, et al. CT imaging in adults with neurofibromatosis-1: frequent asymptomatic plexiform lesions. Neurology 1998;50(6): 1755–60.

65. Waggoner DJ, Towbin J, Gottesman G, et al. Clinic-based study of plexiform neurofibromas in neurofibromatosis 1. Am J Med Genet 2000;92(2):132–5.

66. Korf BR. Plexiform neurofibromas. Am J Med Genet 1999;89(1):31–7.

67. Needle MN, Cnaan A, Dattilo J, et al. Prognostic signs in the surgical management of plexiform neurofibroma: the Children's Hospital of Philadelphia experience, 1974–1994. J Pediatr 1997; 131(5):678–82.

68. Hsu CH, Lee CM, Wang FC, et al. Neurofibroma with increased uptake of [F-18]-fluoro-2 deoxy-D-glucose

interpreted as a metastatic lesion. Ann Nucl Med 2003;17(7):609–11.

69. Son JM, Ahn MI, Cho KD, et al. Varying degrees of FDG uptake in multiple benign neurofibromas on PET/CT. Br J Radiol 2007;80(957):e222–6.

70. Brinkman JM, Bron JL, Wuisman PI, et al. The correlation between clinical, nuclear and histologic findings in a patient with Von Recklinghausen's disease. World J Surg Oncol 2007;5:130.

71. Lim R, Jaramillo D, Poussaint TY, et al. Superficial neurofibroma: a lesion with unique MRI characteristics in patients with neurofibromatosis type 1. AJR Am J Roentgenol 2005;184(3):962–8.

72. Dombi E, Solomon J, Gillespie AJ, et al. NF1 plexiform neurofibroma growth rate by volumetric MRI: relationship to age and body weight. Neurology 2007;68(9):643–7.

73. Fisher MJ, Basu S, Dombi E, et al. The role of [18F]-fluorodeoxyglucose positron emission tomography in predicting plexiform neurofibroma progression. J Neurooncol 2008;87(2):165–71.

74. Avril NE, Weber WA. Monitoring response to treatment in patients utilizing PET. Radiol Clin North Am 2005;43(1):189–204.

75. Westerterp M, van Westreenen HL, Reitsma JB, et al. Esophageal cancer: CT, endoscopic US, and FDG PET for assessment of response to neoadjuvant therapy–systematic review. Radiology 2005;236(3):841–51.

76. Jones DN, McCowage GB, Sostman HD, et al. Monitoring of neoadjuvant therapy response of soft-tissue and musculoskeletal sarcoma using fluorine-18-FDG PET. J Nucl Med 1996;37(9):1438–44.

77. Schulte M, Brecht-Krauss D, Werner M, et al. Evaluation of neoadjuvant therapy response of osteogenic sarcoma using FDG PET. J Nucl Med 1999; 40(10):1637–43.

78. Gutmann DH, Rasmussen SA, Wolkenstein P, et al. Gliomas presenting after age 10 in individuals with neurofibromatosis type 1 (NF1). Neurology 2002; 59(5):759–61.

79. Cnossen MH, de Goede-Bolder A, van den Broek KM, et al. A prospective 10 year follow up study of patients with neurofibromatosis type 1. Arch Dis Child 1998;78(5):408–12.

80. Creange A, Zeller J, Rostaing-Rigattieri S, et al. Neurological complications of neurofibromatosis type 1 in adulthood. Brain 1999;122(Pt 3):473–81.

81. Guillamo JS, Creange A, Kalifa C, et al. Prognostic factors of CNS tumours in Neurofibromatosis 1 (NF1): a retrospective study of 104 patients. Brain 2003;126(Pt 1):152–60.

82. Vinchon M, Soto-Ares G, Ruchoux MM, et al. Cerebellar gliomas in children with NF1: pathology and surgery. Childs Nerv Syst 2000;16(7):417–20.

83. Blazo MA, Lewis RA, Chintagumpala MM, et al. Outcomes of systematic screening for optic pathway tumors in children with Neurofibromatosis Type 1. Am J Med Genet A 2004;127A(3):224–9.

84. Czyzyk E, Jozwiak S, Roszkowski M, et al. Optic pathway gliomas in children with and without neurofibromatosis 1. J Child Neurol 2003;18(7):471–8.

85. Listernick R, Charrow J, Greenwald M, et al. Natural history of optic pathway tumors in children with neurofibromatosis type 1: a longitudinal study. J Pediatr 1994;125(1):63–6.

86. Listernick R, Charrow J, Greenwald MJ, et al. Optic gliomas in children with neurofibromatosis type 1. J Pediatr 1989;114(5):788–92.

87. Hoffman HJ, Humphreys RP, Drake JM, et al. Optic pathway/hypothalamic gliomas: a dilemma in management. Pediatr Neurosurg 1993;19(4): 186–95.

88. Laithier V, Grill J, Le Deley MC, et al. Progression-free survival in children with optic pathway tumors: dependence on age and the quality of the response to chemotherapy–results of the first French prospective study for the French Society of Pediatric Oncology. J Clin Oncol 2003;21(24): 4572–8.

89. Sutton LN, Molloy PT, Sernyak H, et al. Long-term outcome of hypothalamic/chiasmatic astrocytomas in children treated with conservative surgery. J Neurosurg 1995;83(4):583–9.

90. Chateil JF, Soussotte C, Pedespan JM, et al. MRI and clinical differences between optic pathway tumours in children with and without neurofibromatosis. Br J Radiol 2001;74(877):24–31.

91. Deliganis AV, Geyer JR, Berger MS. Prognostic significance of type 1 neurofibromatosis (von Recklinghausen disease) in childhood optic glioma. Neurosurgery 1996;38(6):1114–8 [discussion: 8–9].

92. Kornreich L, Blaser S, Schwarz M, et al. Optic pathway glioma: correlation of imaging findings with the presence of neurofibromatosis. AJNR Am J Neuroradiol 2001;22(10):1963–9.

93. Opocher E, Kremer LC, Da Dalt L, et al. Prognostic factors for progression of childhood optic pathway glioma: a systematic review. Eur J Cancer 2006; 42(12):1807–16.

94. Blatt J, Jaffe R, Deutsch M, et al. Neurofibromatosis and childhood tumors. Cancer 1986;57(6):1225–9.

95. Ferner RE, Huson SM, Thomas N, et al. Guidelines for the diagnosis and management of individuals with neurofibromatosis 1. J Med Genet 2007; 44(2):81–8.

96. Friedman JM, Birch PH. Type 1 neurofibromatosis: a descriptive analysis of the disorder in 1,728 patients. Am J Med Genet 1997;70(2):138–43.

97. Bilaniuk LT, Molloy PT, Zimmerman RA, et al. Neurofibromatosis type 1: brain stem tumours. Neuroradiology 1997;39(9):642–53.

98. Molloy PT, Bilaniuk LT, Vaughan SN, et al. Brainstem tumors in patients with neurofibromatosis

type 1: a distinct clinical entity. Neurology 1995;
45(10):1897–902.

99. Pollack IF, Shultz B, Mulvihill JJ. The management
of brainstem gliomas in patients with neurofibromatosis 1. Neurology 1996;46(6):1652–60.

100. Pirotte B, Acerbi F, Lubansu A, et al. PET imaging in
the surgical management of pediatric brain tumors.
Childs Nerv Syst 2007;23(7):739–51.

101. Deshmukh A, Scott JA, Palmer EL, et al. Impact of
fluorodeoxyglucose positron emission tomography
on the clinical management of patients with glioma.
Clin Nucl Med 1996;21(9):720–5.

102. Di Chiro G, Oldfield E, Wright DC, et al. Cerebral
necrosis after radiotherapy and/or intraarterial
chemotherapy for brain tumors: PET and neuro-
pathologic studies. AJR Am J Roentgenol 1988;
150(1):189–97.

103. Langleben DD, Segall GM. PET in differentiation of
recurrent brain tumor from radiation injury. J Nucl
Med 2000;41(11):1861–7.

104. Ogawa T, Kanno I, Shishido F, et al. Clinical value of
PET with 18F-fluorodeoxyglucose and L-methyl-
11C-methionine for diagnosis of recurrent brain
tumor and radiation injury. Acta Radiol 1991;
32(3):197–202.

105. Tsuyuguchi N, Takami T, Sunada I, et al. Methionine
positron emission tomography for differentiation of
recurrent brain tumor and radiation necrosis after
stereotactic radiosurgery–in malignant glioma.
Ann Nucl Med 2004;18(4):291–6.

106. Levivier M, Massager N, Wikler D, et al. Use of
stereotactic PET images in dosimetry planning of
radiosurgery for brain tumors: clinical experience
and proposed classification. J Nucl Med 2004;
45(7):1146–54.

107. Levivier M, Wikler D Jr, Massager N, et al. The
integration of metabolic imaging in stereotactic
procedures including radiosurgery: a review.
J Neurosurg 2002;97(Suppl 5):542–50.

108. Nuutinen J, Sonninen P, Lehikoinen P, et al. Radiotherapy treatment planning and long-term follow-
up with [(11)C]methionine PET in patients with
low-grade astrocytoma. Int J Radiat Oncol Biol
Phys 2000;48(1):43–52.

109. Tralins KS, Douglas JG, Stelzer KJ, et al. Volumetric analysis of 18F-FDG PET in glioblastoma
multiforme: prognostic information and possible
role in definition of target volumes in radiation
dose escalation. J Nucl Med 2002;43(12):
1667–73.

110. Chao RC, Pyzel U, Fridlyand J, et al. Therapy-
induced malignant neoplasms in Nf1 mutant
mice. Cancer Cell 2005;8(4):337–48.

111. Sharif S, Ferner R, Birch JM, et al. Second primary
tumors in neurofibromatosis 1 patients treated for
optic glioma: substantial risks after radiotherapy.
J Clin Oncol 2006;24(16):2570–5.

112. Grill J, Couanet D, Cappelli C, et al. Radiation-
induced cerebral vasculopathy in children with
neurofibromatosis and optic pathway glioma. Ann
Neurol 1999;45(3):393–6.

113. Kestle JR, Hoffman HJ, Mock AR. Moyamoya
phenomenon after radiation for optic glioma.
J Neurosurg 1993;79(1):32–5.

114. Hyman SL, Gill DS, Shores EA, et al. T2 hyperintensities in children with neurofibromatosis
type 1 and their relationship to cognitive func-
tioning. J Neurol Neurosurg Psychiatr 2007;
78(10):1088–91.

115. Rosenbaum T, Engelbrecht V, Krolls W, et al. MRI abnormalities in neurofibromatosis type 1 (NF1): a study of
men and mice. Brain Dev 1999;21(4):268–73.

116. DiMario FJ Jr, Ramsby G. Magnetic resonance
imaging lesion analysis in neurofibromatosis
type 1. Arch Neurol 1998;55(4):500–5.

117. DiPaolo DP, Zimmerman RA, Rorke LB, et al.
Neurofibromatosis type 1: pathologic substrate of
high-signal-intensity foci in the brain. Radiology
1995;195(3):721–4.

118. Balestri P, Lucignani G, Fois A, et al. Cerebral
glucose metabolism in neurofibromatosis type 1
assessed with [18F]-2-fluoro-2-deoxy-D-glucose
and PET. J Neurol Neurosurg Psychiatr 1994;
57(12):1479–83.

119. Kaplan AM, Chen K, Lawson MA, et al. Positron
emission tomography in children with neurofi-
bromatosis-1. J Child Neurol 1997;12(8):
499–506.

120. Borgwardt L, Hojgaard L, Carstensen H, et al.
Increased fluorine-18 2-fluoro-2-deoxy-D-glucose
(FDG) uptake in childhood CNS tumors is correlated with malignancy grade: a study with FDG
positron emission tomography/magnetic resonance imaging coregistration and image fusion.
J Clin Oncol 2005;23(13):3030–7.

121. De Witte O, Goldberg I, Wikler D, et al. Positron
emission tomography with injection of methionine
as a prognostic factor in glioma. J Neurosurg
2001;95(5):746–50.

122. Delbeke D, Meyerowitz C, Lapidus RL, et al.
Optimal cutoff levels of F-18 fluorodeoxyglucose
uptake in the differentiation of low-grade from
high-grade brain tumors with PET. Radiology
1995;195(1):47–52.

123. Di Chiro G, DeLaPaz RL, Brooks RA, et al. Glucose
utilization of cerebral gliomas measured by [18F]
fluorodeoxyglucose and positron emission tomography. Neurology 1982;32(12):1323–9.

124. Herholz K, Holzer T, Bauer B, et al. 11C-methionine
PET for differential diagnosis of low-grade gliomas.
Neurology 1998;50(5):1316–22.

125. Ogawa T, Shishido F, Kanno I, et al. Cerebral
glioma: evaluation with methionine PET. Radiology
1993;186(1):45–53.

126. Padma MV, Said S, Jacobs M, et al. Prediction of pathology and survival by FDG PET in gliomas. J Neurooncol 2003;64(3):227–37.

127. Utriainen M, Metsahonkala L, Salmi TT, et al. Metabolic characterization of childhood brain tumors: comparison of 18F-fluorodeoxyglucose and 11C-methionine positron emission tomography. Cancer 2002;95(6):1376–86.

128. Chung JK, Kim YK, Kim SK, et al. Usefulness of 11C-methionine PET in the evaluation of brain lesions that are hypo- or isometabolic on 18F-FDG PET. Eur J Nucl Med Mol Imaging 2002; 29(2):176–82.

129. Derlon JM, Petit-Taboue MC, Chapon F, et al. The in vivo metabolic pattern of low-grade brain gliomas: a positron emission tomographic study using 18F-fluorodeoxyglucose and 11C-L-methylmethionine. Neurosurgery 1997;40(2):276–87 [discussion: 87–8].

130. Kaschten B, Stevenaert A, Sadzot B, et al. Preoperative evaluation of 54 gliomas by PET with fluorine-18-fluorodeoxyglucose and/or carbon-11-methionine. J Nucl Med 1998;39(5):778–85.

131. Pirotte B, Goldman S, David P, et al. Stereotactic brain biopsy guided by positron emission tomography (PET) with [F-18]fluorodeoxyglucose and [C-11]methionine. Acta Neurochir Suppl 1997;68: 133–8.

132. Sasaki M, Kuwabara Y, Yoshida T, et al. A comparative study of thallium-201 SPET, carbon-11 methionine PET and fluorine-18 fluorodeoxyglucose PET for the differentiation of astrocytic tumours. Eur J Nucl Med 1998;25(9):1261–9.

133. Alavi JB, Alavi A, Chawluk J, et al. Positron emission tomography in patients with glioma. A predictor of prognosis. Cancer 1988;62(6):1074–8.

134. De Witte O, Lefranc F, Levivier M, et al. FDG-PET as a prognostic factor in high-grade astrocytoma. J Neurooncol 2000;49(2):157–63.

135. Holzer T, Herholz K, Jeske J, et al. FDG-PET as a prognostic indicator in radiochemotherapy of glioblastoma. J Comput Assist Tomogr 1993; 17(5):681–7.

136. Patronas NJ, Di Chiro G, Kufta C, et al. Prediction of survival in glioma patients by means of positron emission tomography. J Neurosurg 1985;62(6): 816–22.

137. Spence AM, Muzi M, Graham MM, et al. 2-[(18)F]Fluoro-2-deoxyglucose and glucose uptake in malignant gliomas before and after radiotherapy: correlation with outcome. Clin Cancer Res 2002; 8(4):971–9.

138. De Witte O, Levivier M, Violon P, et al. Prognostic value positron emission tomography with [18F]fluoro-2-deoxy-D-glucose in the low-grade glioma. Neurosurgery 1996;39(3):470–6 [discussion: 6–7].

139. Kim S, Chung JK, Im SH, et al. 11C-methionine PET as a prognostic marker in patients with glioma: comparison with 18F-FDG PET. Eur J Nucl Med Mol Imaging 2005;32(1):52–9.

140. Torii K, Tsuyuguchi N, Kawabe J, et al. Correlation of amino-acid uptake using methionine PET and histological classifications in various gliomas. Ann Nucl Med 2005;19(8):677–83.

141. Kato T, Shinoda J, Oka N, et al. Analysis of 11C-methionine uptake in low-grade gliomas and correlation with proliferative activity. AJNR Am J Neuroradiol 2008;29(10):1867–71.

142. Ribom D, Eriksson A, Hartman M, et al. Positron emission tomography (11)C-methionine and survival in patients with low-grade gliomas. Cancer 2001;92(6):1541–9.

143. Ribom D, Engler H, Blomquist E, et al. Potential significance of (11)C-methionine PET as a marker for the radiosensitivity of low-grade gliomas. Eur J Nucl Med Mol Imaging 2002;29(5):632–40.

144. Ribom D, Schoenmaekers M, Engler H, et al. Evaluation of 11C-methionine PET as a surrogate endpoint after treatment of grade 2 gliomas. J Neurooncol 2005;71(3):325–32.

145. Smits A, Westerberg E, Ribom D. Adding (11)C-methionine PET to the EORTC prognostic factors in grade 2 gliomas. Eur J Nucl Med Mol Imaging 2008;35(1):65–71.

146. Goldman S, Levivier M, Pirotte B, et al. Regional glucose metabolism and histopathology of gliomas. A study based on positron emission tomography-guided stereotactic biopsy. Cancer 1996;78(5):1098–106.

147. Francavilla TL, Miletich RS, Di Chiro G, et al. Positron emission tomography in the detection of malignant degeneration of low-grade gliomas. Neurosurgery 1989;24(1):1–5.

148. Fulham MJ, Melisi JW, Nishimiya J, et al. Neuroimaging of juvenile pilocytic astrocytomas: an enigma. Radiology 1993;189(1):221–5.

149. Hoffman JM, Hanson MW, Friedman HS, et al. FDG-PET in pediatric posterior fossa brain tumors. J Comput Assist Tomogr 1992;16(1):62–8.

150. Roelcke U, Radu EW, Hausmann O, et al. Tracer transport and metabolism in a patient with juvenile pilocytic astrocytoma. A PET study. J Neurooncol 1998;36(3):279–83.

151. Hustinx R, Alavi A. SPECT and PET imaging of brain tumors. Neuroimaging Clin N Am 1999;9(4):751–66.

152. Derlon JM, Bourdet C, Bustany P, et al. [11C]L-methionine uptake in gliomas. Neurosurgery 1989;25(5):720–8.

153. Popperl G, Kreth FW, Mehrkens JH, et al. FET PET for the evaluation of untreated gliomas: correlation of FET uptake and uptake kinetics with tumour grading. Eur J Nucl Med Mol Imaging 2007; 34(12):1933–42.

154. Moulin-Romsee G, D'Hondt E, de Groot T, et al. Non-invasive grading of brain tumours using dynamic amino acid PET imaging: does it work for 11C-methionine? Eur J Nucl Med Mol Imaging 2007;34(12):2082–7.

155. Paulus W, Peiffer J. Intratumoral histologic heterogeneity of gliomas. A quantitative study. Cancer 1989;64(2):442–7.

156. Floeth FW, Pauleit D, Wittsack HJ, et al. Multimodal metabolic imaging of cerebral gliomas: positron emission tomography with [18F]fluoroethyl-L-tyrosine and magnetic resonance spectroscopy. J Neurosurg 2005;102(2):318–27.

157. Massager N, David P, Goldman S, et al. Combined magnetic resonance imaging- and positron emission tomography-guided stereotactic biopsy in brainstem mass lesions: diagnostic yield in a series of 30 patients. J Neurosurg 2000;93(6):951–7.

158. Pirotte B, Goldman S, Brucher JM, et al. PET in stereotactic conditions increases the diagnostic yield of brain biopsy. Stereotact Funct Neurosurg 1994;63(1–4):144–9.

159. Pirotte B, Goldman S, Massager N, et al. Combined use of 18F-fluorodeoxyglucose and 11C-methionine in 45 positron emission tomography-guided stereotactic brain biopsies. J Neurosurg 2004; 101(3):476–83.

160. Pirotte B, Goldman S, Massager N, et al. Comparison of 18F-FDG and 11C-methionine for PET-guided stereotactic brain biopsy of gliomas. J Nucl Med 2004;45(8):1293–8.

161. Pauleit D, Floeth F, Hamacher K, et al. O-(2-[18F]fluoroethyl)-L-tyrosine PET combined with MRI improves the diagnostic assessment of cerebral gliomas. Brain 2005;128(Pt 3):678–87.

162. Miwa K, Shinoda J, Yano H, et al. Discrepancy between lesion distributions on methionine PET and MR images in patients with glioblastoma multiforme: insight from a PET and MR fusion image study. J Neurol Neurosurg Psychiatr 2004;75(10):1457–62.

163. Pirotte B, Goldman S, Dewitte O, et al. Integrated positron emission tomography and magnetic resonance imaging-guided resection of brain tumors: a report of 103 consecutive procedures. J Neurosurg 2006;104(2):238–53.

164. Pirotte B, Goldman S, Van Bogaert P, et al. Integration of [11C]methionine-positron emission tomographic and magnetic resonance imaging for image-guided surgical resection of infiltrative low-grade brain tumors in children. Neurosurgery 2005;57(Suppl 1):128–39 [discussion: 39].

165. Duncan JD, Moss SD, Bandy DJ, et al. Use of positron emission tomography for presurgical localization of eloquent brain areas in children with seizures. Pediatr Neurosurg 1997;26(3):144–56.

166. Kaplan AM, Bandy DJ, Manwaring KH, et al. Functional brain mapping using positron emission tomography scanning in preoperative neurosurgical planning for pediatric brain tumors. J Neurosurg 1999;91(5):797–803.

167. Macdonald DR. Low-grade gliomas, mixed gliomas, and oligodendrogliomas. Semin Oncol 1994;21(2):236–48.

168. Pollack IF, Claassen D, al-Shboul Q, et al. Low-grade gliomas of the cerebral hemispheres in children: an analysis of 71 cases. J Neurosurg 1995; 82(4):536–47.

169. Sutton LN, Cnaan A, Klatt L, et al. Postoperative surveillance imaging in children with cerebellar astrocytomas. J Neurosurg 1996;84(5):721–5.

170. Khan RB, Sanford RA, Kun LE, et al. Morbidity of second-look surgery in pediatric central nervous system tumors. Pediatr Neurosurg 2001;35(5): 225–9.

171. Palma L, Celli P, Mariottini A. Long-term follow-up of childhood cerebellar astrocytomas after incomplete resection with particular reference to arrested growth or spontaneous tumour regression. Acta Neurochir (Wien) 2004;146(6):581–8 [discussion: 8].

172. Cokgor I, Akabani G, Kuan CT, et al. Phase I trial results of iodine-131-labeled antitenascin monoclonal antibody 81C6 treatment of patients with newly diagnosed malignant gliomas. J Clin Oncol 2000;18(22):3862–72.

173. Pirotte B, Levivier M, Morelli D, et al. Positron emission tomography for the early postsurgical evaluation of pediatric brain tumors. Childs Nerv Syst 2005;21(4):294–300.

174. De Witte O, Hildebrand J, Luxen A, et al. Acute effect of carmustine on glucose metabolism in brain and glioblastoma. Cancer 1994;74(10): 2836–42.

175. Maruyama I, Sadato N, Waki A, et al. Hyperacute changes in glucose metabolism of brain tumors after stereotactic radiosurgery: a PET study. J Nucl Med 1999;40(7):1085–90.

176. Rozental JM, Levine RL, Mehta MP, et al. Early changes in tumor metabolism after treatment: the effects of stereotactic radiotherapy. Int J Radiat Oncol Biol Phys 1991;20(5):1053–60.

177. Spence AM, Mankoff DA, Muzi M. Positron emission tomography imaging of brain tumors. Neuroimaging Clin N Am 2003;13(4):717–39.

178. Brock CS, Young H, O'Reilly SM, et al. Early evaluation of tumour metabolic response using [18F]fluorodeoxyglucose and positron emission tomography: a pilot study following the phase II chemotherapy schedule for temozolomide in recurrent high-grade gliomas. Br J Cancer 2000;82(3): 608–15.

179. Wurker M, Herholz K, Voges J, et al. Glucose consumption and methionine uptake in low-grade gliomas after iodine-125 brachytherapy. Eur J Nucl Med 1996;23(5):583–6.

180. Miyamoto J, Sasajima H, Owada K, et al. Surgical decision for adult optic glioma based on [18F]fluorodeoxyglucose positron emission tomography study. Neurol Med Chir (Tokyo) 2006;46(10):500–3.

181. Peng F, Juhasz C, Bhambhani K, et al. Assessment of progression and treatment response of optic pathway glioma with positron emission tomography using alpha-[(11)C]methyl-L-tryptophan. Mol Imaging Biol 2007;9(3):106–9.

182. Juhasz C, Chugani DC, Muzik O, et al. In vivo uptake and metabolism of alpha-[11C]methyl-L-tryptophan in human brain tumors. J Cereb Blood Flow Metab 2006;26(3):345–57.

183. Molloy PT, Defeo R, Hunter J, et al. Excellent correlation of FDG-PET imaging with clinical outcome in patients with neurofibromatosis type I and low grade astrocytomas. J Nucl Med 1999; 40:129P.

PET/CT in the Evaluation of Neuroblastoma

Susan E. Sharp, MD[a,b], Michael J. Gelfand, MD[a,b],
Barry L. Shulkin, MD, MBA[c,*]

KEYWORDS

• Neuroblastoma • PET • PET/CT • MIBG • FDG

Neuroblastoma is a malignant tumor derived from primitive neural crest cells that normally develop into cells of the sympathetic nervous system. The degree of cellular maturation differentiates neuroblastoma from the closely related ganglioneuroblastoma and the benign neural crest tumor ganglioneuroma. Neuroblastoma most commonly arises in the adrenal gland, but can occur anywhere along the sympathetic chain. Other common sites include the paraspinal ganglia of the posterior mediastinum and retroperitoneum.[1–3]

Neuroblastoma is the most common extracranial solid tumor of the first decade of childhood, comprising 8% to 10% of all neoplasms in that age group. Only childhood leukemia and primary brain tumors occur more commonly. Approximately 600 new cases of neuroblastoma are diagnosed each year in the United States. Median age at presentation is 20 to 30 months with over 90% of cases occurring in children younger than 6 years of age.[1–3]

Neuroblastoma is an unusual tumor in that its prognosis and distribution are variable. Some tumors spontaneously regress or mature, whereas others progress in spite of multimodality therapy. Clinical features of neuroblastoma are frequently age dependent. Children younger than 18 months tend to have a better prognosis and metastatic disease involving bone marrow, liver and skin. Children older than 18 months tend to have a poorer prognosis with metastatic disease involving bone. About 70% of patients have disseminated disease at presentation, most commonly involving bone or bone marrow.[2–4]

Preferred treatment for localized neuroblastoma is surgical excision with preoperative chemotherapy given when local disease is extensive. Treatment for neuroblastoma with distant metastases includes high-dose chemotherapy, radiation therapy, and stem cell transplantation.[3]

The Shimada histopathologic system is used to determine the prognosis of patients with neuroblastoma incorporating patient age, presence or absence of Schwann cell stroma, degree of tumor differentiation, and mitosis-karyorrhexis index.[5] Staging has traditionally been based on the International Neuroblastoma Staging System (INSS), as outlined in **Table 1**.[6] The International Neuroblastoma Risk Group recently published a new staging system (INRGSS) that allows pretreatment staging and risk assessment as outlined in **Table 2**.[7]

The neural crest origin of neuroblastoma can aid in diagnosis and disease surveillance. Clinically, 90% to 95% of neuroblastoma patients will have high levels of urinary catecholamine metabolites, such as vanillylmandelic acid, homovanillic acid, or dopamine. Hypertension can also occur.[8] From an imaging standpoint, functional agents such as metaiodobenzylguanidine (MIBG) use the type 1 catecholamine reuptake system to visualize neuroendocrine tumors.

Functional imaging agents play an important role in the diagnosis and staging of neuroblastoma. They are also used for evaluation of treatment response and detection of disease

[a] Department of Radiology, University of Cincinnati, ML 0761, 234 Goodman Street, Cincinnati, OH 45219, USA
[b] Section of Nuclear Medicine, Department of Radiology, Cincinnati Children's Hospital Medical Center, MLC 5031, 3333 Burnet Avenue, Cincinnati, OH 45229-3039, USA
[c] Nuclear Medicine Division, Department of Radiological Sciences, MS 220, Room I-3128, St. Jude Children's Research Hospital, 262 Danny Thomas Place, Memphis, TN 38105-3678, USA
* Corresponding author.
E-mail address: barry.shulkin@stjude.org (B.L. Shulkin).

PET Clin 3 (2009) 551–561
doi:10.1016/j.cpet.2009.03.006
1556-8598/09/$ – see front matter © 2009 Elsevier Inc. All rights reserved.

Table 1
Summary of the International Neuroblastoma Staging System (INSS)[6]

Stage	Description
1	Localized tumor without regional lymph node involvement
2	Unilateral tumor with either ipsilateral lymph node involvement or incomplete gross resection
3	Tumor that crosses the midline or has contralateral lymph node involvement
4	Tumor with dissemination to distant sites, such as lymph nodes, bone, bone marrow, or liver
4s	Localized tumor in infants *less than 1 year of age* with metastatic involvement only of liver, skin, or bone marrow

recurrence, often guiding therapeutic decisions. MIBG has been the conventional agent used for functional imaging of neuroblastoma. ^{99m}Tc-methylene diphosphonate (MDP) has traditionally been used in neuroblastoma to differentiate bone from bone marrow metastases, which may be important in differentiating Stage 4 from Stage 4S disease in infants.[9] Use of fluorodeoxyglucose (FDG) PET is increasing and recent work has clarified the clinical settings where FDG is likely to be of value. Investigation of new functional imaging agents continues with development of several novel radiopharmaceuticals.

METAIODOBENZYLGUANIDINE

A discussion of MIBG is necessary, not only for its important role in neuroblastoma imaging, but also for its mechanism of uptake, which is shared by most functional agents used in neuroblastoma imaging with the significant exception of FDG. MIBG was originally used for localization of pheochromocytoma[10] with its use in neuroblastoma following shortly thereafter.[11–13] I-131 MIBG was first developed as an imaging agent.[14] MIBG was labeled with I-123 soon after, but for many years I-123 MIBG was not commercially available in

the United States. I-123 MIBG was available in Europe and many US pediatric centers synthesized I-123 MIBG on site for local use.[15] I-123 MIBG is now widely available in the United States and the Food and Drug Administration has recently approved its use in neuroblastoma and pheochromocytoma. Studies have also been performed using I-124 MIBG, although its use has been limited.[16,17]

Radiopharmaceuticals

MIBG can be labeled with I-123, I-131, or I-124. I-123 MIBG gives high-quality images with I-131 MIBG generally considered to be suboptimal in comparison.[18] The administered dose of I-131 MIBG is limited because of its relatively long half-life (8 days), high-energy photon (364 keV), and beta particle, which add to the radiation dose without contributing to imaging. I-123 MIBG has the advantages of a shorter half-life (13 hours), an ideal photon energy (159 keV) for gamma camera and single-photon emission computed tomography (SPECT) imaging, and lack of a beta particle. Given administered doses resulting in the same radiation dose, approximately 10 times as many counts are obtained using I-123 MIBG at 24 hours after administration when compared

Table 2
Summary of the International Neuroblastoma Risk Group Staging System (INRGSS)[7]

Stage	Description
L1	Localized tumor not involving vital structures and confined to one body compartment (neck, chest, abdomen, or pelvis)
L2	Local/regional tumor with one or more image-defined risk factors (ie, involvement of 2 body compartments, encasement of major vascular structures, invasion of adjacent organs, or intraspinal extension)
M	Distant metastatic disease (except stage MS)
MS	Metastatic disease in patients less than 18 months of age with metastases confined to skin, liver, and/or bone marrow

with I-131 MIBG. As a result, I-123 MIBG gives much higher quality images.

I-124 decays by both electron capture (75%) and positron emission (25%). The electron capture mode of decay results in multiple high-energy single photons, which increase radiation dose to the patient. The high-energy photons also increase scatter and detection of random coincidence events, which add to background noise on PET images. The half-life of I-124 (4.2 days) allows imaging over several days, but limits administered activities. These factors limit the practical uses for I-124 MIBG, although its use has been described in treatment planning for I-131 MIBG therapy.[16]

Uptake Mechanism

Functional imaging with MIBG takes advantage of the adrenergic origin of neuroblastoma. The sensitivity of MIBG in the detection of neuroblastoma is about 90% with specificity nearly 100%. MIBG enters neuroblastoma cells using the type 1 catecholamine reuptake system. MIBG is then concentrated within both the cytoplasm and specialized norepinephrine storage granules. Norepinephrine, dopamine, and serotonin transporters have considerable similarities, a fact that may be used when developing novel radiopharmaceuticals.

Acquisition Protocol

Administered doses of I-123 MIBG are generally determined using weight (0.14 mCi/kg or 5.18 mBq/kg) or body surface area (BSA) (10 mCi/1.7 m^2 BSA or 370 mBq/1.7 m^2 BSA), with a maximum administered dose of 10 mCi (370 mBq). Saturated solution of potassium iodide (SSKI) is given before radiopharmaceutical injection to block thyroid uptake. Patient medications should be reviewed, as type 1 catecholamine reuptake is blocked by a number of drugs (including phenylephrine, pseudoephedrine, cocaine, tricyclic antidepressants, and labetalol).[19]

Planar and SPECT I-123 MIBG images are usually obtained 24 hours after radiopharmaceutical injection with supplemental planar images sometimes acquired at 48 hours. SPECT has aided MIBG diagnosis of neuroblastoma, improving anatomic localization.[20–22] Continued improvements are expected with the advent of SPECT/CT.[23,24]

FLUORODEOXYGLUCOSE

FDG PET is well established as an important tool for the management of adult oncology patients. Many adult tumors (including lung, esophageal, colon, and breast cancers) are well demonstrated by FDG PET. Most pediatric tumors, including neuroblastoma, are also metabolically active and thus concentrate FDG. The diagnostic utility of FDG PET and its impact on patient management have also been reported for many pediatric cancers.[25–35]

Uptake Mechanism

FDG is a glucose analog that is concentrated in tumor cells by the glucose transporter. Because most tumors preferentially use glucose for energy, FDG is concentrated within most tumors. FDG is therefore a less specific agent for neuroblastoma than MIBG and other radiopharmaceuticals that use the type 1 catecholamine reuptake system.

Acquisition Protocol

Administered doses of FDG are generally determined using weight (0.14 to 0.15 mCi/kg or 5.18 to 5.55 mBq/kg), with a maximum dosage of 12 mCi (444 mBq). Patients undergo standard preparation, including a 4-hour or overnight fast and avoidance of intravenous glucose. Imaging is performed approximately 1 hour after radiopharmaceutical injection. In contrast to MIBG, FDG allows injection and imaging on the same day, which is often more convenient for patients and their families.

FLUORODEOXYGLUCOSE VERSUS METAIODOBENZYLGUANIDINE

Shulkin and colleagues[36] initially compared FDG PET with MIBG scintigraphy in 1996. They studied 17 patients (20 scans) with neuroblastoma. In 16 of 17 neuroblastoma patients, FDG uptake in tumor was readily identified. FDG compared favorably with MIBG in patients studied before therapy. In seven patients studied before therapy, FDG allowed ready visualization of the primary tumor with uptake that was usually intense (mean SUV 2.8 ± 0.7). Depiction of the primary tumor was better with FDG in two patients, better with MIBG in three patients, and equal with FDG and MIBG in two patients. Six of seven patients had diffuse FDG and MIBG uptake in bone marrow with tumor involvement confirmed by bone marrow biopsy.

On the other hand, FDG PET compared less favorably when patients were studied during or following therapy. FDG uptake in tumor sites was found in 9 of 10 patients studied during or following therapy; however, depiction of residual or recurrent disease was better with MIBG in 8 of 11 scans. FDG was deemed superior to MIBG in only two scans, with FDG and MIBG considered equivalent in one scan. FDG clearly defined tumor sites in a single patient with neuroblastoma that did not concentrate MIBG.

The authors concluded that most neuroblastomas are metabolically active and can be detected using FDG PET. Despite the differences in imaging technology, which favor PET over planar scintigraphy and SPECT because of the considerably higher counts acquired in PET and its intrinsic tomographic basis, they found that FDG is often inferior to MIBG in the evaluation of neuroblastoma. This was largely because of lower tumor to nontumor uptake ratios (especially after therapy) and because of FDG uptake in nontumor sites (such as bone marrow, thymus, and bowel) causing potential false positive or false negative results. They found FDG most beneficial in tumors that failed to or weakly accumulated MIBG.[36]

Kushner and colleagues[37] studied 51 patients (92 scans) with neuroblastoma undergoing staging evaluations to monitor treatment effect and disease status. FDG PET was performed in conjunction with MIBG scans, bone scans, CT (and/or MR imaging), urine catecholamines, and bone marrow examinations. Serial FDG PET scans accurately depicted treatment effects and disease evolution documenting progressive disease, stable disease, and complete and partial remissions. FDG findings correlated well with disease status determined by conventional imaging studies and urinary catecholamine levels. Kushner and colleagues[37] stated that the higher spatial resolution of FDG PET aided in localization of disease sites and diagnosis of small lesions. They also stated that FDG PET might be better for the detection of liver metastases because of the normal intense hepatic uptake of MIBG, which has been shown to complicate detection of hepatic neuroblastoma involvement.[38] Both FDG PET and MIBG depicted widespread bone metastases. They concluded that FDG PET and bone marrow sampling are sufficient to monitor for progressive disease in neuroblastoma patients once the primary tumor has been resected and cranial vault lesions are absent or resolved.

It is important to note that the studies performed by Shulkin and colleagues[36] in 1996 and Kushner and colleagues[37] in 2001 used PET only scanners. Attenuation correction was performed using rotating or fixed rod transmission sources and emission scans were reconstructed using filtered back projection. MIBG was labeled with either ^{131}I or [123]I.

More recently, Sharp and colleagues[39] reviewed 60 patients (113 scans) with neuroblastoma. This study included patients with different stages of neuroblastoma at many points of therapy. There was consistent use of I-123 MIBG planar/SPECT imaging and also extensive use of PET/CT (as opposed to PET only). FDG PET and MIBG planar/SPECT imaging techniques were therefore largely optimized by current standards.

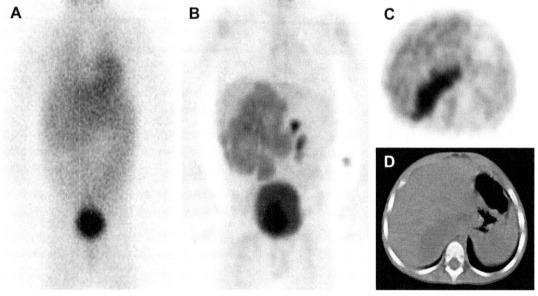

Fig. 1. A 2-year-old boy with stage 2 neuroblastoma imaged 2 months after resection of primary right retroperitoneal tumor without further treatment. (A) Anterior planar MIBG image demonstrates no significant uptake. (B) Anterior MIP FDG PET, (C) axial FDG PET, and (D) localization CT images demonstrate extensive uptake in right retroperitoneal tumor.

In Stage 1 and 2 disease (10 patients/13 scans), FDG was superior in depicting disease sites. FDG depicted more primary tumor and/or local/regional metastases in six patients (nine scans). FDG and ^{123}I-MIBG scans were equivalent in one patient (one scan). FDG and ^{123}I-MIBG scans were negative in three patients (three scans).

In Stage 3 disease (10 patients/15 scans), results were less consistent. MIBG depicted more extensive primary tumor and/or local/regional metastases in four patients (five scans). FDG depicted more extensive primary tumor and/or local/regional metastases in four patients (four scans). MIBG and FDG were equivalent in two patients (two scans). MIBG and FDG scans were negative in three patients (four scans).

In Stage 4 disease (40 patients/85 scans), MIBG was found to be overall superior. MIBG depicted more neuroblastoma sites in 22 patients (44 scans). FDG depicted more neuroblastoma sites in eight patients (11 scans). MIBG and FDG were equivalent in nine patients (10 scans). MIBG and FDG were complementary in two patients (three scans). MIBG and FDG scans were negative in 14 patients (17 scans).

The authors therefore concluded that FDG is superior in depicting Stage 1/2 neuroblastoma, although they state that MIBG may be needed to exclude higher stage disease. They also state that FDG provided important information in tumors that weakly accumulate MIBG and at major decision points during therapy (ie, before stem cell

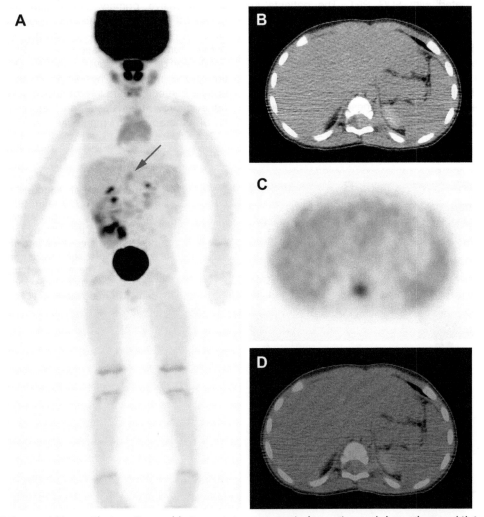

Fig. 2. A 2-year-old boy with stage 3 neuroblastoma status post surgical resection and chemotherapy. (*A*) Anterior MIP FDG PET image demonstrates focal uptake in the upper abdomen (*arrow*), as well as physiologic activity in thymus, bowel, and bladder. (*B*) Localization CT image demonstrates residual hyperdense tumor in the spinal canal with corresponding increased FDG uptake on (*C*) axial FDG and (*D*) axial fusion images.

transplantation or before surgery). FDG also better delineated disease extent in the chest, abdomen, and pelvis. They found MIBG to be overall superior in the evaluation of Stage 4 neuroblastoma, especially during initial chemotherapy. This was primarily attributable to better detection of bone/marrow metastases. They commented on the fact that recent granulocyte colony-stimulating factor (GCSF) therapy can cause diffuse FDG uptake in bone marrow, which can mimic or obscure metastatic disease. However, they warned that generalized statements regarding the use of MIBG and FDG PET in neuroblastoma will often have exceptions that could significantly affect clinical management of individual patients.[39]

Colavolpe and colleagues[40] and McDowell and colleagues[41] recently reported cases of MIBG-negative recurrent neuroblastoma that were well demonstrated with FDG PET. The patients in both reports had MIBG-positive disease at diagnosis that was MIBG-negative at relapse. In the report by Colavolpe and colleagues,[40] relapsed disease was suspected owing to persistent bone pain and elevated urine catecholamines. In the report by McDowell and colleagues,[41] relapsed disease was found by CT. These cases emphasize the importance of FDG imaging when MIBG reveals less disease that suspected by clinical symptoms or conventional imaging modalities, such as CT or MR.

Given these studies, it seems unlikely that FDG PET will fully replace MIBG scintigraphy in the diagnosis and management of patients with neuroblastoma. The decreased specificity of FDG PET relative to MIBG is also a drawback. However, FDG has been shown to be useful in patients with early stage disease and in tumors that weakly accumulate MIBG or do not accumulate MIBG (**Fig. 1**). FDG can also play an important role in recurrent neuroblastoma when MIBG reveals less disease than suspected by clinical evaluation or conventional imaging modalities. The spatial resolution of FDG PET/CT also aids in disease delineation in the chest, abdomen, and pelvis; this is true in both small tumors (**Fig. 2**) and extensive primary tumor and metastatic disease (**Fig. 3**). In patients with neuroblastoma, sites of FDG uptake do not always represent primary tumor or metastatic disease. Physiologic uptake can be seen in bowel, urinary tract, thymus, and bone marrow. Physiologic bone marrow uptake can complicate interpretation when bone/bone marrow metastases are subtle (**Fig. 4**). GCSF therapy can markedly increase bone

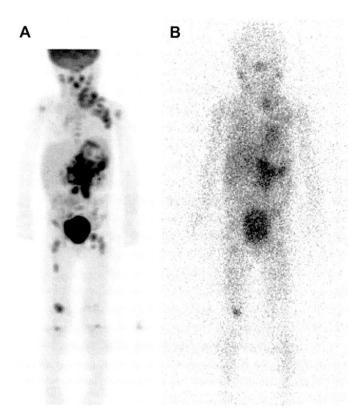

A   B

Fig. 3. A 3-year-old girl with stage 4 neuroblastoma at diagnosis. (A) Anterior MIP FDG PET and (B) anterior planar MIBG images demonstrate uptake within the primary retroperitoneal tumor, metastatic left neck mass, and multiple soft tissue and bone metastases. The extent of tumor and number of metastases are better demonstrated with FDG PET.

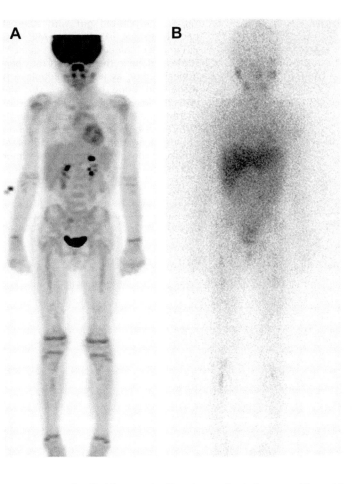

Fig. 4. A 5-year-old boy with stage 4 neuroblastoma after chemotherapy and bone marrow transplantation. (*A*) Anterior MIP FDG PET image demonstrates uptake in bone marrow, which could largely be considered physiologic. (*B*) Anterior planar MIBG image demonstrates uptake in the proximal femurs and tibias, consistent with metastatic disease.

marrow uptake limiting evaluation for metastatic disease (**Fig. 5**). Pathologic uptake in the skin, pleura, and lungs can be seen after radiation therapy. Pathologic uptake is also encountered in areas of inflammation/infection and at sites of prior trauma or surgery.

NOVEL POSITRON-EMITTING TRACERS

Positron-emitting radiopharmaceuticals have potential advantages over conventional agents, such as I-123 MIBG. These include improved resolution of PET when compared with SPECT, accurate quantification of uptake, and short uptake times allowing injection and imaging in a single visit. Potential tracers may be labeled with either C-11 or F-18. However, the short half-life of C-11 requires on-site cyclotron synthesis, which limits the practical use of radiopharmaceuticals with this label. The longer half-life and broader availability of F-18 make use of its radiopharmaceuticals more reasonable. The PET chemistry expertise needed for radiopharmaceutical synthesis and regulatory concerns limit availability of all novel tracers.

Neuroblastoma has been studied with C-11 hydroxyephedrine (HED) and C-11 epinephrine. HED has been shown to be highly concentrated in pheochromocytoma, leading to examination of its uptake in neuroblastoma. Shulkin and colleagues[42] studied seven neuroblastoma patients, each of whom had HED uptake into tumor sites identified by MIBG. Uptake was rapid with 80% of uptake occurring by 2 minutes. In most patients, relatively high retention of HED was also demonstrated. Initial prominence of hepatic and renal activity was seen, with increasing tumor-to-liver ratios noted as hepatic activity declined and tumor activity remained relatively fixed.

C-11 epinephrine is also concentrated by pheochromocytomas[43] and its uptake in neuroblastoma has also been investigated. Shulkin and colleagues[44] studied 20 neuroblastoma patients using C-11 epinephrine PET. PET studies were performed dynamically immediately following injection with distinction of neuroblastoma uptake from background activity by 2 minutes after injection. Retention of C-11 epinephrine in neuroblastoma sites generally increased in intensity as

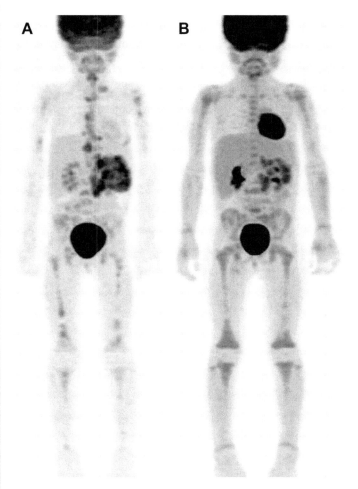

Fig. 5. A 4-year-old girl with stage 4 neuroblastoma. (*A*) Anterior MIP FDG PET image obtained at diagnosis demonstrates uptake in the large left retroperitoneal tumor, as well as multiple soft tissue and bone metastases. (*B*) MIP FDG PET image obtained after chemotherapy and GCSF administration reveals diffuse bone marrow uptake obscuring or mimicking bony metastatic disease. Uptake in the left retroperitoneal tumor and soft tissue metastases has decreased.

background activity declined. However, C-11 epinephrine uptake was seen in only one half to two thirds of neuroblastomas, whereas MIBG uptake was seen in all of the neuroblastomas studied.

Several novel F-18 agents may act as positron-emitting analogs of MIBG with applications for the functional imaging of neuroblastoma. 4-[F-18]-fluoro-3-iodobenzylguanidine (FIBG) has been shown to bind in vitro to human neuroblastoma cells.[45] P-[F-18]-fluorobenzylguanidine (PFBG) has been studied in two dogs with pheochromocytoma.[46] It is hypothesized that these agents could be used in neuroblastoma imaging, although no in vivo human studies have yet been reported.

F-18 dihydroxyphenylalanine (DOPA) uptake can be seen in neuroendocrine tumors that concentrate, decarboxylate, and store amino acids and their biogenic amines. In vitro studies (performed by Shulkin in 2003, currently unpublished), suggest that type 1 catecholamine uptake of F-18 DOPA may also occur. DOPA has been shown to be concentrated in pheochromocytomas.[47]

Tzen and colleagues[48] performed F-18 DOPA PET/CT studies on seven patients imaged 90 minutes after injection with 4 MBq/kg BW of F-18 DOPA. All patients were premedicated with 2 mg/kg BW of oral carbidopa 60 minutes before radiopharmaceutical injection. Three patients with uptake of F-18 DOPA were diagnosed with ganglioneuroma or ganglioneuroblastoma at surgery. One patient with F-18 DOPA uptake was diagnosed with a large neuroblastoma (without DOPA uptake) and a small ganglioneuroma (with DOPA uptake). Four patients with no uptake of F-18 DOPA all had poorly differentiated neuroblastoma cells in their tumors. Tzen and colleagues[48] suggested that F-18 DOPA positivity indicates a well differentiated tumor or tumor component, which may indicate better prognosis, although the clinical significance needs further investigation. This study suggests that F-18 DOPA may demonstrate well differentiated tumors adequately, but may not be useful in the general population of neuroblastoma patients.

F-18 agents can also take advantage of the similarities among the norepinephrine, dopamine, and serotonin transporters. 6-[F-18]-Fluorodopamine (F-18 DA) has been used in pheochromocytoma patients with successful localization of metastatic tumor sites.[49] No F-18 DA studies have yet been reported in neuroblastoma.

F-18 fluorothymidine (FLT) assesses cellular proliferation and is based on a nucleoside that is incorporated into DNA. It has been studied in mice inoculated with human neuroblastoma cells.[50] FLT visualized tumor in 70% of cases, whereas FDG visualized tumor in only 40% of cases. This agent could be especially useful in determining the response of tumors to therapy; however, no correlation between the cell proliferation rate and FLT uptake was detected.

In vitro studies of various tracers, including those based on amino acids and nucleosides, have been performed to assess their potential for neuroblastoma imaging in vivo.[51] Many of these tracers show uptake greater than that of MIBG with the highest uptake seen with the essential amino acids, threonine and methionine. Although promising in vitro, in vivo experiments using animal tumor models or human patients are needed to assess the clinical utility of these agents. Hepatic, renal, pancreatic, or bone marrow activity could potentially be high enough to limit evaluation of tumor relative to background.

SUMMARY

Functional imaging plays an important role in the assessment of neuroblastoma. I-123 MIBG remains the most commonly used agent for neuroblastoma imaging; it is used to define the extent of disease at diagnosis, follow response to treatment, and localize residual and recurrent disease. Use of FDG is increasing and studies continue to clarify its role in the diagnosis and management of neuroblastoma patients. FDG has been shown to be useful in patients with early stage disease and in tumors that weakly accumulate MIBG. FDG should be used when MIBG demonstrates less disease than suspected by clinical symptoms or conventional imaging. The spatial resolution of FDG PET/CT also aids in disease delineation in the chest, abdomen, and pelvis. FDG remains a less specific imaging agent than MIBG with physiologic and non-neoplastic pathologic sites of uptake frequently complicating image interpretation. Several novel positron-emitting radiopharmaceuticals labeled with C-11 or F-18 show potential for neuroblastoma imaging, although further studies are needed and availability is limited.

REFERENCES

1. Shulkin BL. Neuroblastoma. In: Charron M, editor. Pediatric PET imaging. New York: Springer; 2006. p. 243–55.
2. Donnelly LF. Pediatric Imaging: The Fundamentals. Pennsylvania: Saunders; 2009.
3. Jadvar H, Connolly LP, Fahey FH, et al. PET and PET/CT in pediatric oncology. Semin Nucl Med 2007;37(5):316–31.
4. Cohn SL, Pearson AD, London WB, et al. The international neuroblastoma risk group (INRG) classification system: an INRG task force report. J Clin Oncol 2009;27(2):289–97.
5. Shimada H, Chatten J, Newton WA Jr, et al. Histopathologic prognostic factors in neuroblastic tumors: definition of subtypes of ganglioneuroblastoma and an age-linked classification of neuroblastomas. J Natl Cancer Inst 1984;73(2):405–16.
6. Brodeur GM, Pritchard J, Berthold F, et al. Revisions of the international criteria for neuroblastoma diagnosis, staging, and response to treatment. J Clin Oncol 1993;11(8):1466–77.
7. Monclair T, Brodeur GM, Ambros PF, et al. The International Neuroblastoma Risk Group (INRG) staging system: an INRG task force report. J Clin Oncol 2009;27(2):298–303.
8. Brodeur GM, Castleberry RP. Neuroblastoma. In: Pizzo PA, Poplack DG, editors. Principles and practice of pediatric oncology. 3rd edition. Philadelphia: Lippincott-Raven; 1997. p. 761–97.
9. Labreveux de Cervens C, Hartmann O, Bonnin F, et al. What is the prognostic value of osteomedullary uptake on MIBG scan in neuroblastoma patients under one year of age? Med Pediatr Oncol 1994; 22(2):107–14.
10. Sisson JC, Frager MS, Valk TW, et al. Scintigraphic localization of pheochromocytoma. N Engl J Med 1981;305(1):12–7.
11. Treuner J, Feine U, Niethammer D, et al. Scintigraphic imaging of neuroblastoma with [131-I]iodobenzylguanidine. Lancet 1984;1(8372):333–4.
12. Sisson JC, Shulkin BL. Nuclear medicine imaging of pheochromocytoma and neuroblastoma. Q J Nucl Med 1999;43(3):217–23.
13. Englaro EE, Gelfand MJ, Harris RE, et al. I-131 MIBG imaging after bone marrow transplantation for neuroblastoma. Radiology 1992;182(2):515–20.
14. Wieland DM, Wu J, Brown LE, et al. Radiolabeled adrenergi neuron-blocking agents: adrenomedullary imaging with [131I]iodobenzylguanidine. J Nucl Med 1980;21(4):349–53.
15. Paltiel HJ, Gelfand MJ, Elgazzar AH, et al. Neural crest tumors: I-123 MIBG imaging in children. Radiology 1994;190(1):117–21.
16. Ott RJ, Tait D, Flower MA, et al. Treatment planning for 131I-mIBG radiotherapy of neural crest tumours

using 124I-mIBG positron emission tomography. Br J Radiol 1992;65(777):787–91.

17. Moroz MA, Serganova I, Zanzonico P, et al. Imaging hNET reporter gene expression with 124I-MIBG. J Nucl Med 2007;48(5):827–36.

18. Gelfand MJ. I-123-MIBG and I-131-MIBG imaging in children with neuroblastoma [abstract]. J Nucl Med 1996;37:35.

19. Khafagi FA, Shapiro B, Fig LM, et al. Labetalol reduces iodine-131 MIBG uptake by pheochromocytoma and normal tissues. J Nucl Med 1989;30(4):481–9.

20. Gelfand MJ, Elgazzar AH, Kriss VM, et al. Iodine-123-MIBG SPECT versus planar imaging in children with neural crest tumors. J Nucl Med 1994;35(11):1753–7.

21. Vik T, Pfluger T, Kadota R, et al. 123I-MIBG scintigraphy in patients with known or suspected neuroblastoma: results from a prospective multi-center trial. [abstract]. J Nucl Med 2008;49(Suppl 1):238.

22. Serafini A, Heiba SI, Tumeh SS, et al. Influence of SPECT on interpretation of 123I-MIBG scintigraphy in patients with known or suspected pheochromocytoma and neuroblastoma [abstract]. J Nucl Med 2008;49(Suppl 1):239.

23. Bar-Sever Z, Steinmetz A, Ash S, et al. The role of MIBG SPECT/CT in children with neuroblastoma. [abstract]. J Nucl Med 2008;49(Suppl 1):84.

24. Rozovsky K, Koplewitz BZ, Krausz Y, et al. Added value of SPECT/CT for correlation of MIBG scintigraphy and diagnostic CT in neuroblastoma and pheochromocytoma. AJR Am J Roentgenol 2008;190(4):1085–90.

25. Franzius C, Schober O. Assessment of therapy response by FDG PET in pediatric patients. Q J Nucl Med 2003;47(1):41–5.

26. Wegner EA, Barrington SF, Kingston JE, et al. The impact of PET scanning on management of paediatric oncology patients. Eur J Nucl Med Mol Imaging 2005;32(1):23–30.

27. Pacak K, Ilias I, Chen CC, et al. The role of [(18)F]fluorodeoxyglucose positron emission tomography and [(111)In]-diethylenetriaminepentaacetate-D-Phe-pentetreotide scintigraphy in the localization of ectopic adrenocorticotropin-secreting tumors causing Cushing's syndrome. J Clin Endocrinol Metab 2004;89(5):2214–21.

28. Figarola MS, McQuiston SA, Wilson F, et al. Recurrent hepatoblastoma with localization by PET-CT. Pediatr Radiol 2005;35(12):1254–8.

29. Kinoshita H, Shimotake T, Furukawa T, et al. Mucoepidermal carcinoma of the lung detected by positron emission tomography in a 5-year-old girl. J Pediatr Surg 2005;40(4):E1–3.

30. Philip I, Shun A, McCowage G, et al. Positron emission tomography in recurrent hepatoblastoma. Pediatr Surg Int 2005;21(5):341–5.

31. McCarville MB, Christie R, Daw NC, et al. PET/CT in the evaluation of childhood sarcomas. AJR Am J Roentgenol 2005;184(4):1293–304.

32. Sasi OA, Sathiapalan R, Rifai A, et al. Colonic neuroendocrine carcinoma in a child. Pediatr Radiol 2005;35(3):339–43.

33. Buchler T, Cervinek L, Belohlavek O, et al. Langerhans cell histiocytosis with central nervous system involvement: follow-up by FDG-PET during treatment with cladribine. Pediatr Blood Cancer 2005;44(3):286–8.

34. Mackie GC, Shulkin BL, Ribeiro RC, et al. Use of [18F]fluorodeoxyglucose positron emission tomography in evaluating locally recurrent and metastatic adrenocortical carcinoma. J Clin Endocrinol Metab 2006;91(7):2665–71.

35. Mody RJ, Pohlen JA, Malde S, et al. FDG PET for the study of primary hepatic malignancies in children. Pediatr Blood Cancer 2006;47(1):51–5.

36. Shulkin BL, Hutchinson RJ, Castle VP, et al. Neuroblastoma: positron emission tomography with 2-[fluorine-18]-fluoro-2-deoxy-D-glucose compared with metaiodobenzylguanidine scintigraphy. Radiology 1996;199(3):743–50.

37. Kushner BH, Yeung HW, Larson SM, et al. Extending positron emission tomography scan utility to high-risk neuroblastoma: fluorine-18 fluorodeoxyglucose positron emission tomography as sole imaging modality in follow-up of patients. J Clin Oncol 2001;19(14):3397–405.

38. Dessner DA, DiPietro MA, Shulkin BL. MIBG detection of hepatic neuroblastoma: correlation with CT, US and surgical findings. Pediatr Radiol 1993;23(4):276–80.

39. Sharp SE, Shulkin BL, Furman WL, et al. I-123-MIBG scintigraphy and {F-18}FDG PET in neuroblastoma. [abstract]. J Nucl Med 2008;49(Suppl 1):84.

40. Colavolpe C, Guedj E, Cammilleri S, et al. Utility of FDG-PET/CT in the follow-up of neuroblastoma which became MIBG-negative. Pediatr Blood Cancer 2008;51(6):828–31.

41. McDowell HM, Losty P, Barnes N, et al. Utility of FDG-PET/CT in the follow-up of neuroblastoma which became MIBG-negative [letter]. Pediatr Blood Cancer 2009;52(4):552.

42. Shulkin BL, Wieland DM, Baro ME, et al. PET hydroxyephedrine imaging of neuroblastoma. J Nucl Med 1996;37(1):16–21.

43. Shulkin BL, Wieland DM, Sisson JC. PET studies of pheochromocytoma with C-11 epinephrine. Radiology 1994;193:273.

44. Shulkin BL, Wieland DM, Castle VP, et al. Carbon-11 epinephrine PET imaging of neuroblastoma. J Nucl Med 1999;40(5):129.

45. Vaidyanathan G, Affleck DJ, Zalutsky MR. (4-[18F]fluoro-3-iodobenzyl)guanidine, a potential MIBG analogue for positron emission tomography. J Med Chem 1994;37(21):3655–62.

46. Berry CR, DeGrado TR, Nutter F, et al. Imaging of pheochromocytoma in 2 dogs using p-[18F] fluorobenzylguanidine. Vet Radiol Ultrasound 2002;43(2):183–6.

47. Hoegerle S, Nitzsche E, Altehoefer C, et al. Pheochromocytomas: detection with 18F DOPA whole body PET—initial results. Radiology 2002;222(2):507–12.

48. Tzen K, Wang L, Lu M. Characterization of neuroblastic tumors using F-18 DOPA, PET. [abstract]. J Nucl Med 2007;48(Suppl 2):117.

49. Ilias I, Yu J, Carrasquillo JA, et al. Superiority of 6-[18F]-fluorodopamine positron emission tomography versus [131I]-metaiodobenzylguanidine scintigraphy in the localization of metastatic pheochromocytoma. J Clin Endocrinol Metab 2003; 88(9):4083–7.

50. Krieger-Hinck N, Gustke H, Valentiner U, et al. Visualisation of neuroblastoma growth in a Scid mouse model using [18F]FDG and [18F]FLT-PET. Anticancer Res 2006;26(5A):3467–72.

51. Goodwill T, Shulkin BL, Schumacher K, et al. Metabolic characterization of neuroblastoma [abstract]. J Nucl Med 2002;43(5):36.

PET and PET/CT in Pediatric Sarcomas

M. Beth McCarville, MD

KEYWORDS

- Pediatric • Sarcomas • Positron emission tomography
- Computed tomography • Bone scan
- Magnetic resonance imaging

Childhood cancers, in general, are relatively rare. Among children, the hematologic malignancies (leukemias and lymphomas) and brain tumors comprise the majority of malignancies and account for about half of all cancer diagnoses. Sarcomas, malignancies that arise from mesenchymal cells that normally mature into skeletal muscle, smooth muscle, fat, fibrous tissue, bone, or cartilage, represent less than 6% of all childhood cancers.[1] In children, the most common sarcomas are the primary bone tumors—osteosarcoma and Ewing sarcoma—and rhabdomyosarcoma, a tumor that may arise from any tissue except bone.[2–4] In the United States, the annual incidence of osteosarcoma is 4.8 per million, the annual incidence of Ewing sarcoma is 2.9 per million, and the annual incidence of rhabdomyosarcoma is 4.3 per million.[1] The treatment and survival of these children hinges on accurate pathologic grading of the primary tumor and identification of sites of metastatic disease. Approximately 25% to 35% of children and adolescents who have sarcomas experience tumor recurrence after treatment. Thus, patients are followed clinically and radiographically for 3 to 5 years after completion of therapy, and diagnostic imaging plays a pivotal role in their management.[2–4]

MR imaging of primary childhood bone and soft tissue sarcomas is indispensable for determining tumor site, size, margins, and involvement of the neurovascular bundle, features that determine tumor resectability and influence therapeutic options and prognosis. Childhood sarcomas spread via lymphatic and hematogenous routes, and the presence of metastatic disease is an important prognostic variable that significantly affects management. Consequently, an appropriate metastatic investigation must precede the definitive approach to the primary tumor. The lung is the first site of metastatic disease in children who have sarcomas, and lung metastasis is seen in 20% to 25% of patients at diagnosis. Local-regional nodal spread is rare in osteosarcoma and Ewing sarcoma but occurs in up to 20% of children who have rhabdomyosarcoma. Bone marrow metastases occur in 20% to 30% of patients who have rhabdomyosarcoma and in less than 10% of patients who have Ewing sarcoma. Bone metastases occur in 10% of patients who have rhabdomyosarcoma and patients who have osteosarcoma.[2–4] Therefore, the conventional imaging evaluation also includes MR imaging or CT of local-regional nodal beds, CT of the chest to assess for pulmonary metastases, and ^{99m}technetium methyl diphosphonate (^{99m}Tc MDP) nuclear scintigraphy to detect bone metastases.

Most children who have cancer, including children who have sarcomas, are treated on clinical trials designed to evaluate the toxicity or effectiveness of innovative cancer therapies. The Response Evaluation Criteria in Solid Tumors (RECIST) were introduced in 2000 as an alternative to the World Health Organization (WHO) criteria to provide a standard, reproducible, and objective method of assessing the efficacy of experimental solid tumor therapies.[5] These criteria incorporate important advances in imaging technology and simplify the WHO methodology but rely on changes in axial, unidimensional tumor measurements to define tumor response or progression. A limitation of the RECIST criteria is that solid malignancies, such as bone sarcomas and cystic soft tissue sarcomas, may respond well to

Department of Radiological Sciences, St. Jude Children's Research Hospital, 262 Danny Thomas Place, Memphis, TN 38105, USA

E-mail address: beth.mccarville@stjude.org

PET Clin 3 (2009) 563–575

doi:10.1016/j.cpet.2009.04.007

chemotherapy without changing substantially in size. Also, sarcomas do not shrink or grow in a uniform manner, and unidimensional measurements restricted to the axial plane may not reflect tumor response or progression accurately. Tumors that respond poorly to therapy may be followed for months before a significant increase in a unidimensional measurement occurs. Such patients are exposed to the toxicity of ineffective chemotherapy and probably have a diminished likelihood of survival.[6] Furthermore, anatomic changes in tumors are inadequate for evaluating newer therapies, such as cytostatic anti-angiogenic therapies, that were introduced after development of the RECIST criteria and that are not intended to cause tumor shrinkage.

The ideal evaluation of response would use reliable, reproducible, noninvasive techniques to identify nonresponding tumors early in the course of therapy to reduce unnecessary toxicity and to tailor management to optimize patient survival. ^{18}F-labeled fluorodeoxyglucose-PET (FDG-PET) capitalizes on the fact that tumors are highly metabolically active and accumulate more glucose (and FDG) than normal tissue.[7,8] Following therapy, a decrease in glucose uptake by tumors has been shown to correlate with a reduction in viable tumor cells.[9–11] Furthermore, FDG-PET can assess tumor glucose metabolism with high reproducibility.[12] Therefore, for some malignancies, FDG-PET is more sensitive to tumor response or progression than conventional, anatomic imaging modalities.

Recently, a group of expert oncologists, radiologists, and nuclear physicians developed recommendations on the use of FDG-PET in the management of patients who have cancer.[13] The panel's recommendations were based on the existing literature and were approved by the Board of Directors of the Society of Nuclear Medicine. They found sufficient evidence to support the use of FDG-PET in a wide variety of malignancies, but they concluded that, because of the rarity of sarcomas, there is a lack of evidence to support the use of FDG-PET in the management of these tumors. Nonetheless, the panel projected that further research is likely to raise confidence about the effectiveness of FDG-PET in managing patients who have sarcoma. Clearly, investigations of the role of this powerful functional imaging modality in managing these rare malignancies should continue. This article reviews the current literature regarding FDG-PET imaging in the management of pediatric sarcomas and presents important pitfalls in PET/CT imaging of these patients that the author, her colleagues, and others have encountered.

IDENTIFYING AN UNKNOWN PRIMARY SITE

Although most sarcomas are apparent on physical examination, approximately 4% of patients who have rhabdomyosarcoma present with metastatic disease and an unknown primary site.[14] Because surgical resection of the primary tumor is crucial in the management of these patients, the imaging evaluation is focused on identifying the primary site and is guided by clinical suspicion. Traditionally such evaluations could require multiple imaging modalities suitable for assessing various anatomic sites. PET and PET/CT allow evaluation of the entire patient in one setting. In adults, PET alone can reveal the location of primary tumors in 21% to 30% of patients who have occult head and neck or breast cancers but also has a false-positive rate of approximately 20%.[15] PET/CT, with the added benefit of anatomic mapping, may reduce this false-positive rate because it allows sites of physiologically increased FDG activity (eg, supraclavicular brown fat) to be localized accurately and distinguished from tumor-based activity. The Society of Nuclear Medicine currently supports the use of PET and PET/CT for the evaluation of adults who have unknown primary malignancies.[13] Although there is little literature regarding the value of PET in assessing children who have unknown primary sites, the author and others have used PET and PET/CT to identify unknown primary sites in children who had widely metastatic rhabdomyosarcoma (**Fig. 1**).[16,17]

DETECTING PULMONARY DISEASE

Patients who have osteosarcoma and pulmonary metastases have little chance for cure unless all metastases are surgically resected.[2] Patients who have Ewing sarcoma and pulmonary metastases may have improved survival if treated with whole-lung irradiation.[3] Therefore, identification of pulmonary disease is crucial to the management and survival of these children. Although chest CT is the reference standard for detecting pulmonary nodules, the author and colleagues[16] found that three experienced pediatric radiologists had limited ability to classify nodules correctly as benign or malignant in 41 children who had solid malignancies and who underwent pulmonary nodule biopsy (a 57%–67% rate of correct classification). They also found a fairly high rate of benign nodule histology in this group of patients: 42% (17/41) had only benign nodules, and 10% (4/41) had both benign and malignant nodules resected. Furthermore, there was only moderate to slight inter-reviewer agreement among the

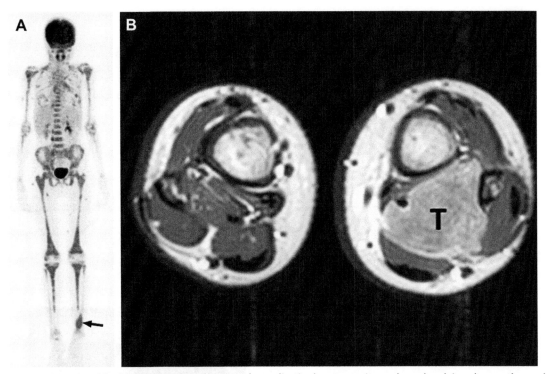

Fig. 1. An 11-year-old girl presented with cervical, mediastinal, retroperitoneal, and pelvic adenopathy and anemia. Burkitt lymphoma was suspected, but bone marrow biopsy revealed metastatic alveolar rhabdomyosarcoma. No primary site was identified on physical examination. PET/CT was performed. (*A*) This maximum intensity projection PET image showed diffuse marrow abnormality and focal abnormality in the left calf (*arrow*). (*B*) MR imaging confirmed that this finding was the primary tumor (T). (*From* McCarville MB, Christie R, Daw NC, et al. PET/CT in the evaluation of childhood sarcomas. AJR Am J Roentgenol 2005;184:1294; with permission.)

radiologists when classifying nodules as benign or malignant based on CT features. Clearly, to reduce undue morbidity associated with thoracotomy when only benign disease is present, the ability to distinguish benign from malignant pulmonary nodules in this patient population must be improved. Franzius and colleagues[18] assessed the value of FDG-PET alone to detect pulmonary metastases in patients who have osteosarcoma or Ewing sarcoma by comparing it with CT, clinical follow-up, and histologic inspection of resected nodules. They found that in 30 FDG-PET scans performed at diagnosis or recurrence (before initiation of therapy) PET had a sensitivity of 14%, a specificity of 91%, and an accuracy of 73%. They also found that the ability to detect pulmonary nodules with FDG-PET improved with increasing nodule size; 12 of 16 nodules 10 mm in diameter or larger were identified, but none smaller than 5 mm was detected (**Fig. 2**). Their results agree with a recent report by Völker and colleagues[19] investigating the value of FDG-PET alone for staging 46 children who had Ewing sarcoma (n = 23), osteosarcoma (n = 11), or rhabdomyosarcoma (n = 12). These investigators

found that 21 of 28 lung metastases detected by CT were missed by FDG-PET, resulting in a sensitivity of 25%. In their study, PET-positive nodules were 8 mm in diameter or larger, and PET-negative nodules were smaller than 7 mm. Gerth and colleagues[20] showed that the fusion modality FDG-PET/CT was superior to PET alone in detecting pulmonary nodules in 53 patients who had Ewing sarcoma because of improved lesion detection by CT. Because PET/CT generally is performed using a low milliampere/second technique for CT scanning, however, image quality may not be sufficient to detect very small pulmonary nodules. Current-generation multislice helical scanners, coupled with the improved accuracy of interpretation when CT imaging is reviewed at picture archiving and communication systems using window and level adjustment and magnification tools allow the detection of increasingly smaller pulmonary nodules. The author and colleagues[16] showed that small pulmonary nodules (< 5 mm) are as likely to be malignant as larger nodules in children who have solid malignancies. Given the need to treat pulmonary metastatic disease aggressively in the pediatric patient who has

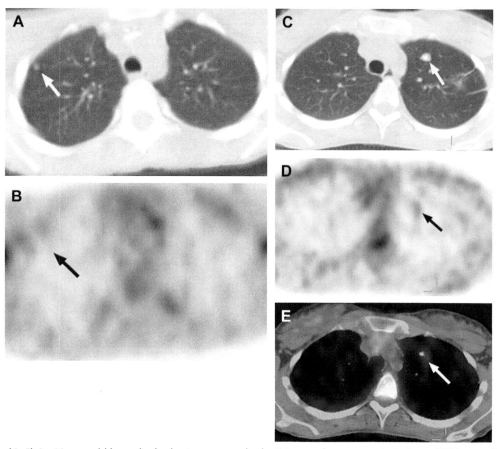

Fig. 2. (*A, B*) An 11-year-old boy who had osteosarcoma had a 0.5-cm pulmonary metastasis on CT (*A, arrow*) that was not evident on the PET image (*B*). (*C–E*) By contrast, a 21-year-old man who had osteosarcoma had a 1.0-cm pulmonary metastasis (*C, arrow*) showing moderate FDG avidity on (*D*) PET and (*E*) fused PET/CT images.

sarcoma, diagnostic chest CT remains an essential part of the metastatic work-up. PET/CT is preferred to PET alone as a potential adjunct to distinguish benign from malignant nodules but should be used with caution and an awareness of the inherent limitations of spatial resolution of both the PET and the CT components of the examination.[18,21] In addition to these limitations, the author and colleagues have found that benign processes, such as active infection, can result in substantial FDG uptake within pulmonary nodules, similar to that seen in metastatic deposits (**Fig. 3**). Further investigation is needed to define better the role of PET imaging in assessing pulmonary nodules in children who have sarcomas.

DETECTING BONE AND BONE MARROW DISEASE

The prognosis of children who have bone or bone marrow metastases from sarcomas is dismal. Approximately 10% of patients who have osteosarcoma develop bone metastases with or without concurrent pulmonary metastases.[2] These patients require surgical resection of all sites of metastases for any chance of cure. Up to 25% of patients who have Ewing sarcoma or rhabdomyosarcoma develop bone or bone marrow metastases. Because Ewing sarcoma is radiosensitive, targeted radiation can be beneficial when there are only few and well circumscribed bone or bone marrow metastases. When more than 50% of the marrow volume is involved, however, irradiation can result in significant myelosuppression and can compound the toxicity of chemotherapy.[3] The prognosis of patients who have rhabdomyosarcoma and bone or bone marrow metastases is not improved by current surgical metastectomy or targeted radiotherapy.[4]

Metastases from osteosarcoma, whether in bone or soft tissue, often contain calcification or ossification. Such metastases therefore are sensitive to detection by the bone-seeking radioisotope, ^{99m}Tc MDP. Franzius and colleagues[22] directly compared FDG-PET with ^{99m}Tc MDP

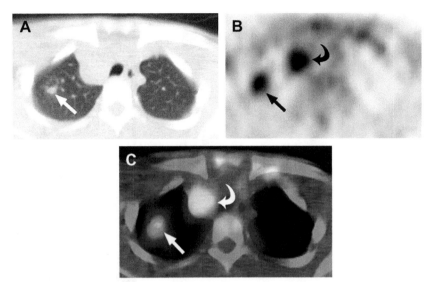

Fig. 3. A 14-year-old boy suspected of having lymphoma underwent PET/CT. (*A*) CT shows an ill-defined, 1.8-cm pulmonary nodule (*arrow*) that was intensely FDG avid on (*B*) PET (*straight arrow*) and (*C*) PET/CT (*straight arrow*). Curved arrows indicate FDG-avid mediastinal adenopathy. Biopsy showed necrotizing granulomatous disease.

bone scintigraphy for the detection of osseous metastases from primary bone tumors, including 32 patients who had osteosarcoma. These investigators found that in two patients who had osteosarcoma with five bone metastases, all foci were evident on ^{99m}Tc MDP bone scan, but none were demonstrated by FDG-PET. Their results were inconclusive, however, because of the small sample size. In the aforementioned study by Völker and colleagues[19] of 12 patients who had osteosarcoma, including 4 who had 31 bone metastases at the time of diagnosis, FDG-PET had a sensitivity of 90%, compared with 81% for ^{99m}Tc MDP scintigraphy; however, the difference was not statistically significant.

FDG-PET is more convincingly superior to ^{99m}Tc MDP scintigraphy in detecting osseous metastases in patients who have Ewing sarcoma. In their study, Franzius and colleagues[22] found that, on 66 paired FDG-PET and ^{99m}Tc MDP bone scans performed to detect osseous metastases before or after initiation of therapy for Ewing sarcoma, FDG-PET had a sensitivity of 100% (19/19), specificity of 96% (45/47), and accuracy of 97% (64/66), compared with 68% (13/19), 87% (41/47), and 82% (54/66), respectively, for ^{99m}Tc MDP scintigraphy. Völker and colleagues[19] substantiated these findings in their study that included 17 patients who had Ewing sarcoma, 6 of whom had 49 osseous metastases. These investigators found that FDG-PET had a sensitivity of 88%, compared with 37% for ^{99m}Tc bone scan (*P* < .01). In their practice, the author and colleagues[16] have found FDG-PET/CT to be more sensitive than ^{99m}Tc bone scan in

detecting osseous metastases in several children who had rhabdomyosarcoma, as well as in Ewing sarcoma (**Fig. 4**). The superiority of FDG-PET to ^{99m}Tc MDP scintigraphy in detecting osseous metastatic disease in patients who have Ewing sarcoma or rhabdomyosarcoma probably is multifactorial. Osseous metastases from Ewing sarcoma and rhabdomyosarcoma frequently arise in and infiltrate the marrow space; for this reason bone marrow aspiration and biopsy are integral in the staging evaluation of patients who have Ewing sarcoma. It is postulated that FDG-PET can depict the increased glucose metabolism of marrow metastases before reactive osteoblastic activity occurs. Detection of bone metastases by ^{99m}Tc bone scintigraphy, on the other hand, depends on the presence of ossification within the metastatic deposit, the degree of associated destruction of normal bone cortex, and the intensity of osteoblastic activity; all of which are greater in bone metastases from osteosarcoma than in those from Ewing sarcoma or rhabdomyosarcoma. Possible cellular differences among these sarcomas in glucose uptake and metabolism also might account for the differences seen on FDG-PET imaging.[22]

Because of the potential risk of ionizing radiation inherent in nuclear imaging, particularly for children, whole-body MR imaging has been investigated as an alternative method of detecting metastatic neoplasia.[23–26] On non–contrast-enhanced MR imaging, bone marrow disease appears as foci exhibiting prolonged T1 and T2 relaxation times, so that metastatic deposits are

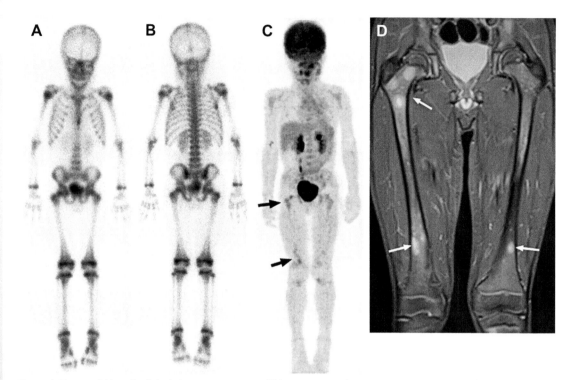

Fig. 4. A 5-year-old boy had rhabdomyosarcoma and biopsy-proven bone marrow metastasis. The patient underwent baseline ^{99m}Tc bone scan and PET/CT. (*A*) Anterior and (*B*) posterior bone scan images were interpreted as normal. (*C*) This maximum intensity projection PET image shows multiple osseous foci of abnormal FDG avidity (*arrows*). (*D*) Several foci in the femora (*arrows*) were confirmed by short tau inversion recovery MR imaging to be metastatic foci.

dark on T1-weighted (T1W) images and bright on T2-weighted (T2W) images. In adults, whole-body MR imaging and FDG-PET have been reported to be highly sensitive in detecting bone metastases and are superior to ^{99m}Tc scintigraphy.[27–30] Children, however, have varying amounts of cellular, hematopoietic bone marrow that may mask metastatic deposits on MR imaging. Daldrup-Link and colleagues[23] compared T1W whole-body MR imaging with the FDG-PET and ^{99m}Tc bone scans of 39 children, aged 2 to 19 years (mean 12.9 years), who had tumors that potentially metastasize to bone. The study included 20 patients who had Ewing sarcoma, 3 who had osteosarcoma, and 3 who had rhabdomyosarcoma. The investigators found that, in 21 patients who had 51 focal bone metastases (proven by biopsy or follow-up), whole-body MR imaging had a sensitivity of 82%, significantly higher than the 71% sensitivity of bone scan ($P < .05$) but significantly lower than the 90% sensitivity of FDG-PET ($P < .05$). Most lesions detected by FDG-PET but missed by whole-body MR imaging, occurred in small or flat bones such as the ribs (n = 3), the skull (n = 2), the distal radius (n = 1), or the carpal bone (n = 1). A potential

limitation of their study was the lack of T2W, short tau inversion recovery MR imaging which, in a small study by Mazumdar and colleagues[24,31] that included two 2 children who had 24 skeletal metastases, was superior to T1W MR imaging in detecting bone lesions. MR imaging techniques, especially those that use rapid imaging sequences to reduce the need for sedation, show promise as a method of detecting skeletal metastases in children and may compare favorably with FDG-PET. Large, comparative, prospective clinical trials are needed to draw meaningful conclusions, however.

In assessing children who have tumors that metastasize to bone, it is important to consider benign processes that can mimic metastatic disease on PET imaging. Akoi and colleagues[32] investigated the value of PET in distinguishing benign (n = 33) from malignant (n = 19) bone tumors in 52 children and adults. These investigators measured the mean standardized uptake value (SUV) within a 1-cm region of interest (ROI) drawn in the area of tumor with maximum FDG accumulation. They found no significant difference between osteosarcomas and giant cell tumors ($P = .171$), between osteosarcomas and fibrous dysplasia ($P = .127$), or between fibrous dysplasia and chondrosarcomas ($P = .667$). Furthermore, they found no statistically significant SUV threshold that reliably distinguished benign from malignant bone lesions. The author and colleagues[16] reviewed imaging of 14 children who had underlying cancers (n = 13) or aggressive fibromatosis (n = 1) who had fibrocortical defects, nonossifying fibromas, or cortical desmoids that were discovered as foci of FDG avidity on PET-CT performed for routine disease evaluation. In some cases, the intense FDG avidity of lesions mimicked the appearance of bony metastatic disease (**Fig. 5**). These relatively common, benign lesions often are discovered incidentally on radiographs of children and young adults. They typically regress spontaneously over time and rarely are seen after the second decade of life. In this study five patients had ^{99m}Tc bone scans performed within 1 month of PET-CT; four showed no abnormal ^{99m}Tc MDP uptake at the site of the lesion, and one showed minimally increased tracer uptake. Therefore, FDG-PET may be more sensitive than ^{99m}Tc MDP scintigraphy in detecting these lesions. Because these lesions have characteristic radiographic features that are well described in the literature, the information gained from correlative CT or plain radiographic imaging

is invaluable in determining whether further imaging or biopsy is necessary.

DETECTING NODAL METASTASES

Although local-regional lymph node metastasis is uncommon in osteosarcoma and Ewing sarcoma, up to 20% of all children who have rhabdomyosarcoma present with nodal disease.[2–4] Importantly, regional nodal spread occurs in approximately half of children who have extremity rhabdomyosarcoma and in older boys ($\geq$ 10 years) who have paratesticular rhabdomyosarcoma. It is more likely to occur with the alveolar rhabdomyosarcoma subtype. In patients who have rhabdomyosarcoma, any palpable or radiographically enlarged lymph node (> 1 cm in largest cross-sectional diameter) at any site requires surgical resection and pathologic inspection. All patients who have extremity rhabdomyosarcoma tumors require aggressive regional lymph node sampling, and boys 10 years of age or older who have paratesticular rhabdomyosarcoma should undergo ipsilateral retroperitoneal lymph node dissection. When lymph node metastasis is present in these children, chances of survival can be improved by intensification of chemotherapy and application

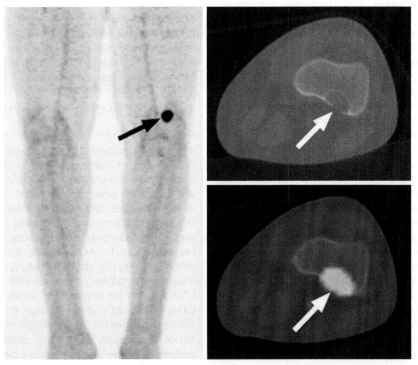

Fig. 5. A 19-year-old man who had metastatic paraganglioma underwent PET/CT. (*Left*) The maximum intensity projection PET image shows a focus of intense activity above the left knee (*arrow*). (*Right*) This focus of activity corresponds to a benign fibrocortical defect (*arrows*) on CT (*upper image*) and PET/CT fusion (*lower image*).

of radiation therapy to the affected region.[4] Therefore, identifying sites of lymph node involvement in children who have rhabdomyosarcoma is crucial to patient management and outcome.

Klem and colleagues[33] investigated the value of FDG-PET in detecting metastases during the baseline staging of 24 patients who had rhabdomyosarcoma (median age, 13 years) by comparing it with CT, MR imaging, clinical assessment, and histology of resected lesions. They measured the SUV of suspicious foci and considered it abnormal when it was greater than background tissue and not caused by a normal physiologic process. Six patients had biopsy-proven lymph node metastases. All six had increased SUVs in the involved nodal sites. The nodes were seen on conventional imaging, but the authors did not provide size measurements or specify whether the nodes were considered pathologically enlarged. An additional patient in their study, who had a lower extremity tumor, had a baseline PET that was "suspicious" for inguinal lymph node involvement. Because a CT of the inguinal area was unrevealing, chemotherapy was initiated after resection of the primary tumor without inguinal node sampling. The patient subsequently developed progression of tumor in the involved inguinal node that became evident on physical examination, FDG-PET, and MR imaging and was confirmed by biopsy. The authors concluded that had the suspicious inguinal nodes been confirmed by biopsy at diagnosis, the patient might have benefited from more aggressive therapy.

In the study by Völker and colleagues,[19] 20 presumed lymphatic metastases were identified in 46 children who had bone and soft tissue sarcomas. These metastases occurred in eight patients: one had osteosarcoma, one had Ewing sarcoma, and six had rhabdomyosarcoma. Fourteen of the 20 nodal metastases occurred in patients who had rhabdomyosarcoma. A lesion-based analysis showed that FDG-PET was more sensitive (95%, 19/20) than CT (25%, 5/20) in detecting these nodes. Among four patients who had extremity rhabdomyosarcoma who underwent regional lymph node sampling, the conventional imaging, PET imaging, and biopsy were concordantly negative in one patient. In one patient the sampled lymph node was biopsy positive, was falsely negative by conventional imaging, and was truly positive by PET. In the two remaining patients, conventional imaging, PET and histology were concordantly positive. Limitations of their study were that no size criteria were provided for defining abnormal nodes by conventional imaging and many (16/20) of the presumed sites of nodal metastases were not confirmed pathologically.

In a small case series by Ben Arush and colleagues,[34] three children who had alveolar rhabdomyosarcoma underwent PET/CT and conventional imaging for baseline staging. Two patients had moderately FDG-avid regional lymph nodes that were biopsied. In one, the node was positive for tumor; in the other, the node showed no evidence of malignancy. The third patient had mild FDG avidity within a regional node that was not resected. High-risk therapy was initiated. On scheduled follow-up the patient presented with palpable adenopathy in the area of the previously seen, mildly FDG-avid node. Lymph node biopsy revealed recurrent alveolar rhabdomyosarcoma.

Consistent with these reports, the author and colleagues have found that, in patients who have extremity sarcomas, benign processes such as reactive hyperplasia, rather than metastatic disease, can cause regional nodes to be enlarged (> 1 cm in largest cross-sectional diameter) and FDG avid on PET imaging (**Fig. 6**). The existing evidence suggests that FDG-PET may identify sites of nodal disease overlooked by conventional imaging modalities, but care should be used in interpreting the PET findings associated with lymph nodes. In children who have sarcomas, metastatic lymph nodes may demonstrate only mild FDG avidity, whereas nonmetastatic nodes may show intense avidity. When there are discordant findings between imaging modalities or between imaging and clinical findings, and when the presence of nodal disease will affect patient management and outcome, biopsy of suspicious lymph nodes should be considered to confirm the presence or absence of metastatic disease.

ASSESSING TUMOR RESPONSE TO THERAPY

Patients who have nonmetastatic osteosarcoma and Ewing sarcoma are treated with neoadjuvant therapy before surgical resection of the primary tumor and adjuvant therapy. Chances of survival are improved when the resected tumor is 90% or more necrotic and resection margins are negative for residual tumor.[2,3] Because osteosarcoma and Ewing sarcoma arise in bone, tumors may respond well to neoadjuvant therapy without much change in size. Therefore, conventional imaging modalities, such as MR imaging and CT, that rely on anatomic changes have limited value in assessing the response of these tumors. Factors that predict the histologic response of the tumor to neoadjuvant therapy could help predict patient outcome and distinguish between candidates for limb-sparing surgery versus amputation or early resection, thereby allowing tailored clinical management.[35] In these malignancies,

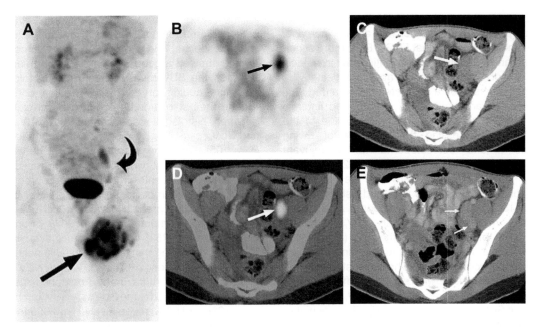

Fig. 6. A 20-year-old woman had malignant peripheral nerve sheath tumor. (*A*) The maximum intensity projection PET image shows the primary left thigh tumor (straight *arrow*) and several foci of increased FDG activity in the left pelvis (*curved arrow*). (*B–D*) PET/CT images localized the activity to enlarged left iliac nodes (*arrow*). (*E*) Contrast-enhanced, diagnostic-quality CT better demonstrates enlarged nodes (*arrows*) that were proven by biopsy to be reactive hyperplasia. (*From* McCarville MB, Christie R, Daw NC, et al. PET/CT in the evaluation of childhood sarcomas. AJR Am J Roentgenol 2005;184:1296; with permission.)

a reliable, noninvasive method, such as FDG-PET, for assessing tumor metabolism and viability would permit the oncologist and surgeon to individualize management of tumors that are aggressive, respond poorly, or arise in surgically challenging sites.

The FDG-PET SUV offers a semiquantitative measure of tumor metabolic activity that shows potential as a method of assessing tumor response to therapy. In general, the SUV is obtained from a single static image of an ROI centered on the tumor. The measured SUV is corrected for the injected radioactivity per kilogram body weight. Two types of SUV may be obtained that represent different biologic information. The first type, the average tumor SUV, is the mean of all pixel-related SUVs within the ROI and is a statistical measure of tumor metabolism in general. The second type, the maximum SUV, is the highest single SUV obtained within an ROI.[36]

Osteogenic sarcoma and Ewing sarcoma are metabolically heterogeneous tumors. Because tumor histologic grade and patient outcome are determined by the percent of viable tumor after preoperative radiotherapy and chemotherapy, the maximum tumor SUV (SUV_{max}) is thought to provide the most accurate assessment of tumor grade. In a study of 29 patients who had

osteosarcoma, Franzius and colleagues[37] showed that, when measured before administration of chemotherapy, a tumor-to-nontumor SUV_{max} ratio (T/NT SUV_{max}) that was at the median for the cohort (12.6) or higher significantly correlated with poorer overall survival ($P < .05$) and event-free survival ($P < .005$). Their findings suggest that the T/NT SUV_{max} at diagnosis reflects tumor aggressiveness, and patients who have more aggressive tumors (higher T/NT SUV_{max}) are more likely than others to fail therapy. In another small study by these investigators, 17 patients who had primary bone tumors (6 who had Ewing sarcoma and 11 who had osteosarcoma) had ^{99m}Tc MDP bone scans and FDG-PET at diagnosis and at completion of neoadjuvant therapy. All patients (n = 15) who had a good histologic response (tumor $\geq$ 90% necrotic) had at least a 30% reduction in the average PT/NT ratio, on PET imaging, from baseline to post therapy time points.[9] Of the two patients who had a poor histologic response (< 90% necrotic tumor), the PT/NT ratio increased in one patient and decreased by only 11% in the other. In contrast, eight patients who had a good histologic response had either increasing PT/NT by ^{99m}Tc MDP bone scan (n = 3) or a reduction of less than 30% (n = 5). Of the two patients who had a poor response, one had a 19% decrease in T/NT on ^{99m}Tc MDP scintigraphy, and the other had an 8% increase. The findings suggest that FDG-PET is more sensitive than ^{99m}Tc MDP bone scintigraphy in detecting tumor response to therapy in patients who have Ewing sarcoma and osteosarcoma (**Fig. 7**).

Hawkins and colleagues[10,11] reported findings from two studies investigating the value of the SUV$_{max}$ in assessing the response of Ewing sarcoma and osteosarcoma to neoadjuvant therapy. The first study, published in 2002, examined the correlation between the histologic response of 18 patients who had osteosarcoma and 13 who had Ewing sarcoma and tumor SUV$_{max}$ measured at diagnosis (SUV$_{max1}$) and at the end of neoadjuvant therapy (SUV$_{max2}$).[10] They found no difference in baseline SUV$_{max1}$ values between patients who had osteosarcoma and those who had Ewing sarcoma. After neoadjuvant therapy, however, the mean SUV$_{max2}$ and the ratio of SUV$_{max2}$/SUV$_{max1}$ were significantly higher in patients who had osteosarcoma than in patients who had Ewing sarcoma ($P = .01$ and $P = .048$, respectively). The mean percentage of necrosis was significantly lower in resected osteosarcoma tumors than in Ewing sarcoma tumors ($P < .001$).

All the Ewing sarcoma tumors but only 28% of osteosarcoma tumors showed a favorable histologic response. Because all Ewing sarcoma tumors showed a good response, the correlation between the SUV measurements and histologic response could not be made for this cohort. Among the osteosarcoma cohort, the correlation between histologic response and the SUV$_{max2}$ and SUV$_{max2}$/SUV$_{max1}$ ratio were significant (both $P = .05$). There was no correlation between SUV$_{max1}$ and tumor necrosis within the resected specimen for patients who had osteosarcoma. For all patients combined, an SUV$_{max2}$ lower than 2 had a positive predictive value (PPV) of 93% for identifying tumors that were 90% or more necrotic and a 75% negative predictive value (NPV) for identifying those less than 90% necrotic (unfavorable response). The PPV and NPV for a favorable and unfavorable response using a cut-off point of 0.5 for the SUV$_{max2}$/SUV$_{max1}$ ratio were 78% and 63%, respectively.[10] In 2005 these investigators reported similar findings from a follow-up study of 36 patients who had Ewing sarcoma who had FDG-PET imaging at diagnosis and after neoadjuvant therapy. Among the 32 patients who underwent surgical resection of the

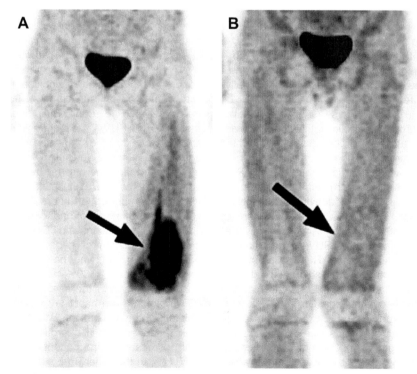

Fig. 7. An 8-year-old boy had osteosarcoma of distal left femur. (*A*) Maximum intensity projection PET image, obtained before neoadjuvant therapy, shows intense FDG avidity within primary tumor (*arrow*). (*B*) A maximum intensity projection PET image at completion of neoadjuvant therapy shows a lack of tumor FDG avidity (*arrow*). The resected tumor was more than 90% necrotic.

primary tumor, a SUV_{max2} lower than 2.5 gave a PPV of 79% for a favorable histologic response and an NPV of 40% for an unfavorable response. The PPV and NPV for a SUV_{max2}/SUV_{max1} ratio 0.5 or less for favorable and unfavorable responses were 77% and 33%, respectively. A SUV_{max2} lower than 2.5 also was associated with improved 4-year progression-free survival for all 36 patients ($P = .006$) and for those without metastatic disease at diagnosis (n = 24, $P = .036$). Neither the SUV_{max1} or an SUV_{max2}/SUV_{max1} ratio of 0.5 or lower was associated with progression-free survival in this cohort. These findings corroborate those of Franzius and colleagues[37] and suggest that the maximum SUV of primary osteosarcoma and Ewing sarcoma tumors, measured after neoadjuvant therapy, can predict tumor histologic response and patient outcome. Further studies are needed to determine whether the SUV can allow nonresponding or poorly responding tumors to be identified earlier in the course of neoadjuvant therapy, before local control, to alter patient management and improve chances of survival.

SUMMARY

Because of the rarity of pediatric bone and soft tissue malignancies, it is difficult to validate the role of emerging imaging technologies in their management. The growing body of literature regarding the use of PET and PET/CT in children supports the continued investigation of this modality in the management of pediatric sarcomas. PET and PET/CT have shown value in detecting unknown primary sites in children who have widely metastatic rhabdomyosarcoma. PET/CT may provide valuable information regarding pulmonary nodules in children who have sarcomas, but its limitations must be recognized when interpreting findings. Small pulmonary nodules may be malignant but below the level of resolution by FDG-PET. Conversely, larger nodules that are benign may show intense FDG avidity. The potential value of PET/CT in the management of pulmonary nodules in children who have sarcomas requires further investigation. FDG-PET seems to be superior to ^{99m}Tc bone scintigraphy in evaluating osseous metastases in children who have Ewing sarcoma and rhabdomyosarcoma because these tumors tend to metastasize to the bone marrow before causing cortical destruction and the resultant osteoblastic reaction. On the other hand, the bone-seeking radiotracer ^{99m}Tc MDP may be superior to FDG in detecting the lytic and ossifying bone metastases often associated with osteosarcoma. When

PET is used to detect bone metastasis in children, an awareness of the commonly occurring benign bone lesions in this age group is essential, because these lesions can appear intensely FDG avid and may mimic metastatic disease. In such cases the correlative CT imaging obtained during PET/CT or plain-film radiography is instrumental in determining the need for further imaging or biopsy. Ssites of local-regional nodal FDG uptake should be interpreted with care in children who have bone and soft tissue sarcomas. Biopsy of suspicious lymph nodes probably is warranted when there are conflicting findings between imaging modalities or between imaging and physical examination. Last, because bone tumors do not change substantially in size in response to neoadjuvant therapy, CT and MR imaging are of limited value for assessing the primary tumor response. Because FDG-PET reflects the metabolic activity of tumors, and because the activity can be measured semi-quantitatively using the SUV, PET holds great promise as an alternative method of assessing the therapeutic response of these tumors. To allow early intervention when tumors are responding poorly and thus to enhance patient survival, additional studies are needed to elucidate better the optimal timing of PET during neoadjuvant therapy.

REFERENCES

1. Gurney JG, Young Jr JL, Roffers SD, et al. Soft tissue sarcomas, 111–1223, 1999. National Cancer Institute. Cancer incidence and survival among children and adolescents: United States SEER Program 1975–1995.
2. Link MP, Gebhardt M, Meyers P. Osteosarcoma. In: Pizzo P, Poplack D, editors. Principles and practice of pediatric oncology. 5th edition. Philadelphia: Lippincott Williams & Wilkins; 2006. p. 1074–115.
3. Bernstein M, Kovar H, Paulussen M, et al. Ewing sarcoma family of tumors: Ewing sarcoma of bone and soft tissue and the peripheral primitive neuroectodermal tumors. In: Pizzo P, Poplack D, editors. Principles and practice of pediatric oncology. 5th edition. Philadelphia: Lippincott, Williams & Wilkins; 2006. p. 1002–32.
4. Wexler L, Meyer W, Helman L. Rhabdomyosarcoma and the undifferentiated sarcomas. In: Pizzo PA, Poplack DG, editors. Principles and practice of pediatric oncology. 5th editon. Philadelphia: Lippincott, Williams & Wilkins; 2006. p. 971–1001.
5. Therasse P, Arbuck S, Eisenhauer E, et al. New guidelines to evaluate the response to treatment in solid tumors. J Natl Cancer Inst 2000;92: 205–16.

6. Fournier LS, Cuénod CA, Clément O, et al. Imaging of response to treatment in oncology. J Radiol 2007; 88:829–43 [in French].

7. Rohren EM, Turkington TG, Coleman RE. Clinical applications of PET in oncology. Radiology 2004; 231:305–32.

8. Kostakoglu L, Agress H Jr, Goldsmith SJ. Clinical role of FDG-PET in evaluation of cancer patients. Radiographics 2003;23:315–40.

9. Franzius C, Sciuk J, Brinkschmidt C, et al. Evaluation of chemotherapy response in primary bone tumors with F-18 FDG positron emission tomography compared with histologically assessed tumor necrosis. Clin Nucl Med 2000;25:874–81.

10. Hawkins DS, Rajendran JG, Conrad EU, et al. Evaluation of chemotherapy response in pediatric bone sarcomas by [F-18]-fluorodeoxy-D-glucose positron emission tomography. Cancer 2002;94: 3277–84.

11. Hawkins DS, Schuetze SM, Butrynski JE, et al. [18F]Fluorodeoxyglucose positron emission tomography predicts outcome for Ewing sarcoma family of tumors. J Clin Oncol 2005;23:8828–34.

12. Schuetze SM, Baker LH, Benjamin RS, et al. Selection of response criteria for clinical trials of sarcoma treatment. Oncologist 2008;13(Suppl 2): 32–40.

13. Fletcher JW, Djulbegovic B, Soares HP, et al. Recommendations on the use of 18F-FDG-PET in oncology. J Nucl Med 2008;49:480–508.

14. Etcubanas E, Peiper S, Stass S, et al. Rhabdomyosarcoma, presenting as disseminated malignancy from an unknown primary site: a retrospective study of ten pediatric cases. Med Pediatr Oncol 1989;17: 39–44.

15. Varadhachary GR, Abbruzzese JL, Lenzi R. Diagnostic strategies for unknown primary cancer. Cancer 2004;100:1776–85.

16. McCarville MB, Christie R, Daw NC, et al. PET/CT in the evaluation of childhood sarcomas. AJR Am J Roentgenol 2005;184:1293–304.

17. Seshadri N, Wright P, Balan KK. Rhabdomyosarcoma with widespread bone marrow infiltration: beneficial management role of F-18 FDG-PET. Clin Nucl Med 2007;32:787–9.

18. Franzius C, Drup-Link HE, Sciuk J, et al. FDG-PET for detection of pulmonary metastases from malignant primary bone tumors: comparison with spiral CT. Ann Oncol 2001;12:479–86.

19. Volker T, Denecke T, Steffen I, et al. Positron emission tomography for staging of pediatric sarcoma patients: results of a prospective multicenter trial. J Clin Oncol 2007;25:5435–41.

20. Gerth HU, Juergens KU, Dirksen U, et al. Significant benefit of multimodal imaging: PET/CT compared with PET alone in staging and follow-up of patients with Ewing tumors. J Nucl Med 2007;48:1932–9.

21. Iagaru A, Quon A, McDougall IR, et al. F-18 FDG-PET/CT evaluation of osseous and soft tissue sarcomas. Clin Nucl Med 2006;31:754–60.

22. Franzius C, Sciuk J, Drup-Link HE, et al. FDG-PET for detection of osseous metastases from malignant primary bone tumours: comparison with bone scintigraphy. Eur J Nucl Med 2000;27:1305–11.

23. Daldrup-Link HE, Franzius C, Link TM, et al. Whole-body MR imaging for detection of bone metastases in children and young adults: comparison with skeletal scintigraphy and FDG-PET. AJR Am J Roentgenol 2001;177:229–36.

24. Mazumdar A, Siegel MJ, Narra V, et al. Whole-body fast inversion recovery MR imaging of small cell neoplasms in pediatric patients: a pilot study. AJR Am J Roentgenol 2002;179:1261–6.

25. Kellenberger CJ, Epelman M, Miller SF, et al. Fast STIR whole-body MR imaging in children. Radiographics 2004;24:1317–30.

26. Goo HW, Choi SH, Ghim T, et al. Whole-body MRI of paediatric malignant tumours: comparison with conventional oncological imaging methods. Pediatr Radiol 2005;35:766–73.

27. Flickinger FW, Sanal SM. Bone marrow MRI: techniques and accuracy for detecting breast cancer metastases. Magn Reson Imaging. 1994;12:829–35.

28. Frank JA, Ling A, Patronas NJ, et al. Detection of malignant bone tumors: MR imaging vs scintigraphy. AJR Am J Roentgenol 1990;155:1043–8.

29. Eustace S, Tello R, DeCarvalho V, et al. A comparison of whole-body turboSTIR MR imaging and planar 99mTc-methylene diphosphonate scintigraphy in the examination of patients with suspected skeletal metastases. AJR Am J Roentgenol 1997;169:1655–61.

30. Gosfield E III, Alavi A, Kneeland B. Comparison of radionuclide bone scans and magnetic resonance imaging in detecting spinal metastases. J Nucl Med 1993;34:2191–8.

31. Darge K, Jaramillo D, Siegel MJ. Whole-body MRI in children: current status and future applications. Eur J Radiol 2008;68:289–98.

32. Aoki J, Watanabe H, Shinozaki T, et al. FDG-PET of primary benign and malignant bone tumors: standardized uptake value in 52 lesions. Radiology 2001;219:774–7.

33. Klem ML, Grewal RK, Wexler LH, et al. PET for staging in rhabdomyosarcoma: an evaluation of PET as an adjunct to current staging tools. J Pediatr Hematol Oncol 2007;29:9–14.

34. Ben Arush MW, Bar SR, Postovsky S, et al. Assessing the use of FDG-PET in detecting regional and metastatic nodes in alveolar rhabdomyosarcoma of extremities. J Pediatr Hematol Oncol 2006;28: 440–5.

35. Malawer MM, Link M, Donaldson S. Cancer. In: DeVita VT, Hellman S, Rosenberg SA, editors. Principles and practice of oncology. 6th edition.

Philadelphia: Lippincott Williams & Wilkins; 2001. p. 1891–935.

36. Brenner W, Bohuslavizki KH, Eary JF. PET imaging of osteosarcoma. J Nucl Med 2003;44:930–42.

37. Franzius C, Bielack S, Flege S, et al. Prognostic significance of (18)F-FDG and (99m)Tc-methylene diphosphonate uptake in primary osteosarcoma. J Nucl Med 2002;43:1012–7.

Fluorine-18 DOPA-PET and PET/CT Imaging in Congenital Hyperinsulinism

Mohamed Houseni, MD[a,b], Wichana Chamroonrat, MD[a],
Hongming Zhuang, MD, PhD[a], MiGuel Hernandez-Pampolini, MD[a],
Abass Alavi, MD, MD (Hon), PhD (Hon), DSc (Hon)[a,c],*

KEYWORDS

• Congenital hyperinsulinism • Persistent hypoglycemia
• PET • FDOPA • PET/CT

Hyperinsulinism is the most common cause of transient and permanent neonatal disorders of hypoglycemia.[1,2] It has the incidence of 1 in 30,000 to 50,000 live births.[3] Hypoglycemia in infancy and early childhood may lead to a variety of manifestations, ranging from poor feeding and lethargy to seizures, delayed milestones, and permanent neurologic damage.[4,5] Hyperinsulinism in infancy represents a group of clinically, genetically, morphologically, and functionally heterogeneous disorders. It is characterized by inappropriate insulin secretion for the level of glycemia.[6,7]

Mutations in six genes have been involved in congenital hyperinsulinism (**Table 1**). The most common forms of mutation occur in both potassium inwardly rectifying channel and ATP-binding cassette genes located on chromosome 11p.[8–11] This is associated with alteration in the function of ATP-sensitive potassium channels.[12] Closure of the channel by high ATP following stimulation with glucose leads to depolarization of the membrane and activation of a voltage-gated calcium channel that results in exocytosis of insulin granules.[13] Loss of either gene results in

a recessive form of hyperinsulinism, with severe symptoms that often need surgery. Milder mutations lead to hypoglycemia, which may be controlled medically.[14,15] However, despite advances in genetics, many patients studied do not have a definable genetic abnormality.[4,16,17]

In addition to genetic disorders, hyperinsulinism in infants can occur in the setting of maternal diabetes, rhesus incompatibility, and perinatal stresses.[18–20] Secondary causes of hyperinsulinism include neonatal panhypopituitarism, congenital disorders of glycosylation, fatty-acid oxidation deficiency, drug-induced hypoglycemia, anti-insulin and insulin-receptor stimulating antibodies, Beckwith-Wiedemann Syndrome, Perlman syndrome, and Sotos syndrome.[6,12]

The diagnosis of hyperinsulinism can be established by means of biochemical, genotype, clinical investigations, and pancreatic imaging. Laboratory findings include a persistent blood-glucose level less than 2.6 mmol/liter, detectable insulin at the point of hypoglycemia with raised C peptide, and inappropriately low-blood free fatty acid and ketone body concentrations. A glucose requirement of 16 mg/kg to 8 mg/kg per minute to

M. Houseni and W. Chamroonrat contributed equally to this manuscript.
[a] Division of Nuclear Medicine, Department of Radiology, The Children's Hospital of Philadelphia, PA, USA
[b] Department of Radiology, National Liver Institute, Egypt
[c] Department of Radiology, Hospital of University of Pennsylvania, University of Pennsylvania School of Medicine, 34th & Spruce Street, Philadelphia, PA 19104, USA
* Corresponding author. Department of Radiology, Hospital of University of Pennsylvania, University of Pennsylvania School of Medicine, PA.
E-mail address: abass.alavi@uphs.upenn.edu (A. Alavi).

PET Clin 3 (2009) 577–585
doi:10.1016/j.cpet.2009.04.002
1556-8598/09/$ – see front matter © 2009 Elsevier Inc. All rights reserved.

Table 1
Genes involved in congenital hyperinsulinism

Gene Name	Symbol	Aliases	Chromosome	Autosomal Inheritance
ATP-binding cassette, subfamily C (CFTR/ MRP), member 8[11]	ABCC8	SUR1	11p15.1	Dominant/Recessive
Potassium inwardly rectifying channel, subfamily J, member 11[10]	KCNJ11	Kir6.2, BIR	11p15.1	Dominant/Recessive
Glucokinase (hexokinase 4)[74]	GCK	HK4	7p15.3-p15.1	Dominant
Glutamate dehydrogenase 1[75]	GLUD1	GDH	10q21.1-q24.3	Dominant
Hydroxyacyl-Coenzyme A dehydrogenase[76]	HADH	SCHAD	4q22-q26	Recessive
Solute carrier family 16, member 1 (monocarboxylic acid transporter 1)[77]	SLC16A1	MCT1	1p12	Dominant

maintain blood glucose less than 2.6 mmol to 3 mmol per liter is a key for the diagnosis, as well as treatment of hyperinsulinism.[4,6] Facial dysmorphism with high forehead, large bulbous nose with short columella, smooth philtrum, and thin upper lip are often observed in hyperinsulinism.[21]

Histologic differentiation of hyperinsulinism includes focal adenomatous hyperplasia, diffuse disorder, atypical diffuse form, bifocal, and multifocal forms.[22–24] Rarely, extra-pancreatic ectopic focal hyperinsulinism may occur.[25,26]

Focal adenomatous hyperplasia is a poorly delineated lesion, usually less than 10 mm in diameter, characterized by the presence of a confluent proliferation of β-cell clusters.[27,28] Retaining relatively normal histology outside the focal lesion is essential for the diagnosis.[29] Focal hyperplasia is associated non-Mendelian mode of inheritance of ATP-sensitive potassium channel dysfunction and β-cell hyperplasia.[28,30] The epigenetic phenomena comprise of gene silencing with loss of heterozygosity of a region of the maternal chromosome 11p15 and a reduction to homozygosity of paternally derived genes, resulting in a somatic lesion of defective β-cells within the pancreas.[6,31]

Diffuse hyperinsulinism is characterized by the presence of β-cells with abundant cytoplasm and a large nucleus throughout the pancreas.[32,33] Diffuse forms are predominantly linked with autosomal recessive inheritance of gene mutations; however, autosomal dominant mutations have been described.[34]

The molecular pathophysiology of the atypical form is unclear. The pattern of pancreatic involvement is of the diffuse type, demonstrating β-cell nuclear enlargement but confined to a discrete area of the pancreas.[22,23] The bifocal form is rare. Molecular biology analysis shows that the length of the deletions on the maternal chromosome 11p differs in the two foci, suggesting that the bifocal form is attributable to two independent hits.[12,23]

MANAGEMENT
Initial Stabilization

Immediate treatment should be commenced to prevent long-term neurologic complications. There should be constant administration of glucose or enteral feeds aiming to maintain the plasma glucose levels above 70 mg/dL.[2] Glucagon infusion may be added if blood-glucose levels are unstable, despite high-glucose administration. Glucagon increases glycogenolysis and gluconeogenesis; however, it is insulin secretagogue.[35]

Medical Therapy

Diazoxide is a key medicine in hyperinsulinism. It inhibits insulin release by activating potassium channels, thus functional channels are required for diazoxide to be effective. Chlorothiazide is given in combination to overcome the fluid-retaining effect of diazoxide.[4] The success rate is 15%

to 60%, depending on patient selection.[36,37] Neonates and cases with recessive inheritance showed resistance to this line of therapy.[37]

Octreotide, a long-acting somatostatin analog that inhibits insulin secretion distal to potassium channels, is another line of treatment for cases unresponsive to diazoxide.[38] It should be noted that tachyphylaxis may develop to octreotide.[2]

Nifedipine, a calcium channel-blocker agent, has been shown to decrease insulin secretion. It was introduced to avoid the side effects of diazoxide or somatostatin. It has been reported that nifedipine can be effective as a long-term therapy.[39,40]

Surgery

Surgery is required for cases with intractable hypoglycemia that is not responding to medical therapy, especially in cases with focal disease. A significant proportion of cases requiring surgery may develop diabetes mellitus, which is related to age at surgery and extent of the pancreatectomy. There is also risk of persistent hypoglycemia.[41] Surgery planning is based on laboratory evaluation, genetic testing, and imaging.[2]

Near total pancreatectomy is performed in infants with diffuse disease and not responding to medical treatment.[42] Infants with focal disease, accounting for approximately 40% to 60% of cases with potassium inwardly rectifying channel and ATP-binding cassette gene mutations,[2] can be cured with limited pancreatectomy, preserving the normal pancreatic tissue. Successful surgery should be preceded with accurate localization of the focal pancreatic lesions. Partial pancreatectomy is usually aided by frozen section histologic examination to determine the extent of resection.[36]

Infants with hyperinsulinism require long-term management, including medical, nutritional, neurologic, and psychologic care. Unfortunately, even with adequate treatment, there is a high incidence of neurologic damage, ranging from the subtle to the severe, with an incidence range of 25% to 50%.[4,5]

Preoperative Planning and Localization of Focal Lesions

When surgery is indicated, it is critical to identify cases with focal disease and precisely localize the focal mass. Efforts to image focal lesions using CT, MR imaging, ultrasound, and radio-labeled octreotide scans have not been successful.[43]

Selective pancreatic, arterial-calcium stimulation with hepatic vein sampling is effectively used to map the portion of the pancreas that contains diseased tissue. A diseased area gives a twofold or greater increase in plasma insulin in response to calcium stimulation, with a reported sensitivity reaching 73%.[44] However, it is an invasive procedure, technically difficult, and requires special preparations.[45] Transhepatic catheterization of the portal and pancreatic veins is a similar invasive method for pre-operative resection planning.[36]

A noninvasive method to differentiate diffuse from focal form is the use of PET/CT utilizing 18F-fluoro-L-dihydroxyphenylalanine (FDOPA). This method has been used successfully to localize focal lesions in hyperinsulinism.[46–51]

FDOPA-PET
Pathophysiology of FDOPA-PET Scanning

Dopamine receptors are expressed on β-cells and dopamine can be generated by β-cells from its precursor L-DOPA through the action of L-DOPA decarboxylase.[52,53]

Dopamine concentration regulates insulin secretion in vitro through inhibiting the glucose-stimulated insulin secretion by specific receptor-receptor interactions.[53] However, the link between dopamine and insulin secretion is not fully understood.[54] Electron microscopy shows dopamine to be present in the soluble part of secretory granules. Enhanced-dopamine metabolism in abnormal β-cells of diseased areas in hyperinsulinism could be related to dopamine-carrier defect, reducing its reuptake.[23] Furthermore, the diseased area is abnormally rich in L-DOPA decarboxylase. These factors lead to FDOPA accumulation in the affected regions.[49]

In focal hyperinsulinism, there is greater FDOPA uptake in the lesion (**Fig. 1**) than in the remainder of the pancreas where islets of Langerhans are dispersed. In diffuse disease, there is diffuse increased FDOPA uptake with slightly more activity in the head than the other parts of the pancreas (**Fig. 2**).[49]

Patient Selection

Patients with persistent hyperinsulinemic hypoglycemia and requiring surgery will benefit from FDOPA-PET scanning. Documented loss of heterozygosity of a region of the maternal chromosome 11p15 and a reduction to homozygosity of paternally derived genes is highly suggestive of focal forms. FDOPA-PET imaging could be the only noninvasive method available for localizing focal lesions.[55]

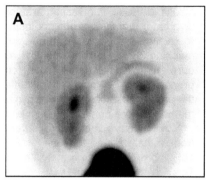
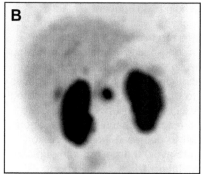

Fig. 1. FDOPA-PET images of patients with typical diffuse hypeinsulinism (*A*) and focal hyperinsulinism (*B*).

Patient Preparation

Informed consent and ethical approval should be provided. Medications, especially glucagon and carbidopa, might be adjusted or stopped 2 to 3 days before the imaging; however, Ribeiro and colleagues[56] reported that diazoxide and octreotide cessation is unnecessary. Fasting for 6 hours together with glucose infusion and blood-glucose monitoring during the scan are important to ensure euglycemia.[43] Further preparation include a sheet wrapped around the body, sand bags or holding devices for immobilization, reliable intravenous access, and bladder catheterization to avoid discomfort.[57,58] Anesthesia may be achieved by intravenous propofol infusion or inhalational anesthesia via a tracheal tube.[43] Parents may accompany their child.[59]

Image Acquisition and Interpretation

A PET/CT scanner is preferred, as anatomical correlation is essential. The FDOPA intravenous injection dose is 0.08 mCi/kg to 0.16 mCi/kg (3 MBq/kg –6 MBq/kg).[47,51] The child is positioned in the way that the whole pancreas can be easily seen in a single-axial reformatted image. Dynamic data acquisition starts from 5 to 60 minutes after injection, with a sequence of 5- to 10-minute frames. Images are viewed in axial, coronal, and sagittal plans.[55]

Physiologic uptake of FDOPA occurs in the basal ganglia of brain, growth plates, and the urinary collection system. Mild uptake is seen in the liver, pancreas, and brain cortex.[26] Gall bladder visualization may occur because of biliary excretion of FDOPA.[60]

Localizing the focal lesion within the pancreas can be achieved visually by assessing FDOPA uptake in the pancreas and correlating the abnormality to the corresponding CT images.[49] Extrapancreatic focal FDOPA uptake has been observed and should be excluded. Furthermore, measuring the standardized uptake value is suggestive of focal disease when there is more than 1.5-fold localized FDOPA uptake compared to that remaining in the pancreas.[48,55]

Radiation Dosimetry

Harvey and colleagues and Dhawan and colleagues developed a biokinetic data table for FDOPA assuming its homogenous distribution in the body and its elimination by kidneys and biliary tracts. Radiation doses of selected organs are presented in **Table 2**. The bladder wall is the target

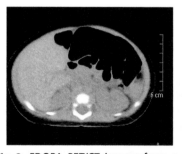
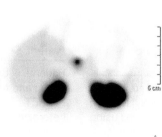
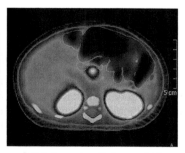

Fig. 2. FDOPA PET/CT images from a patient suffering focal form of congenital hyperinsulinism, which was confirmed by surgical pathological examination. The CT image (*left*) is unremarkable. However, the PET (*middle*) and fused-PET/CT (*right*) images clearly demonstrated the abnormally increased FDOPA activity in the head of the pancreas.

Table 2
Estimated radiation doses of F-DOPA in children

Organ	Estimated Dose (mGy/MBq)	
	Age 1-year	Age 5-year
Bladder wall	1	0.56
Brain	0.044	0.024
Heart	0.05	0.027
Liver	0.052	0.028
Kidney	0.11	0.063
Adrenals	0.055	0.03
Lung	0.46	0.024
Pancreas	0.56	0.03
Red marrow	0.47	0.026
Estimated dose (mSv/MBq)	0.1	0.056

organ. Absorbed dose per unit in different organs of infants is higher than that reported in adults.[61–63]

Considering PET/CT, the radiation dose of the CT using 80 mAs and 140 KV is 3 mSv to 5 mSv. The effective dose from a diagnostic CT scan is estimated to be 1 mSv to 10 mSv. The calculated risk of eventual death from radiation-induced malignancy by an effective dose of 10 mSv was estimated to be 1 in 1,000.[64] In addition, CT is often performed using adult exposure settings, which resulted in high radiation exposure.[65] Intelligent dose reduction based on the principles of as low as reasonably achievable is essential for the safest possible care of children.[66]

FDOPA-PET Performance and Correlation to Management

FDOPA-PET imaging has been shown to accurately distinguish focal from diffuse hyperinsulinism (see **Fig. 1**), and its coregistration with CT images allows precise localization of focal lesions.[47,49,50,56] Until now, the sensitivity of PET scanners in detecting focal lesions is directly related to the lesion size. The smallest reported focal lesion on FDOPA has measured 4 mm by 5 mm.[50] The reported sensitivity and specificity of FDOPA, in the detection of focal lesions, approach 94% and 100%, respectively.[49,50,56] However, because of patient selection and absence of histopathology in some cases, the authors assume a mild degree of statistical over-estimation.

In a series of 50 cases with uncontrolled hyperinsulinism, FDOPA identified 75% (18 out of 24) of patients with focal disease with 100% specificity, 100% positive and 81% negative predictive values. In addition, it accurately localized the

lesions in all the cases with focal disease detected by PET imaging. Limited pancreatectomy had been done in most of these patients and surgery was guided by PET results.[47] Similar results have been reported by Otonkoski and colleagues.[50] In another study by Ribeiro and colleagues, FDOPA diagnosed focal lesions in 15 patients; focal disease was proven in 14 of them, with a positive predictive value of 93%. Limited pancreatectomy with clinical remission has been achieved in all the 14 patients. Furthermore, PET had correctly localized 92% of cases with focal disease.[51] In a recent study using PET/CT, 9 of 10 children with focal FDOPA uptake exactly correlated to the intraoperative site of disease (see **Fig. 2**). A limited resection of the pancreas has been curative in all nine cases.[46] The high rate of accurate localization of focal lesions allows potentials of laparoscopic surgery with the benefit of low morbidity and better postoperative care.[67]

Atypical disease with diffuse pattern confined to discrete regions of the pancreas usually reveals diffuse FDOPA uptake.[22,47] Partial pancreatectomy with follow-up could be curative for the atypical form; however, some cases require postsurgery medical control or repeated surgery with near total pancreatectomy.[23] Extensive focal disease is another challenge: it appears as diffuse FDOPA uptake and near total pancreatectomy is indicated. On the other hand, small focal lesions in the tail of the pancreas can be overlooked because of their proximity to the kidney; however, when detected it allows laparoscopic limited pancreatectomy.[47]

Bifocal and multifocal forms are rare. It is difficult to distinguish multiple foci on PET imaging if they occur in the same area. A second focal disease should be considered in patients suffering hypoglycemic episodes after limited partial pancreatectomy. Bifocal, focal, and multifocal forms have to be differentiated from incompletely removed focal disease, requiring different surgical approaches.[23,68]

Ectopic pancreatic tissue may occur in the stomach, duodenum, jejunum, and ileum.[69] Although rare, hyperinsulinism has been reported to be caused by ectopic pancreatic tissue, and repeated surgery without identifying the ectopic disease will not control hypoglycemia. A FDOPA scan can also accurately localized ectopic focal lesion (**Fig. 3**). A focal hyperinsulinism in the wall of the duodenum detected by FDOPA-PET has been reported, in which PET results would have changed the surgical approach.[26] Similarly, Peranteau and colleagues[25] reported multiple ectopic lesions of focal islet adenomatosis in the jejunum in a case with postsurgical persistent

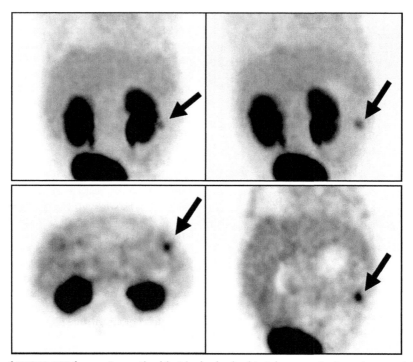

Fig. 3. Images of FDOPA-PET from a 2-month-old girl who had subtotal pancreatectomy in an outside institution for her congenital hyperinsulinemia but was still hypoglycemic. The images (*upper left*, anterior maximum intensity projection image; *upper right*, left anterior oblique maximum intensity projection image; *lower left*, trans-axial; *lower right*, coronal) revealed a remaining abnormal focus of increased tracer uptake (*arrows*) outside the normal pancreas bed and its proved-to-be abnormal islet pancreatic tissue in the jejunum. After resection of the jejunum, the patient turned diabetic, which was controlled by insulin.

hypoglycemia. FDOPA imaging has precisely localized the disease sites, and targeted further resection corrected the hypoglycemia. Furthermore, these two reports demonstrated the usefulness of FDOPA-PET in cases with postsurgical persistent or recurrent hypoglycemia.[25,26]

The FDOPA-PET results have been shown to be comparable, even better by some reports, to both selective pancreatic, arterial calcium stimulation with hepatic vein sampling and transhepatic catheterization of the portal and pancreatic veins. The reported sensitivity for both procedures were 73% and 89%, respectively.[36,44] However, PET imaging is preferable, being noninvasive, simpler, and likely without complications.

LIMITATIONS AND PITFALLS

Small and thin lesions may not accumulate enough FDOPA to be detectable. The smallest lesion reported in the literature has measured 5 mm in diameter.[50] Conservative interpretation has been shown to underestimate the diagnosis of focal lesions. FDOPA-PET imaging for surgery planning should direct the surgeon to areas with suspicious abnormalities, even if those regions are questionable on imaging.[47] Moreover, it could be difficult to identify two or more focal lesions in the same area.[23,68] In addition, focal lesions have ill-defined borders; therefore, multiple frozen sections from the remaining pancreatic tissue might be necessary.[70–72] Postsurgical PET/CT imaging is another challenge, because of distortion of the anatomy, and requires careful interpretation.[25,26]

The head of the pancreas contains about 50% of the pancreatic tissue; this leads to more FDOPA activity in the pancreatic head compared to the body and tail. Diffuse hyperinsulinism with gradient adenomatosis having more affected cells in the head can give a false impression of focal hyperinsulinism.[46]

FDOPA excretion occurs mainly through the kidneys; however, elimination may occur in the liver where activity is seen in the biliary tract, gall bladder, and duodenum. Pancreatic lesions near the left kidney, gall bladder, or the duodenum could be missed, especially when small in size.[46,51] On the other hand, FDOPA accumulation in the gall bladder or alimentary tract can be confused with pancreatic focal lesion.[60] Dynamic imaging may help to clear this issue and a late-appearing focal FDOPA uptake is considered positive when identified at the same location on a second scan with at least a 15-minute time interval.[46]

Ectopic focal hyperinsulinism has been reported in the alimentary tract.[69] If ectopic lesions are suspected, gastrointestinal preparation and oral contrast agent will be helpful in the localization using PET/CT images. It has been shown that negative oral-contrast material delineates intestinal structures and overcomes contrast-induced PET artifacts.[73]

SUMMARY

Congenital hyperinsulinism is the main cause of persistent hypoglycemia during infancy and childhood. Early detection and appropriate management is critical to avoid neurologic complications. Distinguishing diffuse from focal forms fundamentally change the management approach. FDOPA-PET imaging has been shown to be accurate and precise in identification and localization of focal hyperinsulinism, allowing curative limited targeted surgery. Partial pancreatectomy saves the normal pancreatic tissue and function. In addition, FDOPA may localize extra-pancreatic ectopic focal hyperinsulinism. As a noninvasive and accurate modality, FDOPA-PET is becoming a powerful tool in the management of congenital hyperinsulinism.

REFERENCES

1. Soltesz G, Jenkins PA, Aynsley-Green A. Hyperinsulinaemic hypoglycaemia in infancy and childhood: a practical approach to diagnosis and medical treatment based on experience of 18 cases. Acta Paediatr Hung 1984;25(4):319–32.
2. Palladino AA, Bennett MJ, Stanley CA. Hyperinsulinism in infancy and childhood: when an insulin level is not always enough. Clin Chem 2008;54(2):256–63.
3. Dekelbab BH, Sperling MA. Recent advances in hyperinsulinemic hypoglycemia of infancy. Acta Paediatr 2006;95(10):1157–64.
4. Aynsley-Green A, Hussain K, Hall J, et al. Practical management of hyperinsulinism in infancy. Arch Dis Child Fetal Neonatal Ed 2000;82(2):F98–107.
5. Steinkrauss L, Lipman TH, Hendell CD, et al. Effects of hypoglycemia on developmental outcome in children with congenital hyperinsulinism. J Pediatr Nurs 2005;20(2):109–18.
6. Cosgrove KE, Shepherd RM, Fernandez EM, et al. Genetics and pathophysiology of hyperinsulinism in infancy. Horm Res 2004;61(6):270–88.
7. Hussain K. Insights in congenital hyperinsulinism. Endocr Dev 2007;11:106–21.
8. Nestorowicz A, Inagaki N, Gonoi T, et al. A nonsense mutation in the inward rectifier potassium channel gene, Kir6.2, is associated with familial hyperinsulinism. Diabetes 1997;46(11):1743–8.
9. Nestorowicz A, Wilson BA, Schoor KP, et al. Mutations in the sulonylurea receptor gene are associated with familial hyperinsulinism in Ashkenazi Jews. Hum Mol Genet 1996;5(11):1813–22.
10. Thomas P, Ye Y, Lightner E. Mutation of the pancreatic islet inward rectifier Kir6.2 also leads to familial persistent hyperinsulinemic hypoglycemia of infancy. Hum Mol Genet 1996;5(11):1809–12.
11. Thomas PM, Cote GJ, Wohllk N, et al. Mutations in the sulfonylurea receptor gene in familial persistent hyperinsulinemic hypoglycemia of infancy. Science 1995;268(5209):426–9.
12. Giurgea I, Bellanne-Chantelot C, Ribeiro M, et al. Molecular mechanisms of neonatal hyperinsulinism. Horm Res 2006;66(6):289–96.
13. Meissner T, Mayatepek E. Clinical and genetic heterogeneity in congenital hyperinsulinism. Eur J Pediatr 2002;161(1):6–20.
14. Stanley CA. Advances in diagnosis and treatment of hyperinsulinism in infants and children. J Clin Endocrinol Metab 2002;87(11):4857–9.
15. Pinney SE, MacMullen C, Becker S, et al. Clinical characteristics and biochemical mechanisms of congenital hyperinsulinism associated with dominant KATP channel mutations. J Clin Invest 2008;118(8):2877–86.
16. Cosgrove KE, Shepherd RM, Hashmi MN, et al. The role of calcium ions in determining insulin hypersecretion in patients with persistent hyperinsulinaemic hypoglycaemia of infancy. Horm Res 1999;55:15P.
17. Natarajan G, Aggarwal S, Merritt TA. A novel mutation associated with congenital hyperinsulinism. Am J Perinatol 2007;24(7):401–4.
18. Christesen HB, Feilberg-Jorgensen N, Jacobsen BB. Pancreatic beta-cell stimulation tests in transient and persistent congenital hyperinsulinism. Acta Paediatr 2001;90(10):1116–20.
19. Clark W, O'Donovan D. Transient hyperinsulinism in an asphyxiated newborn infant with hypoglycemia. Am J Perinatol 2001;18(4):175–8.
20. Parviainen AM, Puolakka J, Kirkinen P. Antepartum findings and obstetric aspects in pregnancies followed by neonatal persistent hyperinsulinemic hypoglycemia. Am J Perinatol 2002;19(3):163–8.
21. de Lonlay P, Cormier-Daire V, Amiel J, et al. Facial appearance in persistent hyperinsulinemic hypoglycemia. Am J Med Genet 2002;111(2):130–3.
22. Hussain K, Flanagan SE, Smith VV, et al. An ABCC8 gene mutation and mosaic uniparental isodisomy resulting in atypical diffuse congenital hyperinsulinism. Diabetes 2008;57(1):259–63.

23. Delonlay P, Simon A, Galmiche-Rolland L, et al. Neonatal hyperinsulinism: clinicopathologic correlation. Hum Pathol 2007;38(3):387–99.

24. Goossens A, Gepts W, Saudubray JM, et al. Diffuse and focal nesidioblastosis. A clinicopathological study of 24 patients with persistent neonatal hyperinsulinemic hypoglycemia. Am J Surg Pathol 1989; 13(9):766–75.

25. Peranteau WH, Bathaii SM, Pawel B, et al. Multiple ectopic lesions of focal islet adenomatosis identified by positron emission tomography scan in an infant with congenital hyperinsulinism. J Pediatr Surg 2007;42(1):188–92.

26. Hussain K, Seppanen M, Nanto-Salonen K, et al. The diagnosis of ectopic focal hyperinsulinism of infancy with [18F]-dopa positron emission tomography. J Clin Endocrinol Metab 2006;91(8): 2839–42.

27. Kloppel G, Reinecke-Luthge A, Koschoreck F. Focal and diffuse beta cell changes in persistent hyperinsulinemic hypoglycemia of infancy. Endocr Pathol 1999;10(4):299–304.

28. Verkarre V, Fournet JC, de Lonlay P, et al. Paternal mutation of the sulfonylurea receptor (SUR1) gene and maternal loss of 11p15 imprinted genes lead to persistent hyperinsulinism in focal adenomatous hyperplasia. J Clin Invest 1998;102(7):1286–91.

29. Sempoux C, Guiot Y, Rahier J. The focal form of persistent hyperinsulinemic hypoglycemia of infancy. Diabetes 2001;50(Suppl 1):S182–3.

30. Fournet JC, Mayaud C, de Lonlay P, et al. Loss of imprinted genes and paternal SUR1 mutations lead to focal form of congenital hyperinsulinism. Horm Res 2000;53(Suppl 1):2–6.

31. Suchi M, MacMullen CM, Thornton PS, et al. Molecular and immunohistochemical analyses of the focal form of congenital hyperinsulinism. Mod Pathol 2006;19(1):122–9.

32. Rahier J, Falt K, Muntefering H, et al. The basic structural lesion of persistent neonatal hypoglycaemia with hyperinsulinism: deficiency of pancreatic D cells or hyperactivity of B cells? Diabetologia 1984;26(4):282–9.

33. Sempoux C, Guiot Y, Lefevre A, et al. Neonatal hyperinsulinemic hypoglycemia: heterogeneity of the syndrome and keys for differential diagnosis. J Clin Endocrinol Metab 1998;83(5):1455–61.

34. Glaser B, Thornton P, Otonkoski T, et al. Genetics of neonatal hyperinsulinism. Arch Dis Child Fetal Neonatal Ed 2000;82(2):F79–86.

35. Mohnike K, Blankenstein O, Pfuetzner A, et al. Long-term non-surgical therapy of severe persistent congenital hyperinsulinism with glucagon. Horm Res 2008;70(1):59–64.

36. de Lonlay-Debeney P, Poggi-Travert F, Fournet JC, et al. Clinical features of 52 neonates with hyperinsulinism. N Engl J Med 1999;340(15):1169–75.

37. Touati G, Poggi-Travert F, Ogier de Baulny H, et al. Long-term treatment of persistent hyperinsulinaemic hypoglycaemia of infancy with diazoxide: a retrospective review of 77 cases and analysis of efficacy-predicting criteria. Eur J Pediatr 1998;157(8): 628–33.

38. Kane C, Lindley KJ, Johnson PR, et al. Therapy for persistent hyperinsulinemic hypoglycemia of infancy. Understanding the responsiveness of beta cells to diazoxide and somatostatin. J Clin Invest 1997;100(7):1888–93.

39. Bas F, Darendeliler F, Demirkol D, et al. Successful therapy with calcium channel blocker (nifedipine) in persistent neonatal hyperinsulinemic hypoglycemia of infancy. J Pediatr Endocrinol Metab 1999; 12(6):873–8.

40. Muller D, Zimmering M, Roehr CC. Should nifedipine be used to counter low blood sugar levels in children with persistent hyperinsulinaemic hypoglycaemia? Arch Dis Child 2004;89(1):83–5.

41. Jack MM, Greer RM, Thomsett MJ, et al. The outcome in Australian children with hyperinsulinism of infancy: early extensive surgery in severe cases lowers risk of diabetes. Clin Endocrinol (Oxf) 2003; 58(3):355–64.

42. Fekete CN, de Lonlay P, Jaubert F, et al. The surgical management of congenital hyperinsulinemic hypoglycemia in infancy. J Pediatr Surg 2004;39(3): 267–9.

43. Hardy OT, Litman RS. Congenital hyperinsulinism—a review of the disorder and a discussion of the anesthesia management. Paediatr Anaesth 2007; 17(7):616–21.

44. Stanley CA, Thornton PS, Ganguly A, et al. Preoperative evaluation of infants with focal or diffuse congenital hyperinsulinism by intravenous acute insulin response tests and selective pancreatic arterial calcium stimulation. J Clin Endocrinol Metab 2004;89(1):288–96.

45. Cucchiaro G, Markowitz SD, Kaye R, et al. Blood glucose control during selective arterial stimulation and venous sampling for localization of focal hyperinsulinism lesions in anesthetized children. Anesth Analg 2004;99(4):1044–8 table of contents.

46. Barthlen W, Blankenstein O, Mau H, et al. Evaluation of [18F]fluoro-L-DOPA positron emission tomography-computed tomography for surgery in focal congenital hyperinsulinism. J Clin Endocrinol Metab 2008;93(3):869–75.

47. Hardy OT, Hernandez-Pampaloni M, Saffer JR, et al. Accuracy of [18F]fluorodopa positron emission tomography for diagnosing and localizing focal congenital hyperinsulinism. J Clin Endocrinol Metab 2007;92(12):4706–11.

48. Kapoor RR, Gilbert C, Mohnike K, et al. Congenital hyperinsulinism: [18F]DOPA PET/CT scan of a focal

lesion in the head of the pancreas. Arch Dis Child Fetal Neonatal Ed 2008;93(2):F166.

49. Mohnike K, Blankenstein O, Minn H, et al. [18F]-DOPA positron emission tomography for preoperative localization in congenital hyperinsulinism. Horm Res 2008;70(2):65–72.

50. Otonkoski T, Nanto-Salonen K, Seppanen M, et al. Noninvasive diagnosis of focal hyperinsulinism of infancy with [18F]-DOPA positron emission tomography. Diabetes 2006;55(1):13–8.

51. Ribeiro MJ, Boddaert N, Bellanne-Chantelot C, et al. The added value of [18F]fluoro-L-DOPA PET in the diagnosis of hyperinsulinism of infancy: a retrospective study involving 49 children. Eur J Nucl Med Mol Imaging 2007;34(12):2120–8.

52. Borelli MI, Villar MJ, Orezzoli A, et al. Presence of DOPA decarboxylase and its localisation in adult rat pancreatic islet cells. Diabetes Metab 1997; 23(2):161–3.

53. Rubi B, Ljubicic S, Pournourmohammadi S, et al. Dopamine D2-like receptors are expressed in pancreatic beta cells and mediate inhibition of insulin secretion. J Biol Chem 2005;280(44): 36824–32.

54. Bello NT, Hajnal A. Alterations in blood glucose levels under hyperinsulinemia affect accumbens dopamine. Physiol Behav 2006;88(1–2):138–45.

55. Mohnike K, Blankenstein O, Christesen HT, et al. Proposal for a standardized protocol for 18F-DOPA-PET (PET/CT) in congenital hyperinsulinism. Horm Res 2006;66(1):40–2.

56. Ribeiro MJ, De Lonlay P, Delzescaux T, et al. Characterization of hyperinsulinism in infancy assessed with PET and 18F-fluoro-L-DOPA. J Nucl Med 2005;46(4):560–6.

57. Gordon I. Issues surrounding preparation, information and handling the child and parent in nuclear medicine. J Nucl Med 1998;39(3):490–4.

58. Shulkin BL. PET imaging in pediatric oncology. Pediatr Radiol 2004;34(3):199–204.

59. Shulkin BL. PET applications in pediatrics. Q J Nucl Med 1997;41(4):281–91.

60. Balan KK. Visualization of the gall bladder on F-18 FDOPA PET imaging: a potential pitfall. Clin Nucl Med 2005;30(1):23–4.

61. Montravers F, Grahek D, Kerrou K, et al. Can fluorodihydroxyphenylalanine PET replace somatostatin receptor scintigraphy in patients with digestive endocrine tumors? J Nucl Med 2006; 47(9):1455–62.

62. Dhawan V, Belakhlef A, Robeson W, et al. Bladder wall radiation dose in humans from fluorine-18-FDOPA. J Nucl Med 1996;37(11):1850–2.

63. Harvey J, Firnau G, Garnett ES. Estimation of the radiation dose in man due to 6-[18F]fluoro-L-dopa. J Nucl Med 1985;26(8):931–5.

64. Brenner D, Elliston C, Hall E, et al. Estimated risks of radiation-induced fatal cancer from pediatric CT. Am J Roentgenol 2001;176(2):289–96.

65. Paterson A, Frush DP, Donnelly LF. Helical CT of the body: are settings adjusted for pediatric patients? Am J Roentgenol 2001;176(2):297–301.

66. Shah NB, Platt SL. ALARA: is there a cause for alarm? Reducing radiation risks from computed tomography scanning in children. Curr Opin Pediatr 2008;20(3):243–7.

67. Bax KN, van der Zee DC. The laparoscopic approach toward hyperinsulinism in children. Semin Pediatr Surg 2007;16(4):245–51.

68. Giurgea I, Sempoux C, Bellanne-Chantelot C, et al. The Knudson's two-hit model and timing of somatic mutation may account for the phenotypic diversity of focal congenital hyperinsulinism. J Clin Endocrinol Metab 2006;91(10):4118–23.

69. Cagirici U, Ozbaran M, Veral A, et al. Ectopic mediastinal pancreas. Eur J Cardiothorac Surg 2001; 19(4):514–5.

70. Adzick NS, Thornton PS, Stanley CA, et al. A multidisciplinary approach to the focal form of congenital hyperinsulinism leads to successful treatment by partial pancreatectomy. J Pediatr Surg 2004;39(3): 270–5.

71. Cretolle C, Fekete CN, Jan D, et al. Partial elective pancreatectomy is curative in focal form of permanent hyperinsulinemic hypoglycaemia in infancy: a report of 45 cases from 1983 to 2000. J Pediatr Surg 2002;37(2):155–8.

72. Suchi M, Thornton PS, Adzick NS, et al. Congenital hyperinsulinism: intraoperative biopsy interpretation can direct the extent of pancreatectomy. Am J Surg Pathol 2004;28(10):1326–35.

73. Antoch G, Kuehl H, Kanja J, et al. Dual-modality PET/CT scanning with negative oral contrast agent to avoid artifacts: introduction and evaluation. Radiology 2004;230(3):879–85.

74. Glaser B, Kesavan P, Heyman M, et al. Familial hyperinsulinism caused by an activating glucokinase mutation. N Engl J Med 1998;338(4):226–30.

75. Stanley CA, Lieu YK, Hsu BY, et al. Hyperinsulinism and hyperammonemia in infants with regulatory mutations of the glutamate dehydrogenase gene. N Engl J Med 1998;338(19):1352–7.

76. Clayton PT, Eaton S, Aynsley-Green A, et al. Hyperinsulinism in short-chain L-3-hydroxyacyl-CoA dehydrogenase deficiency reveals the importance of beta-oxidation in insulin secretion. J Clin Invest 2001;108(3):457–65.

77. Otonkoski T, Jiao H, Kaminen-Ahola N, et al. Physical exercise-induced hypoglycemia caused by failed silencing of monocarboxylate transporter 1 in pancreatic beta cells. Am J Hum Genet 2007; 81(3):467–74.

Pediatric Cardiac PET Imaging

Amol Takalkar, MD[a,b,*], MiGuel Hernandez-Pampaloni, MD[c,d],
Gang Cheng, MD[c,d], Hongming Zhuang, MD, PhD[c,d],
Abass Alavi, MD, MD (Hon), PhD (Hon), DSc (Hon)[c,d]

KEYWORDS
- PET • FDG • Pediatric cardiac PET • PET MPI
- Cardiac flow reserve • Myocardial viability

There has been significant progress in understanding the pathophysiology of various pediatric heart diseases. Moreover, significant progress has been made in the surgical and medical management of these conditions leading to improved outcomes and increasing number of children surviving with congenital or acquired heart diseases. These children are at risk for development of posttreatment myocardial ischemia and hence need to be evaluated periodically to detect this potentially reversible condition.[1,2] Consequently, a noninvasive and reliable imaging technique that can accurately assess the pediatric heart (perfusion, function, viability, and structure) would be extremely beneficial in such patient population. Since this patient population is special (pediatric) and is expected to survive long term, any imaging modality that has potential serious adverse effects especially with repeated testing (like cumulative radiation exposure over time) is an obvious concern in this subgroup.

Fortunately, cardiac imaging has also evolved significantly over the past few decades with tremendous advances in nuclear cardiology, computerized tomography (CT) and magnetic resonance imaging (MR imaging) imaging of the heart. The phenomenal progress in CT technology now allows us to obtain extremely high resolution structural images of the heart within a few seconds. The anatomic and structural information provided by CT imaging in exquisite detail is extremely useful in the management of pediatric heart diseases. However, it is associated with significant radiation exposure and there are concerns about the long-term effects of cumulative radiation exposure in children with repeated CT imaging. MR imaging provides a comprehensive cardiac evaluation without any ionizing radiation and with high temporal and contrast resolution. Its spatial resolution is suboptimal compared with CT, but is improving. Although it was echocardiography that revolutionized the imaging approach to congenital heart disease, MR imaging has been shown to have tremendous incremental advantages over echocardiography and allows a more comprehensive assessment of cardiac morphology and function (including heart, valves, and major vessels). In spite of its considerable advantages, cardiac MR imaging remains a quite labor- and time-intensive procedure. It requires direct hands-on protocol decision making and supervision by a qualified pediatric radiologist experienced in cardiac MR imaging, and intravenous sedation or endotracheal intubation in many pediatric patients.[3]

Nuclear cardiology has also progressed from simple planar cardiac imaging to more advanced single-photon emission computed tomography (SPECT) with ECG-gating and attenuation correction. For some time, SPECT myocardial perfusion

[a] PET Imaging Center, Research Foundation of Northwest Louisiana, 1505 Kings Highway, Shreveport, LA 71103, USA
[b] Department of Radiology, LSUHSC-S, 1501 Kings Highway, Shreveport, LA 71103, USA
[c] Department of Radiology, Children's Hospital of Philadelphia, Philadelphia, PA, USA
[d] Department of Radiology, Hospital of the University of Pennsylvania, Philadelphia, PA, USA
* Corresponding author. PET Imaging Center, Biomedical Research Foundation of Northwest Louisiana, Shreveport, LA.
E-mail address: amoltakalkar@yahoo.com (A. Takalkar).

PET Clin 3 (2009) 587–596
doi:10.1016/j.cpet.2009.03.007

imaging remained the unchallenged imaging modality to assess myocardial perfusion noninvasively and is still routinely used in most places. The technique of positron emission tomography (PET) was developed soon after the SPECT imaging technique was introduced in the 1970s. However, it took almost 2 decades for PET to come to mainstream clinical imaging. Nevertheless, since the late 1990s, there has been a virtual explosion in the use of PET imaging especially for oncologic workup. This has led to widespread availability of PET instrumentation and reduced the cost of PET imaging. Consequently, other indications including cardiac applications of PET imaging have seen increasing use. Presently, there is much literature validating the utility and cost-effectiveness of cardiac PET imaging for various indications like myocardial perfusion and viability evaluations. However, most of the data in current literature focuses on the adult population. Data about the value of cardiac PET imaging in pediatric population remain sparse, although not completely nonexistent. Pediatric cardiac conditions are usually addressed in specialized medical centers that have the requisite expertise to effectively treat these complex disease entities. Hence, cardiac PET imaging has remained restricted to such advanced medical and research centers. Although underused, cardiac PET has been proven to be useful in detecting myocardial ischemia and viability in pediatric patients.

ADVANTAGES OF PET OVER SINGLE-PHOTON EMISSION COMPUTED TOMOGRAPHY

SPECT myocardial perfusion imaging is a proven reliable and cost-effective technique. However, it has several limitations, some specifically related to the pediatric population subgroup. Compared with CT (and also PET), SPECT has suboptimal spatial resolution. This assumes more significance in pediatric patients with small hearts. Attenuation correction is also suboptimal with SPECT compared with PET. Dosimetric concerns restrict the use of thallium radionuclides for SPECT myocardial perfusion and viability studies in pediatric population. Moreover, technetium-based agents suffer from high liver activity that severely affects evaluation of the inferior wall in pediatric patients.[4] SPECT studies also take a comparatively longer time to complete during which the child needs to remain still/motionless necessitating sedation in most patients. Another significant issue with SPECT studies is the inability to provide absolute quantification of regional radiotracer uptake.

In contrast, PET offers superior spatial and temporal resolution as well as better attenuation correction. Dosimetric considerations are more favorable with PET because it uses radiopharmaceuticals with significantly shorter half-lives and allows for more efficient protocols.[5,6] Hence, PET protocols are also completed much faster compared with SPECT studies. Moreover, it is possible to get absolute quantification of regional radiotracer uptake with PET that facilitates obtaining absolute values of myocardial biochemical processes like regional myocardial blood flow and glucose metabolism. In fact, techniques for obtaining quantification of myocardial blood flow with PET have been validated since the early 1990s.[7,8] The availability of integrated PET/CT scanners makes the studies even shorter with better attenuation correction along with anatomic localization but adds additional radiation exposure from the CT portion of the study. If the CT performed is dedicated CT with contrast enhancement, it is feasible to obtain additional high-resolution structural details including CT angiography (CTA) but adds even more radiation and risks of contrast administration. So although PET/CT (with or without dedicated contrast-enhanced CT studies) offers certain advantages, there is concern over potential long-term consequences with repeated use. To minimize unnecessary radiation exposure in children, the dedicated PET scanner at Children's Hospital of Philadelphia has the unique capability of using either CT or regular transmission scanning for attenuation correction, so that the CT portion is applied only when absolutely essential. On most PET/CT scanners, there is no alternative capability for attenuation correction other than the CT scan, but CT for attenuation correction may not be absolutely essential/advisable in all pediatric PET imaging studies.

PET INSTRUMENTATION

A typical PET scanner is a cylindrical assembly of numerous block detectors in a ring configuration for optimal spatial resolution. Several scintillators such as Sodium Iodide (NaI), Bismuth Germanium Oxide (BGO), Lutetium OxyorthoSilicate (LSO), Gadolinium OxyorthoSilicate (GSO), and the newer Lutetium-Yttrium OxyorthoSilicate (LYSO) can detect the radioactive events occurring in PET imaging. PET radiopharmaceuticals contain a positron emitter that undergoes positron (β^+) decay, emitting a positron (β^+) and a neutrino (ν). The emitted positron travels a very short distance in surrounding tissue and then combines with an electron to annihilate and release a pair of 511

KeV photons at almost exactly 180° apart. It is these photons (and not the actual positrons) that are almost simultaneously detected by the scintillation detectors in PET scanners as coincidence events and millions of such coincidences are acquired and stored in sinogram form as Lines of Responses (LORs) that basically connect the detector pair in which the coincidence occurs. This emission data are then digitally reconstructed and attenuation correction algorithms are applied to generate high-resolution tomographic images depicting the radiopharmaceutical biodistribution.

CARDIAC PET RADIOPHARMACEUTICALS

Several PET radiopharmaceuticals have been evaluated to assess various myocardial biochemical parameters including perfusion, glucose and oxidative metabolism, hypoxia, autonomic innervation, and others. Currently, Rb-82 chloride and N-13 ammonia are approved by the Food and Drug Administration and used clinically for myocardial perfusion studies and F-18 fluorodeoxyglucose (FDG) is used for evaluating myocardial glucose metabolism. Other PET radiopharmaceuticals are not routinely used clinically but are widely used in the research realm. These include O-15 water and C-11 acetate. O-15 water used for evaluating myocardial perfusion is considered an ideal perfusion agent as it is freely diffusible and metabolically inert, but requires complex mathematical algorithms and generates images that are too noisy for visual interpretation. C-11 acetate can reliably assess myocardial oxidative metabolism but is not useful in ischemic myocardium and use is further hampered by difficulty in optimal delivery/distribution from cyclotron site to imaging center owing to its short half-life and relatively long synthesis time for C-11 tagged radiopharmaceuticals. Several other agents to assess cardiac autonomic nervous system, cardiac receptors, cardiac hypoxia, and cardiac gene therapy assessment are also in the research or translational environment.

N-13, a cyclotron-produced radioisotope, has relatively optimal physical characteristics and biologic properties to generate excellent PET images (9.9-minute half-life, 1.19 MeV average positron energy, and about 0.4-mm average positron range). It shows prolonged myocardial retention as a result of its high extraction rate and metabolic trapping via the glutamine synthetase pathway. Although it is feasible to perform exercise stress perfusion studies with N-13 ammonia in contrast to Rb-82 chloride (which allows only pharmaceutical stressing), this is not a substantial advantage in the pediatric population (especially younger children).

Rb-82, a generator-produced radioisotope, has slightly less favorable physical characteristics (higher positron energy of 3.15 MeV and longer average positron range of about 2.8 mm), that slightly hinders its inherent spatial resolution. Its ultra-short half-life of 75 seconds enables the study to be completed very fast (within 1 hour or less) but also necessitates administration of higher doses of the radiopharmaceutical. In addition, the extremely short half-life of Rb-82 allows (or rather necessitates) imaging almost during effect of the pharmacologic stressing agent, thus acquiring "pure" stress images (and not poststress images) not contaminated by residual radiotracer from the rest injection and with minimal background activity. Although Rb-82 does not require an in-house cyclotron because it is generator produced and each generator can be used for up to a month, the generator itself is quite expensive, dictating a certain number of minimum studies to justify its use financially. Rb-82 chloride shows pharmacologically similar behavior to potassium and thallium-201 and needs an active Na/K-ATPase pump for intracellular transport.

F-18 FDG, by far remains the most widely used PET radiopharmaceutical. F-18 is a cyclotron-produced radioisotope with a half-life of 110 minutes. This obviates the need for an on-site cyclotron, as it is feasible to transport the radiopharmaceutical to imaging centers located 2 to 3 hours away from the cyclotron site. The half-life also eases time frame restrictions on study protocols but is low enough not to cause prolonged exposure. Moreover, its optimal physical characteristics (0.63-MeV average positron energy and 0.3-mm average positron range) produce high-resolution PET images. Glucose transporters (mainly GLUT-1 and GLUT-4) are responsible for intracellular transport of FDG wherein it undergoes phosphorylation to FGD-6-phosphate by the enzyme hexokinase. However, FDG-6-phosphate is not a good substrate for enzymes phosphohexose isomerase or glucose-6-phosphate dehydrogenase and hence it does not undergo further metabolism. FDG-6-phosphate cannot diffuse out of the cells and it remains metabolically trapped within the cells (Fig. 1). Cells and tissues with higher rates of glucose metabolism show up-regulation of glucose transporters and increased glucose (and consequently FDG) uptake. All the activity on FDG PET imaging represents FDG-6-phosphate alone and the images represent a map of glucose metabolism in the body as there is no further metabolism of FDG-6-phosphate and there is no further radioactive

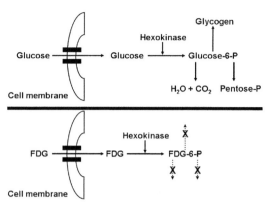

Fig. 1. Schema for FDG metabolic-trapping in cardiac myocytes.

decay of F-18 to any daughter molecules. Cells and tissues with higher rates of glucose metabolism show up-regulation of glucose transporters and increased glucose (and consequently FDG) uptake. Areas with increased FDG uptake represent areas with high glucose metabolism (like cancer cells, inflammatory cells, or other cells with high glucose metabolism like gray matter cells in brain or cardiac myocytes under certain circumstances). The substrate preferred by myocardium for its energy needs is highly variable and several factors including the hormonal milieu and available substrate concentration affect it substantially. A fasting environment with low plasma glucose as well as insulin levels but high plasma free fatty acid (FFA) levels promotes FFA as the preferred myocardial substrate. On the other hand, in a postprandial setting with increased plasma glucose and consequently increased insulin levels, as well as under ischemic and hypoxic conditions, glucose is favored over FFA as the preferred substrate by the myocytes.[9–18] This is the underlying basis for using FDG to assess myocardial glucose metabolism (and C-11 acetate to assess myocardial oxidative metabolism). **Table 1** summarizes the commonly used cardiac PET radiopharmaceuticals in the pediatric population.

CARDIAC PET PROTOCOLS

The PET imaging protocol depends on the indication for the study and the radiopharmaceutical being used. PET myocardial perfusion imaging (MPI) protocol is slightly different using Rb-82 chloride versus N-13 ammonia. With N-13 ammonia, typically a rest-stress protocol is followed consisting of transmission scan followed by an initial set of rest emission images of the heart obtained 5 minutes after the intravenous administration of N-13 ammonia. After an interval of about 50 to 60 minutes during which the tracer is allowed to decay completely, either pharmacologic (more common) or exercise (technically challenging but feasible; may not be practical in infants and small children) stressing is performed and a subsequent set of stress emission images of the heart are obtained 5 minutes after another intravenous administration of N-13 ammonia followed by a second transmission scan. The protocol using Rb-82 is largely similar except that there is almost no delay between the rest and stress studies in view of the extremely short half-life of Rb-82 (**Fig. 2**). Since the emission images are obtained very shortly (about 1 to 3 minutes) after radiopharmaceutical administration, only pharmacologic stress is feasible with Rb-82 chloride as the perfusion agent.

Absolute quantification of regional myocardial perfusion/blood flow is feasible and validated with PET. This requires the ability to accurately measure the rapid initial changes of radiopharmaceutical occurring in the tissue of interest immediately after radiopharmaceutical administration until a steady-state situation is achieved. The high temporal and spatial resolution of PET imaging coupled with the short half-life of PET radioisotopes allows dynamic acquisition of PET data. Various tracer kinetic models are employed to derive absolute quantification of regional myocardial blood flow.[7,8] However, this is not routinely practiced in the standard clinical setting (usually only static images are obtained) and is more labor intensive, requiring rigorous data reprocessing.

Table 1				
Commonly used cardiac PET radiopharmaceuticals				
Radiopharmaceutical	Radioisotope	Source	Half-life	Utility
C-11 acetate	C-11	Cyclotron	20 min	Cardiac oxidative metabolism
F-18 FDG	F-18	Cyclotron	110 min	Glucose metabolism
N-13 ammonia	N-13	Cyclotron	9.9 min	Myocardial perfusion
Rb-82 chloride	Rb-82	Generator	75 s	Myocardial perfusion

Abbreviation: FDG, fluorodeoxyglucose.

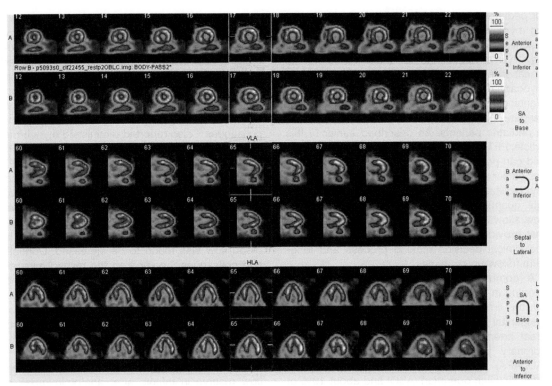

Fig. 2. Rb-82 PET images from a patient using the standard Persantine infusion protocol. PET images were acquired at rest and then at stress on the same day with CT attenuation correction. The study shows moderately decreased tracer uptake in the inferior/posterior walls from the base to the apex with partially reversible perfusion defect, consistent with coronary artery disease in the right coronary artery distribution.

The calculated regional myocardial blood flow is generally provided in terms of mL per minute per 100 g of myocardial tissue.

The protocol to assess myocardial glucose metabolism requires some additional preparation. Cardiac glucose uptake can be highly variable and patients are usually asked to fast for at least 4 hours (preferably overnight) before study. The fasting blood sugar level (BSL) is expected to be less than 110 mg/dL in most patients in this patient population and after checking the fasting BSL, an oral glucose loading dose is given (except in neonates) about 60 minutes before FDG administration to facilitate high FDG uptake by the cardiac myocytes. However, older children with known diabetes may require additional insulin supplementation with the glucose loading dose to maintain a BSL between 110 and 140 mg/dL. After 60 more minutes, dedicated PET images of the heart are obtained. To assess myocardial viability, a myocardial glucose metabolism study is routinely coupled with a myocardial perfusion study (rest only is adequate), if the perfusion study has not been performed recently or is not available for direct comparison with the metabolism images.

Although the pediatric cardiac PET protocols are similar to adult cardiac PET imaging protocols, there are few special considerations. An important issue is dose of the administered radiopharmaceuticals. This usually needs to be adjusted for the child's body weight rather than a standard dose that is usually prescribed in adults. Moreover, because the protocols last for a relatively long time, sedation is necessary in most patients. Several sedation protocols are in clinical use including chloral hydrate, fentanyl, and midazolam[19,20] and it is best to collaborate with a pediatric anesthesiologist to achieve optimal sedation and acquire high-quality images. In addition to sedation, familiarity and experience with handling pediatric concerns and providing an environment that will ease the child's nervousness and keep him or her calm and cooperative also help significantly to achieve optimal results.

CLINICAL APPLICATIONS OF PEDIATRIC CARDIAC PET STUDIES

The applications of pediatric cardiac PET are still evolving. At the current time, the major indications for pediatric cardiac PET studies include assessing myocardial perfusion for ischemia as well as coronary flow reserve and assessing myocardial viability in several congenital and acquired cardiac diseases in children.[21–23] Accurate assessment of myocardial perfusion is important in therapeutic planning as well as posttreatment follow-up of various congenital and acquired heart diseases in pediatric patients. As described earlier in this article, PET offers several advantages over SPECT and can potentially detect myocardial abnormalities earlier allowing earlier therapeutic intervention and facilitate a better outcome. In addition, absolute quantification of regional myocardial blood flow allows assessment of coronary flow reserve that provides supplemental information to aid in the clinical decision making process and long-term follow-up strategies.

A common indication for cardiac perfusion imaging in children is to detect perfusion abnormalities in patients after corrective surgery for congenital heart disorders like transposition of great arteries (TGA) or anomalous origin of left coronary artery from the pulmonary artery (ALCAPA). TGA is now usually corrected by the arterial switch operation (ASO) and about 10% of such patients suffer from adverse events related to coronary perfusion abnormalities (myocardial infarction and sudden death as a result of coronary occlusion).[24,25] Perfusion defects in patients who had undergone ASO were reported by Vogel and colleagues[26] using isoproterenol stress thallium-201 computed scintigraphy. Weindling and colleagues[1] reported regional myocardial ischemia in patients with history of ASO by demonstrating reversible perfusion defects on exercise stress myocardial perfusion imaging with 99m-technetium–labeled sestamibi SPECT technique. Subsequently, several investigators evaluated myocardial perfusion with cardiac PET imaging in this patient population and detected perfusion abnormalities in asymptomatic patients without evidence of contractile dysfunction. Although the incidence of reversible perfusion defects was slightly lower on PET imaging compared with SPECT imaging, there was diminished coronary flow reserve as suggested by lower adenosine-induced hyperemic myocardial blood flow.[27–29] Myocardial flow reserve was also found to be impaired with adenosine stress N13-ammonia PET myocardial perfusion imaging in patients who underwent the earlier Mustard or atrial switch repair for TGA.[30] Bengel and colleagues[27] attributed the impaired coronary flow reserve to possible altered vaso-reactivity or endothelial dysfunction but the long-term prognostic significance of this remained unclear at

that time. However, Hauser and colleagues[31] subsequently reported reduced coronary flow reserve as detected by PET myocardial perfusion imaging correlated significantly with impaired ventricular function in the absence of coronary stenosis by angiography in children late after Fontan-like operations and this was felt to be risk factor for long-term outcome. Singh and colleagues[32] also reported diminished myocardial flow reserve in long-term survivors of ALCAPA repair using adenosine stress N13-ammonia PET myocardial perfusion imaging and suggested that this may limit cardiac output reserve and impair exercise tolerance. In most of the studies mentioned previously, along with the diminished coronary flow reserve, the resting myocardial blood flow was found to be increased. Donnelly and colleagues[33] compared the resting myocardial blood flow and coronary flow reserve in infants who had anatomic repair of a congenital heart lesion with infants who had Norwood palliation for hypoplastic left heart syndrome. Using adenosine stress PET myocardial perfusion imaging with N-13 ammonia, they reported increased resting myocardial blood flow with diminished coronary flow reserve in infants after anatomic repair of a congenital heart lesion but decreased resting as well as maximal (adenosine stimulated) myocardial blood flow leading to diminished coronary flow reserve in infants after Norwood palliation for hypoplastic left heart syndrome. The authors proposed that decreased coronary flow reserve along with reduced oxygen delivery to the ventricular myocardium may partly be responsible for the unfavorable outcome seen after Norwood palliation.

Hernandez-Pampaloni and colleagues[21] have reported significant correlation between PET myocardial perfusion and metabolism imaging and echocardiography, angiography as well histopathology in infants and children with suspected coronary abnormalities. They confirmed that PET perfusion-metabolism imaging can reliably and accurately assess myocardial viability in pediatric population. Rickers and colleagues[34] used information from PET myocardial viability evaluation using gated FDG PET to determine the treatment approach for infants and children with suspected infarction after ASO for TGA. They detected viable myocardium in akinetic or hypokinetic regions with corresponding coronary stenosis/occlusion and chose revascularization as the preferred treatment in this setting. Follow-up revealed recovery of full function in these infants. Patients with impaired glucose metabolism indicating scarring did not undergo revascularization and were steered toward medical management. A few patients had

NH₃

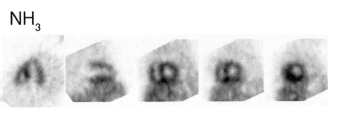

FDG

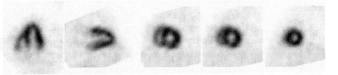

Horizontal Vertical
←—— Long Axis —→ ←—— Short Axis ——→

Fig. 3. PET perfusion-metabolism viability imaging in an infant with history of ASO for TGA. N-13 ammonia perfusion PET demonstrates perfusion defects in the lateral wall, apex, and anterior wall with preserved glucose metabolism in those areas indicating myocardial viability.

normal glucose metabolism in areas that were akinetic or dyskinetic on echocardiography and were also found to have to have no coronary stenosis or occlusion angiographically. These areas were felt to represent myocardial stunning. **Figs. 3** and **4** demonstrate myocardial viability with PET perfusion-metabolism imaging after ASO in patients with TGA.

Another condition that has been relatively well evaluated with cardiac PET imaging is Kawasaki disease. Also known as mucocutaneous lymph node syndrome, it is a disease of unknown etiology characterized by acute vasculitis of mainly medium-sized arteries including the coronaries. Cardiac manifestations of Kawasaki disease are by far the most clinically significant manifestations and are generally caused by involvement of the

coronaries that can progress from vasculitis to aneurysms to stenosis/occlusion leading to myocardial infarction and scarring. In untreated cases, coronary manifestations can occur in up to 40% of patients. Cardiac PET imaging has been shown to be useful in assessing the various coronary manifestations of Kawasaki disease during its natural history of the disease progression. Ohmochi and colleagues[35] demonstrated diminished myocardial flow reserve in the presence of coronary aneurysms associated with Kawasaki disease. Yoshibayashi and colleagues[36] assessed the significance of newly appearing abnormal Q waves and their disappearance in patients with Kawasaki disease with PET perfusion-metabolism myocardial viability imaging. They found that the new appearance of abnormal

NH₃

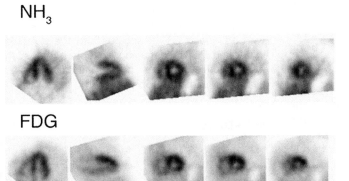

FDG

Horizontal Vertical
←—— Long Axis —→ ←—— Short Axis ——→

Fig. 4. PET perfusion-metabolism viability imaging in an infant with history of ASO for TGA. N-13 ammonia perfusion PET demonstrates perfusion defects in the lateral and inferior walls with decreased glucose metabolism in those areas as well indicating nonviable myocardium/scarring.

Q waves in patients with Kawasaki disease indicates myocardial injury but a large number of them are associated with metabolically active myocardium and their early disappearance is usually associated with viable myocardium. Moreover, myocardial viability evaluation using PET perfusion-metabolism imaging has shown value in assessing treatment. Hwang and colleagues[37] found PET abnormalities in about 60% of patients with acute and subacute phases of Kawasaki disease and in about 40% of patients with convalescent phase of Kawasaki disease. Different therapies during the acute phase of Kawasaki disease were not significantly effective in avoiding or diminishing myocardial injury, notwithstanding the absence of coronary arterial abnormalities. However, the 5-day regimen of intravenous immunoglobulin (IVIG) therapy resulted in significantly lower incidence of PET abnormalities compared with the single-day regimen. Iemura and colleagues[38] investigated the long-term consequences of regressed aneurysms after Kawasaki disease and found persisting abnormal vascular wall morphology and vascular dysfunction at the site of regressed coronary aneurysms in patients with previous Kawasaki disease. Ischemic perfusion defects have been reported on scintigraphic imaging even with normal coronary angiography[39] and hence long-term follow-up is recommended in these patients as they seem to be at risk for developing coronary abnormalities including atherosclerosis in adult life. PET MPI can play a central role in the follow-up of myocardial perfusion status in this setting as it can detect even a small degree of perfusion abnormality. In fact, several investigators have confirmed decreased hyperemic-induced myocardial blood flow and diminished coronary flow reserve in patients with history Kawasaki disease with angiographically normal coronary arteries.[40–43] This is believed to be related to endothelial dysfunction with residual damage in the coronary microcirculation and impaired coronary vasoreactivity. Thus, in addition to being useful in assessing the cardiac perfusion and viability manifestations of the various coronary manifestations occurring in Kawasaki disease, cardiac PET is also valuable in monitoring the consequences of coronary involvement with Kawasaki disease, and long-term follow-up.

Thus, cardiac PET imaging provides a safe, reliable, and accurate means of assessing various myocardial processes including perfusion, flow reserve, and metabolism in a wide range of congenital and acquired heart conditions such as Kawasaki disease, coronary artery anomalies, cardiac transplant vasculopathy, valvular heart disease, and postsurgical correction of various congenital heart diseases like TGA, ALCAPA, and others. It also offers precise assessments of the coronary blood flow and flow reserve over time for long-term follow-up.

SUMMARY

In summary, cardiac PET imaging can play a significant role in assessing and managing children with congenital and acquired heart disorders but remains largely underused for multiple reasons, not related to the accuracy or usefulness of the modality. PET offers several advantages over other imaging modalities in the evaluation of cardiac perfusion and metabolism. The technique for cardiac PET imaging has been validated by several investigators. There is sufficient literature to establish the utility of this imaging modality in the pediatric population and this merits larger prospective studies to confirm the long-term clinical significance of the findings on these highly sophisticated studies. Specifically, the implications of decreased coronary flow reserve and perfusion abnormalities after surgical correction of a congenital heart lesion in the absence of demonstrable coronary stenosis on angiography remain unclear. Further work with cardiac PET may provide a broader understanding of myocardial perfusion and coronary flow reserve in infants. Myocardial perfusion assessment (with SPECT or PET) in combination with myocardial glucose metabolism with FDG PET is the gold standard for evaluating myocardial viability.[44] Current work focusing on evaluation of cardiac innervation, cardiac receptor function and noninvasive cardiac gene therapy assessment with PET imaging has tremendous potential to revolutionize cardiac evaluation. Awareness and widespread availability of PET systems is expected to increase use of cardiac PET applications in the pediatric population. The advent of integrated PET/CT systems with advanced CT technology and the possible integrated PET/MR imaging systems opens even more promising future possibilities for cardiac evaluation in a one-stop approach.

REFERENCES

1. Weindling SN, Wernovsky G, Colan SD, et al. Myocardial perfusion, function and exercise tolerance after the arterial switch operation. J Am Coll Cardiol 1994;23(2):424–33.
2. Bonhoeffer P, Bonnet D, Piéchaud JF, et al. Coronary artery obstruction after the arterial switch operation for transposition of the great arteries in newborns. J Am Coll Cardiol 1997;29(1):202–6.

3. Krishnamurthy R. Pediatric cardiac MRI: anatomy and function. Pediatr Radiol 2008;38(Suppl 2): S192–9.

4. Machac J. Gated positron emission tomography for the assessment of myocardial perfusion and function. In: Germano G, Berman DS, editors. Clinical gated cardiac SPECT. 2nd edition. Malden (MA): Blackwell Futura; 2006. p. 285–316.

5. ICRP Committee 2 Radiation dose to patients from radiopharmaceuticals. A report of a Task Group of Committee 2 of the International Commission on Radiological Protection. Ann ICRP 1987;18:1–377.

6. Hernandez-Pampaloni N. Cardiovascular applications. In: Charron M, editor. Practical pediatric PET imaging. New York: Springer; 2006. p. 407–27.

7. Hutchins GD, Schwaiger M, Rosenspire KC, et al. Noninvasive quantification of regional blood flow in the human heart using N-13 ammonia and dynamic positron emission tomographic imaging. J Am Coll Cardiol 1990;15(5):1032–42.

8. Kuhle WG, Porenta G, Huang SC, et al. Quantification of regional myocardial blood flow using 13N-ammonia and reoriented dynamic positron emission tomographic imaging. Circulation 1992;86(3): 1004–17.

9. Liedtke AJ. Alterations of carbohydrate and lipid metabolism in the acutely ischemic heart. Prog Cardiovasc Dis 1981;23:321–6.

10. Schelbert HR, Henze E, Phelps ME, et al. Assessment of regional myocardial ischemia by positron-emission computed tomography. Am Heart J 1982; 103(4 Pt 2):588–97.

11. Taegtmeyer H. Myocardial metabolism. In: Phelps M, Mazziotta J, Schelbert H, editors. Positron emission tomography and autoradiography: principles and applications for the brain and heart. New York: New York Raven Press; 1986. p. 149–95.

12. Schwaiger M, Fishbein MC, Block M, et al. Metabolic and ultrastructural abnormalities during ischemia in canine myocardium: noninvasive assessment by positron emission tomography. J Mol Cell Cardiol 1987;19:259–69.

13. Kalff V, Schwaiger M, Nguyen N, et al. The relationship between myocardial blood flow and glucose uptake in ischemic canine myocardium determined with fluorine-18-deoxyglucose. J Nucl Med 1992; 33:1346–53.

14. Marwick TH, MacIntyre WJ, Lafont A, et al. Metabolic responses of hibernating and infracted myocardium to revascularization: a follow-up study of regional perfusion, function, and metabolism. Circulation 1992;85:1347–53.

15. Vanoverschelde JL, Wijns W, Depre C, et al. Mechanisms of chronic regional postischemic dysfunction in humans: new insights from the study of noninfarcted collateral-dependent myocardium. Circulation 1993;87:1513–23.

16. Liedtke AJ, Renstrom B, Hacker TA, et al. Effects of moderate repetitive ischemia on myocardial substrate utilization. Am J Phys 1995;269(1 Pt 2):H246–53.

17. Liedtke AJ, Renstrom B, Nellis SH, et al. Mechanical and metabolic functions in pig hearts after 4 days of chronic coronary stenosis. J Am Coll Cardiol 1995; 26:815–25.

18. Liedtke AJ. The origins of myocardial substrate utilization from an evolutionary perspective: the enduring role of glucose in energy metabolism. J Mol Cell Cardiol 1997;29:1073–86.

19. American Academy of Pediatrics Committee on Drugs. Guidelines for monitoring and management of pediatric patients during and after sedation for diagnostic and therapeutic procedures. Pediatrics 1992;89(6 pt 1):1110–5.

20. American Society of Anesthesiologists Task Force on Sedation and Analgesia by Non-Anesthesiologists. Practice guidelines for sedation and analgesia by non-anesthesiologists. Anesthesiology 2002; 96(4):1004–17.

21. Hernandez-Pampaloni M, Allada V, Fishbein MC, et al. Myocardial perfusion and viability by positron emission tomography in infants and children with coronary abnormalities: correlation with echocardiography, coronary angiography, and histopathology. J Am Coll Cardiol 2003;41(4):618–26.

22. Singh TP, Muzik O, Forbes TF, et al. Positron emission tomography myocardial perfusion imaging in children with suspected coronary abnormalities. Pediatr Cardiol 2003;24(2):138–44.

23. Chhatriwalla AK, Prieto LR, Brunken RC, et al. Preliminary data on the diagnostic accuracy of rubidium-82 cardiac PET perfusion imaging for the evaluation of ischemia in a pediatric population. Pediatr Cardiol 2008;29(4):732–8.

24. Tanel RE, Wernovsky G, Landzberg MJ, et al. Coronary artery abnormalities detected at cardiac catheterization following the arterial switch operation for transposition of the great arteries. Am J Cardiol 1995;76(3):153–7.

25. Wernovsky G, Mayer JE Jr, Jonas RA, et al. Factors influencing early and late outcome of the arterial switch operation for transposition of the great arteries. J Thorac Cardiovasc Surg 1995;109(2): 289–301 [discussion 301–2].

26. Vogel M, Smallhorn JF, Gilday D, et al. Assessment of myocardial perfusion in patients after the arterial switch operation. J Nucl Med 1991;32(2):237–41.

27. Bengel FM, Hauser M, Duvernoy CS, et al. Myocardial blood flow and coronary flow reserve late after anatomical correction of transposition of the great arteries. J Am Coll Cardiol 1998;32(7):1955–61.

28. Yates RW, Marsden PK, Badawi RD, et al. Evaluation of myocardial perfusion using positron emission tomography in infants following a neonatal arterial switch operation. Pediatr Cardiol 2000;21(2):111–8.

29. Hauser M, Bengel FM, Kühn A, et al. Myocardial blood flow and flow reserve after coronary reimplantation in patients after arterial switch and ross operation. Circulation 2001;103(14):1875–80.

30. Singh TP, Humes RA, Muzik O, et al. Myocardial flow reserve in patients with a systemic right ventricle after atrial switch repair. J Am Coll Cardiol 2001; 37(8):2120–5.

31. Hauser M, Bengel FM, Kühn A, et al. Myocardial perfusion and coronary flow reserve assessed by positron emission tomography in patients after Fontan-like operations. Pediatr Cardiol 2003;24(4): 386–92.

32. Singh TP, Di Carli MF, Sullivan NM, et al. Myocardial flow reserve in long-term survivors of repair of anomalous left coronary artery from pulmonary artery. J Am Coll Cardiol 1998;31(2):437–43.

33. Donnelly JP, Raffel DM, Shulkin BL, et al. Resting coronary flow and coronary flow reserve in human infants after repair or palliation of congenital heart defects as measured by positron emission tomography. J Thorac Cardiovasc Surg 1998;115(1):103–10.

34. Rickers C, Sasse K, Buchert R, et al. Myocardial viability assessed by positron emission tomography in infants and children after the arterial switch operation and suspected infarction. J Am Coll Cardiol 2000;36(5):1676–83.

35. Ohmochi Y, Onouchi Z, Oda Y, et al. Assessment of effects of intravenous dipyridamole on regional myocardial perfusion in children with Kawasaki disease without angiographic evidence of coronary stenosis using positron emission tomography and H2(15)O. Coron Artery Dis 1995;6(7):555–9.

36. Yoshibayashi M, Tamaki N, Nishioka K, et al. Regional myocardial perfusion and metabolism assessed by positron emission tomography in children with Kawasaki disease and significance of abnormal Q waves and their disappearance. Am J Cardiol 1991;68(17):1638–45.

37. Hwang B, Liu RS, Chu LS, et al. Positron emission tomography for the assessment of myocardial viability in Kawasaki disease using different therapies. Nucl Med Commun 2000;21(7):631–6.

38. Iemura M, Ishii M, Sugimura T, et al. Long term consequences of regressed coronary aneurysms after Kawasaki disease: vascular wall morphology and function. Heart 2000;83(3):307–11.

39. Hamaoka K, Onouchi Z, Ohmochi Y. Coronary flow reserve in children with Kawasaki disease without angiographic evidence of coronary stenosis. Am J Cardiol 1992;69(6):691–2.

40. Muzik O, Paridon SM, Singh TP, et al. Quantification of myocardial blood flow and flow reserve in children with a history of Kawasaki disease and normal coronary arteries using positron emission tomography. J Am Coll Cardiol 1996;28(3):757–62.

41. Furuyama H, Odagawa Y, Katoh C, et al. Assessment of coronary function in children with a history of Kawasaki disease using (15)O-water positron emission tomography. Circulation 2002;105(24):2878–84.

42. Furuyama H, Odagawa Y, Katoh C, et al. Altered myocardial flow reserve and endothelial function late after Kawasaki disease. J Pediatr 2003;142(2): 149–54.

43. Hauser M, Bengel F, Kuehn A, et al. Myocardial blood flow and coronary flow reserve in children with "normal" epicardial coronary arteries after the onset of Kawasaki disease assessed by positron emission tomography. Pediatr Cardiol 2004;25(2): 108–12.

44. Bax JJ, Visser FC, van Lingen A, et al. Metabolic imaging using F18-fluorodeoxyglucose to assess myocardial viability. Int J Cardiovasc Imaging 1997;13(2):145–55 [discussion 157–60].

The Role of PET/CT in the Monitoring and Diagnosis of Pediatric Inflammatory Bowel Disease

Roland Hustinx, MD, PhD[a],*, Edouard Louis, MD, PhD[b]

KEYWORDS

- Crohn's disease • Ulcerative colitis • PET/CT
- FDG • Inflammatory Bowel Disease

Inflammatory bowel diseases (IBD) are chronic immune-mediated inflammatory diseases affecting the gastrointestinal tract. Classically, two subtypes of IBD are recognized: ulcerative colitis (UC), characterized by a continuous mucosal inflammation starting in the rectum and involving a variable part of the colon upward; and Crohn's disease (CD), characterized by focal transmural inflammation involving most often the terminal ileum and parts of the colon, but that could affect any part of the gastrointestinal tract from the mouth to the anus. IBD are multifactorial polygenic diseases. A large number of genes definitely associated with IBD have been discovered, first in CD[1–6] and more recently in UC.[7–9] These genes are mainly involved in mucosal barrier integrity, innate immunity, and adaptative immunity. Environmental factors are also implicated, although they are less well characterized. It is currently thought that IBD are at least partly caused by an abnormal immune and inflammatory reaction to the luminal content of the gastrointestinal tract. Recent data from Europe indicate a steady increase in the incidence and prevalence of IBD, particularly in the pediatric population in which a combined incidence of 5 to 10 out of 100,000 per year has been reported.[10]

IBD are chronic relapsing diseases. In UC, periods of activity and remission are often well delineated, while CD is more often a chronic active disease with a continuous inflammatory process. Also, probably because of its essentially mucosal inflammation, UC is usually not associated with the development of intestinal complications. In contrast, CD is frequently complicated by fibrotic or deeply penetrating lesions, leading to intestinal strictures or fistulas. These complications affect a minority of the patients at the time of diagnosis but can be present in up to 50% to 60% of them after 10 years of evolution.[11] Finally, as it always affects the rectum, UC is much more accessible to surveillance by a simple rectoscopy than CD, which can affect parts of the gastrointestinal tract that are very difficult to reach. For all these reasons, CD is a disease probably much more difficult to monitor than UC.

MONITORING INFLAMMATORY BOWEL DISEASES

Major progresses have been made over the last 10 years in clinical biology, medical imaging, and endoscopy, now giving the clinician a broad range of techniques to optimize disease diagnosis and

[a] Department of Medicine, Division of Nuclear Medicine, University Hospital of Liège, Campus Universitaire du Sart Tilman B35, 4000 Liège, Belgium

[b] Department of Medicine, Division of Gastroenterology, University Hospital of Liège, Campus Universitaire du Sart Tilman B35, 4000 Liège, Belgium

* Corresponding author.

E-mail address: rhustinx@chu.ulg.ac.be (R. Hustinx).

PET Clin 3 (2009) 597–603

doi:10.1016/j.cpet.2009.04.003

monitoring. Even if ileo-colonoscopy has been considered over the last 20 to 30 years as the gold standard, both for diagnosis and monitoring, a series of weaknesses of this technique have been highlighted: it is a rather invasive procedure, often requiring deep sedation, a large part of the small bowel can not be reached, and it only can assess mucosal inflammation while deeper layers are not seen. As previously stated, these limitations only mildly affect UC monitoring because of its pure mucosal character and its systematic distal location. In contrast, they represent serious weaknesses for CD. Fecal markers of inflammation, serologic markers, videocapsule endoscopy, and cross-sectional imaging with CT scanner or MR imaging are now more regularly used to try and remedy this. The most widely studied and currently used fecal marker of inflammation is fecal calprotectin. This is a protein originating form neutrophils granules, which is rather well correlated with the existence and intensity of inflammation in the colon and small bowel. It has a high sensitivity and specificity to differentiate IBD from irritable bowel syndrome, but can not properly distinguish IBD from other organic illnesses of the colon, including colonic cancer.[12–14] It can be used as a first-line test in patients for whom a suspicion of IBD exists, before contemplating endoscopic procedures. It can also have some value in disease monitoring because it is significantly correlated to endoscopic activity of IBD.[15] From this point of view however, the correlation does not appear strong enough for fecal calprotectin to be used as a universal marker with standard thresholds for remission or relapse. The value of this marker could rather be on an individual basis, with longitudinal variation in individual subjects probably being more informative. Serologic markers including anti-glycan and anti-bacterial antibodies are significantly associated with the diagnosis of IBD. Their positive and negative predictive values, however, are too low to be used as a diagnostic test.[16] These markers could have some value in predicting the development of stricturing and fistulizing complications of CD.[17]

Videocapsule endoscopy allows effective noninvasive exploration of the entire small bowel. The diagnostic yield of this procedure in patients presenting with symptoms suggesting CD is higher than the one of other modalities of small bowel exploration.[18,19] Nevertheless, the added value of the diagnosis of tiny erosive lesions of the small bowel, which represent the majority of lesions specifically diagnosed by videocapsule endoscopy, remains to be evaluated. Furthermore, the frequency of capsule impaction in CD is significantly higher than in other indications and

represents an important drawback of the technique that patency capsule may help to solve.[20] Cross-sectional imaging has also made considerable progress, and both MR imaging and CT scanner are now used in routine practice, particularly for the evaluation of perianal CD (MR imaging) and diagnosis of abdominal complications linked to IBD (CT scanner). Entero-scanner and entero-MR imaging are also emerging as very powerful tools to assess both disease extent and activity in small bowel CD.[21,22] A drawback of CT scanner is of course the irradiation, and recent studies have shown a significant increase of the total dose of irradiation over the last 20 years in CD patients in parallel to the increased use of CT scanner. Up to 15% of the CD patients now reach irradiation levels that have been associated with a significant increase in the risk of various cancers.[23] The impact of this irradiation is particularly important in younger patients, and is thus particularly critical in the pediatric setting. MR imaging does not have this disadvantage and the quality of the image definition with new generation MR imaging is now close to the one obtained with CT scanner. For entero-MR imaging and entero-CT scanner, best images throughout the small bowel are currently obtained with an enteroclysis technique, which is not very well tolerated by the patient.[24,25] Ongoing studies are also trying to assess the value of entero-colography with these cross-sectional imaging techniques. This would have the advantage of a one-shot transmural evaluation of the small bowel and the colon. However, this requires a bowel preparation similar to the one needed for colonoscopy.

The ultimate tool for the diagnosis and monitoring of IBD, particularly CD, would be noninvasive, able to assess inflammation throughout the entire gastrointestinal tract, and to quantify its intensity in the various layers of the bowel wall. PET/CT may have such profile, as it can give a whole-body evaluation of inflammation-related increased glucose uptake, without any bowel preparation.

[F-18]2-FLUORO-2-DEOXYGLUCOSE-PET IMAGING

It has long been known that [F-18]2-fluoro-2-deoxyglucose (FDG) uptake is not limited to cancer cells,[26] which has led to a growing interest in evaluating the clinical applications of FDG-PET in inflammatory and infectious diseases.[27] Bicik and colleagues first suggested using FDG-PET in patients with IBD.[28] Skehan and colleagues soon after described, in a short report published in *Lancet* in 1999, the use of FDG-PET in children with IBD.[29] Twenty-five patients, aged 7 to 18 years, were studied, including 15 with CD, 3 with UC, and 7 with nonspecific abdominal pain or diarrhea. Using a four-point scoring system for the PET images, they found a sensitivity of 81% and a specificity of 85% for detecting IBD in a patient per patient analysis. The sensitivity was 71% and the specificity was 81% in the bowel segment per segment analysis, using histology or small bowel follow-through as reference standards. The same group evaluated 65 children with newly diagnosed IBD (37 patients), symptoms suggesting recurrent disease (18 patients), or with recurrent abdominal pain (10 patients).[30] The reference study was colonoscopy or small bowel follow-through with pneumocolon. PET correctly identified active inflammatory disease in 80% of children with IBD (81.5% with CD; 76.4% with UC). None of the children with recurrent abdominal

pain had abnormal PET findings. There was a strong correlation between the PET results and the colonoscopic findings.

Neurath and colleagues studied an equally large population but none of the patients were children.[31] They performed FDG-PET, hydro-MR imaging, and granulocyte antibodies scintigraphy in 59 patients with active CD. Colonoscopy was also performed in 28 patients. All three techniques had a high specificity and FDG-PET was by far the most sensitive method in the subgroup of patients with endoscopic verification. Visual analysis of the PET images provided the best results, as the standardized uptake values (SUVs) were not correlated with any of the other indicators of CD activity, such as the Crohn's Disease Activity Index (CDAI), C-reactive protein (CRP) levels, or inflamed segments visualized at colonoscopy. In a series

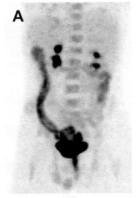

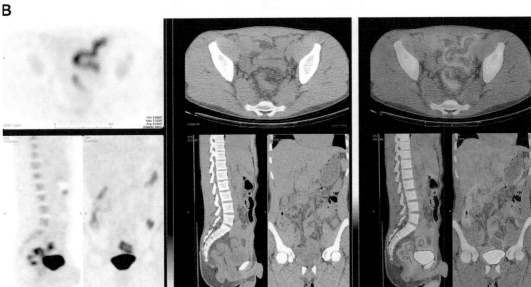

Fig.1. A 16-year-old boy with CD diagnosed 1 year before is re-evaluated before introducing anti-TNFα treatment. Serum biologic markers are markedly increased. PET/CT shows diffusely increased FDG uptake in the descending colon, sigmoid colon, and rectum [(*A*) three-dimensional-projection image, (*left panel* of *B*)], associated with wall thickening and infiltration of the perivisceral fatty tissue on the low-dose CT.

of 23 children aged 2 to 16 years, PET showed a very high sensitivity for identifying diseased segments when histology was the reference standard.[32] This population was somewhat heterogeneous, however, as it comprised 17 patients with CD, 2 patients with UC, and various other conditions. There was no separate analysis for the CD/UC patients. Using a cut-off of 1.2 for the ratio target lesion SUV_{max}/liver SUV, the sensitivity was 98%, the specificity 68%, and the accuracy 83%.

FDG PET/CT IMAGING

All the PET reports point towards a high sensitivity for detecting inflamed bowel segments, regardless of the age of the population studied.[28,29,31,32] The specificity is more variable, which is understandable considering the rather frequent presence of nonspecific bowel uptake, especially in the colon.[33] However, adding the anatomic information provided by the CT part of the PET/CT study may improve the specificity. Indeed, Kamel and colleagues showed that concomitant increased FDG uptake and abnormal soft-tissue density or

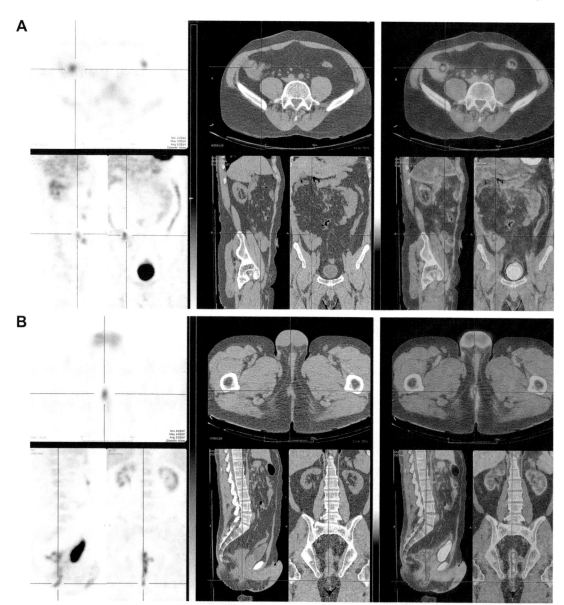

Fig. 2. A 30-year-old patient with a long-standing history of CD is investigated because of clinical signs suggesting disease re-activation. The CRP level is three times the normal level. FDG PET/CT shows focal uptake in the ileocolonic junction (A) (PET, CT, and fused PET/CT images) as well as an inflammatory fistula in the pelvis (B).

bowel wall thickening were strongly indicative of actual lesions, either malignant of inflammatory/infectious.[34] Several groups thus investigated PET/CT in the assessment of IBD. Louis and colleagues performed FDG PET/CT in 22 patients with CD and a clinical or biologic suspicion of active disease.[35] FDG PET/CT and ileocolonoscopy were obtained within 1 week. The CDAI was calculated, and serum CRP and fecal calprotectin were measured before endoscopy. The Crohn's disease endoscopy index of severity (CDEIS) was also recorded. Overall, the sensitivity for detecting all endoscopic lesions was 72.9% (35 of 48 endoscopically affected segments). However, PET/CT detected all the severe endoscopic lesions (14 out of 14 deep ulcers and strictures). The global PET/CT score significantly correlated with the endoscopic score (CDEIS),

clinical score (CDAI), and biologic findings (CRP). A receiver operating characteristic analysis showed that the optimal cut-off for the lesion-to-liver SUV ratio was 1.47. Using this cut-off, the sensitivity for detecting severe endoscopic lesions was 100% and the specificity was 67%. The CT was mostly useful for accurately localizing the areas of increased uptake, but the logistic regression analysis showed that, unlike the SUV, bowel wall thickening was not independently associated with the presence of severe lesions (**Figs. 1–3**).

Similarly, Meisner and colleagues found a significant correlation between disease activity and PET/CT findings in 12 adult patients with IBD, 7 with CD, and 5 with UC.[36] Although the PET/CT approach has yet to be validated in children, the high sensitivity for detecting severe lesions reported in the initial publications is highly

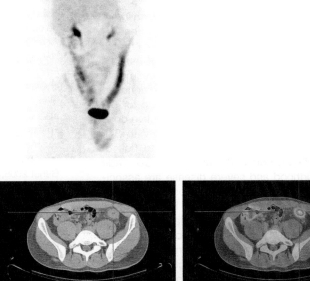

Fig. 3. CD in a 40-year-old patient. The PET shows highly increased uptake in the descending colon. (*A*) three-dimensional-projection image (*left panel* of *B*). The low-dose CT shows circumferential thickening of the same bowel segment.

encouraging. Indeed, PET/CT should not be used as a screening tool in the general population, but it may be proposed in selected patients with proven IBD and signs or symptoms of disease reactivation, as a first-line step. With a negative PET/CT result it might be possible to proceed with a conservative attitude, whereas positive PET findings should be confirmed by endoscopy. Of course, such an algorithm cannot be recommended at this stage and should be tested on a large scale, but it may be of particular interest in children and adolescents who are often very reluctant to undergo endoscopic procedures.

The combination of PET/CT may also be further exploited by performing combined PET and CT enteroclysis in the same procedure. A feasibility study was recently published by Das and colleagues, with encouraging results.[37] It remains to be seen whether the additional discomfort and slightly enhanced radiation dose associated with such a procedure are worth the diagnostic gain.

DOSIMETRY

Radiation dose is of particular concern in children, and it must be taken into account whenever ionizing radiations are being used. IBD are chronic ailments that are highly likely to require multiple explorations throughout the patient's lifetime. In a recent series of 103 patients with CD diagnosed between 1990 and 2001 and followed up for 8.9 years on average, the median total effective dose was 26.6 mSv, and ranged from 0 mSV to 279 mSV.[38] CT examinations contributed to half of the total effective dose. A diagnosis of CD made during childhood and severe disease are associated with a higher cumulative exposure.[23]

The acquisition parameters used in the study by Louis and colleagues led to a radiation dose per procedure that is largely acceptable in an adult population.[35] When the recommended doses of FDG are used in children, the effective dose from the PET procedure varies from 5 mSv in 1-year-old infants to 8.6 mSv in adolescents.[39] Considering the CT procedure, a low-dose CT may decrease by a factor of 2 the exposure, as compared to a diagnostic CT. Furthermore, it is possible that in the setting of IBD, a very low-dose CT, mainly used for attenuation correction, would be sufficient in terms of clinical efficacy. Such very low-exposure CT may decrease the radiation dose to 3% of the level resulting from a conventional CT study.[39]

REFERENCES

1. Duerr RH, Taylor KD, Brant SR, et al. A genome-wide association study identifies *IL23R* as an inflammatory bowel disease gene. Science 2006; 314(5804):1461–3.

2. Hampe J, Franke A, Rosenstiel P, et al. A genome-wide association scan of nonsynonymous SNPs identifies a susceptibility variant for Crohn disease in ATG16L1. Nat Genet 2007;39(2):207–11.

3. Libioulle C, Louis E, Hansoul S, et al. Novel Crohn disease locus identified by genome-wide association maps to a gene desert on 5p13.1 and modulates expression of PTGER4. PLoS Genet 2007; 3(4):0538–43.

4. Parkes M, Barrett JC, Prescott NJ, et al. Sequence variants in the autophagy gene IRGM and multiple other replicating loci contribute to Crohn's disease susceptibility. Nat Genet 2007;39(7):830–2.

5. Rioux JD, Xavier RJ, Taylor KD, et al. Genome-wide association study identifies new susceptibility loci for Crohn disease and implicates autophagy in disease pathogenesis. Nat Genet 2007;39(5):596–604.

6. Barrett JC, Hansoul S, Nicolae DL, et al. Genome-wide association defines more than 30 distinct susceptibility loci for Crohn's disease. Nat Genet 2008;40(8):955–62.

7. Fisher SA, Tremelling M, Anderson CA, et al. Genetic determinants of ulcerative colitis include the ECM1 locus and five loci implicated in Crohn's disease. Nat Genet 2008;40(6):710–2.

8. Franke A, Balschun T, Karlsen TH, et al. Replication of signals from recent studies of Crohn's disease identifies previously unknown disease loci for ulcerative colitis. Nat Genet 2008;40(6):713–5.

9. Franke A, Balschun T, Karlsen TH, et al. Sequence variants in IL10, ARPC2 and multiple other loci contribute to ulcerative colitis susceptibility. Nat Genet 2008;40(11):1319–23.

10. Lakatos PL. Recent trends in the epidemiology of inflammatory bowel diseases: up or down? World J Gastroenterol 2006;12(38):6102–8.

11. Louis E, Collard A, Oger AF, et al. Behaviour of Crohn's disease according to the Vienna classification: changing pattern over the course of the disease. Gut 2001;49(6):777–82.

12. Bunn SK, Bisset WM, Main MJ, et al. Fecal calprotectin: validation as a noninvasive measure of bowel inflammation in childhood inflammatory bowel disease. J Pediatr Gastroenterol Nutr 2001;33(1): 14–22.

13. Tibble JA, Sigthorsson G, Foster R, et al. Use of surrogate markers of inflammation and Rome criteria to distinguish organic from nonorganic intestinal disease. Gastroenterology 2002;123(2):450–60.

14. Konikoff MR, Denson LA. Role of fecal calprotectin as a biomarker of intestinal inflammation in inflammatory bowel disease. Inflamm Bowel Dis 2006; 12(6):524–34.

15. Jones J, Loftus EV Jr, Panaccione R, et al. Relationships between disease activity and serum and fecal

biomarkers in patients with Crohn's disease. Clin Gastroenterol Hepatol 2008;6(11):1218–24.

16. Ferrante M, Henckaerts L, Joossens M, et al. New serological markers in inflammatory bowel disease are associated with complicated disease behaviour. Gut 2007;56(10):1394–403.

17. Dubinsky MC, Kugathasan S, Mei L, et al. Increased immune reactivity predicts aggressive complicating Crohn's disease in children. Clin Gastroenterol Hepatol 2008;6(10):1105–11.

18. Triester SL, Leighton JA, Leontiadis GI, et al. A meta-analysis of the yield of capsule endoscopy compared to other diagnostic modalities in patients with non-stricturing small bowel Crohn's disease. Am J Gastroenterol 2006;101(5):954–64.

19. Shamir R, Eliakim R. Capsule endoscopy in pediatric patients. World J Gastroenterol 2008;14(26):4152–5.

20. Moy L, Levine J. Wireless capsule endoscopy in the pediatric age group: experience and complications. J Pediatr Gastroenterol Nutr 2007;44(4):516–20.

21. Liu YB, Liang CH, Zhang ZL, et al. Crohn disease of small bowel: multidetector row CT with CT enteroclysis, dynamic contrast enhancement, CT angiography, and 3D imaging. Abdom Imaging 2006; 31(6):668–74.

22. Ryan ER, Heaslip IS. Magnetic resonance enteroclysis compared with conventional enteroclysis and computed tomography enteroclysis: a critically appraised topic. Abdom Imaging 2008;33(1):34–7.

23. Desmond AN, O'Regan K, Curran C, et al. Crohn's disease: factors associated with exposure to high levels of diagnostic radiation. Gut 2008;57(11):1524–9.

24. Masselli G, Casciani E, Polettini E, et al. Comparison of MR enteroclysis with MR enterography and conventional enteroclysis in patients with Crohn's disease. Eur Radiol 2008;18(3):438–47.

25. Negaard A, Sandvik L, Berstad AE, et al. MRI of the small bowel with oral contrast or nasojejunal intubation in Crohn's disease: randomized comparison of patient acceptance. Scand J Gastroenterol 2008; 43(1):44–51.

26. Kubota R, Yamada S, Kubota K, et al. Intratumoral distribution of fluorine-18-fluorodeoxyglucose in vivo: high accumulation in macrophages and granulation tissues studied by microautoradiography. J Nucl Med 1992;33(11):1972–80.

27. Zhuang H, Yu JQ, Alavi A. Applications of fluorodeoxyglucose-PET imaging in the detection of infection and inflammation and other benign disorders. Radiol Clin North Am 2005;43(1):121–34.

28. Bicik I, Bauerfeind P, Breitbach T, et al. Inflammatory bowel disease activity measured by positron-emission tomography. Lancet 1997;350(9073):262.

29. Skehan SJ, Issenman R, Mernagh J, et al. 18F-fluorodeoxyglucose positron tomography in diagnosis of paediatric inflammatory bowel disease. Lancet 1999;354(9181):836–7.

30. Lemberg DA, Issenman RM, Cawdron R, et al. Positron emission tomography in the investigation of pediatric inflammatory bowel disease. Inflamm Bowel Dis 2005;11(8):733–8.

31. Neurath MF, Vehling D, Schunk K, et al. Noninvasive assessment of Crohn's disease activity: a comparison of 18F-fluorodeoxyglucose positron emission tomography, hydromagnetic resonance imaging, and granulocyte scintigraphy with labeled antibodies. Am J Gastroenterol 2002;97(8):1978–85.

32. Loffler M, Weckesser M, Franzius C, et al. High diagnostic value of 18F-FDG-PET in pediatric patients with chronic inflammatory bowel disease. Ann N Y Acad Sci 2006;1072:379–85.

33. Cook GJ, Maisey MN, Fogelman I. Normal variants, artefacts and interpretative pitfalls in PET imaging with 18-fluoro-2-deoxyglucose and carbon-11 methionine. Eur J Nucl Med 1999; 26(10):1363–78.

34. Kamel EM, Thumshirn M, Truninger K, et al. Significance of incidental 18F-FDG accumulations in the gastrointestinal tract in PET/CT: correlation with endoscopic and histopathologic results. J Nucl Med 2004;45(11):1804–10.

35. Louis E, Ancion G, Colard A, et al. Noninvasive assessment of Crohn's disease intestinal lesions with (18)F-FDG PET/CT. J Nucl Med 2007;48(7): 1053–9.

36. Meisner RS, Spier BJ, Einarsson S, et al. Pilot study using PET/CT as a novel, noninvasive assessment of disease activity in inflammatory bowel disease. Inflamm Bowel Dis 2007;13(8):993–1000.

37. Das CJ, Makharia G, Kumar R, et al. PET-CT enteroclysis: a new technique for evaluation of inflammatory diseases of the intestine. Eur J Nucl Med Mol Imaging 2007;34(12):2106–14.

38. Peloquin JM, Pardi DS, Sandborn WJ, et al. Diagnostic ionizing radiation exposure in a population-based cohort of patients with inflammatory bowel disease. Am J Gastroenterol 2008;103(8):2015–22.

39. Gelfand MJ, Lemen LC. PET/CT and SPECT/CT dosimetry in children: the challenge to the pediatric imager. Semin Nucl Med 2007;37(5):391–8.

Applications of PET/CT in Pediatric Patients with Fever of Unknown Origin

Mohamed Houseni, MD[a,b], Wichana Chamroonrat, MD[a],
Sabah Servaes, MD[a], Abass Alavi, MD, MD (Hon), PhD (Hon), DSc (Hon)[a],
Hongming Zhuang, MD, PhD[a,*]

KEYWORDS
- Fever of unknown origin • PET/CT
- Infections • Inflammation • Oncology

One common medical problem is prolonged fever, with or without localizing signs of disease. This problem is challenging for physicians, and it has not become less significant over the past decades despite significant development of medical technology.[1] Fever of unknown origin (FUO) in pediatrics is defined by febrile disorders that last for more than 1 week in children or 3 weeks in adolescents with elevated body temperature to measure 101°F (38.3°C) or greater that remain undiagnosed despite comprehensive inpatient and/or outpatient investigations.[2–4] It has been suggested that FUO has to be defined based on time criteria as well as the intensity of diagnostic investigations.[1] Durack and Street[5] subdivided FUO into classic, nosocomial FUO that occurs in hospitalized patients in whom infection was not manifest on admission, neutropenic FUO, and human immune deficiency virus (HIV)-associated FUO. Chronic episodic FUO is a fluctuating fever pattern for more than 4 weeks with a fever-free interval of at least 2 weeks.[6] In literature, this uncommon type of FUO is also called recurrent FUO.[7] FUO can be an atypical presentation of common disorders; however, less frequently can be a typical presentation of familiar diseases, such as rheumatoid arthritis, where diagnosis is possible after a prolonged period of observation.[8,9]

Close attention should be given to FUO, as it may present life-threatening or disabling diseases. Furthermore, fever by itself has associated problems.[8] Febrile seizure is an important problem associated with fever. It affects up to 5% of children with fever.[10,11] In the absence of preexisting neurologic damage, febrile seizures are largely innocuous.[12] In addition, fever increases cardiac function and oxygen consumption.[13] Fever higher than 105.8°F (41°C) carries the risk of brain damage. Moreover, antipyretics overdose may lead to pancreatic and hepatic insult and may impair the immunologic response to infection.[14–16]

DIFFERENTIAL DIAGNOSIS

Many factors influence the etiology of FUO. Age-related immunologic factors play a significant role in increasing susceptibility of children to infections. Bacterial infections are particularly important in the first 2 years of life.[17–20] Children with immunocompromise, sickle cell disease, severe malnutrition, HIV infection, and children on anticancer therapy are more liable to specific and unusual infections.[21–31] Long duration of FUO would suggest chronic infections, autoimmune disorders, or neoplasms. Furthermore, there is an increased chance of failure of diagnosis in

[a] Department of Radiology, The Children's Hospital of Philadelphia, 34th Street and Civic Center Boulevard, Philadelphia, PA 19104, USA
[b] Department of Radiology, National Liver Institute, 1 El-Gizera El-Wousta Street, Zamalek, 11211, Cairo, Egypt
* Corresponding author.
E-mail address: zhuang@email.chop.edu (H. Zhuang).

PET Clin 3 (2009) 605–619
doi:10.1016/j.cpet.2009.04.009

cases with prolonged FUO. The availability of the updated diagnostic tools is an important factor that helps in earlier diagnosis.[9,32] Geographic and climate factors have a strong influence on the pattern of pathogens. For example, group B β-hemolytic streptococci and self-limited viral infections are common in temperate areas.[3,33] On the other hand, malaria is common in the tropical areas.[34,35]

Generally, the main causes of FUO are infectious, rheumatologic, malignant diseases and miscellaneous disorders (**Box 1**). Infection is the most common etiology accounting for 30% to 50% of pediatric cases with FUO. Bacterial infections are the most critical. Other infectious disorders include viral, rickettsial, and parasitic infections.[8,36] Rheumatologic and connective diseases come after infections. Systemic-onset juvenile rheumatoid arthritis and systemic lupus erythematosus are the best examples that may present as FUO. However, Kawasaki disease, Wegener granulomatosis, and other vasculitic syndromes may, uncommonly, emerge as FUO.[36]

Childhood malignancies account for 7% to 13% of pediatric cases with FUO. The typical examples include acute leukemia and non-Hodgkin's lymphoma.[37,38] There are other disorders that may induce FUO as disseminated form of class I Langerhan cell histiocytosis and drug-induced fever.[39]

Chronic episodic FUO may accompany chronic disorders that are associated with fever and a prolonged intermittent course (see **Box 1**). Familial Mediterranean fever and hyper-immunoglobulin D syndrome are classic examples in this group.[36] In contrast to classic FUO, chronic episodic FUO is usually caused by rare diseases.[7] It has been reported that even with intensive investigations for cases with FUO, many children will recover before establishing a diagnosis.[40] However, dire consequence can occur for those children who have persistent fever.

DIAGNOSTIC APPROACH

Comprehensive history and repeated, careful, and targeted physical examination are invaluable to guide the diagnostic procedures. Age and time at onset, the height of the fever and its pattern, and the use of antipyretics should be documented. Cutaneous signs; mucosal, bone and joint involvement; and signs of eyes, lungs, or gastrointestinal tract problems provide important clues.[41,42] Basic laboratory tests include full blood count, C-reactive protein (CRP) and erythrocyte sedimentation rate (ESR), liver function tests, blood cultures, chest x-ray, and ultrasonographic imaging.[43]

Standard investigations and immunologic tests to rule out infection, malignancy, immunodeficiency, and auto-immune diseases have to be done before considering more invasive procedures.[44]

Investigations should be tailored according to the predominant finding of the clinical presentation.[1] Advanced imaging workup in the form of CT, magnetic resonance imaging (MR imaging), and functional scanning should be relevant and focused rather than irrelevant.[44]

CONVENTIONAL IMAGING

The decision to image a pediatric patient with FUO is complex and depends on many factors including the patient's age as well as localizing signs. Many authors suggested that a chest x-ray may help in the initial workup of patients with FUO.[8,45,46] However, some articles emphasized the presence of localizing signs before ordering a chest x-ray in an infant.[47–50] Furthermore, there can be confusion regarding the findings and their significance in infants.[51] Localizing signs are not always present, which adds to the difficulty in deciding how to image these patients.

Ultrasonography can identify masses and collections with the benefit of no ionizing radiation, but the sensitivity is less than CT.[52] Echocardiogram is useful in cases with suspected endocarditis that render negative laboratory results.[53]

CT and MR imaging may reveal unsuspected adenopathy, hepatomegaly, splenomegaly, abscesses, or masses. Cases with sinusitis, osteomyelitis, and vasculitis can be clarified with CT and MR imaging.[46,52,54] With the advent of faster MR imaging sequences, whole body MR imaging has recently been advocated in the identification of multifocal disease and has potential in identifying pathology in the patient with FUO. However, the cause of the abnormal signal cannot be discerned with MR imaging and more data are needed to determine its utility.[55]

Conventional imaging techniques are limited by the presence of substantial structural changes to render detectable abnormalities. Furthermore, discrimination of active lesions from residual post-therapeutic changes is often difficult.[56]

SCINTIGRAPHY

A variety of radiolabeled compounds are used in the detection of infections, inflammatory diseases, and some malignancies. Gallium-67-citrate is commonly used in clinical practice with high sensitivity for infectious and noninfectious inflammatory disorders as well as certain malignancies. However, the quality of Gallium-67 images is

---

Box 1
Differential diagnosis of fever of unknown origin in children

Generalized infections

Brucellosis

Borreliosis

Cat scratch disease

Leptospirosis

Malaria

Mycobacterial

Salmonellosis

Tuberculosis

Toxoplasmosis

Tularemia

Human immunodeficiency virus (HIV)

Viral infections

Localized infections

Bone and joint

Infection endocarditis

Intra-abdominal abscess

Hepatic infection

Respiratory tract infection

Urinary tract infection

Mastoiditis

Noninfectious inflammatory disorders

Juvenile rheumatoid arthritis

Systemic lupus erythematosus

Sarcoidosis

Inflammatory bowel disease

Thyroiditis

Vasculitis

Lymphangiomatosis

Cystic fibrosis

Mastocytosis

Neoplasms

Leukemia

Lymphoma

Neurologic tumors

Sarcomas

Hepatoblastoma

Miscellaneous

Central nervous dysfunction

Diabetes insipidus

Drug fever

Factious fever

Familial dysautonomia

Immunodeficiency

Infantile cortical hyperostosis

Hyperthyroidism

Fabry disease (angiokeratoma corposus diffusum)

Atrial myxoma

Icthyotic disorders

Anhidrotic ectodermal dysplasia

Chronic episodic fever of unknown origin

Familial Mediterranean fever (FMF)

Hyper-IgD and periodic fever syndrome (HIDS)

Familial Hibernian fever

Syndrome of periodic fever, aphthous stomatitis, pharyngitis, and adenitis (PFAPA)

Behçet disease

Cyclical neutropenia

Autosomal dominant FMF-like syndromes

Muckle-Wells syndrome

Familial periodic fever

---

generally poor because of their low resolution and the low contrast of the abnormalities detected. Furthermore, lack of specificity and the required delayed imaging for accurate interpretation are shortcomings for Ga-67.[57,58]

Labeled leukocyte and labeled antigranulocyte antibodies scintigraphy are useful in many acute and some chronic infections; however, they have not been extensively used in patients with FUO. Labeled leukocyte scintigraphy is related to the amount of neutrophile accumulation. In many forms of chronic infection in which very few neutrophiles are involved, such as tuberculosis, labeled leukocyte imaging is not useful. Furthermore, leukocyte imaging has poor results in cases with aseptic inflammation.[59–63]

FLUORODEOXYGLUCOSE POSITRON EMISSION TOMOGRAPHY/COMPUTED TOMOGRAPHY

Fluorodeoxyglucose positron emission tomography/CT (FDG-PET/CT) is one of the major imaging modalities in the field of oncology and it has been recognized in the management of inflammatory and infectious disorders.[64–69] The integration of PET with CT provides a unique tool combining both functional data with precise anatomic details of the body.[70,71] The role of PET/CT in the pediatric population is promising yet it is still evolving.[72–74]

Increased FDG uptake is demonstrated in lesions with a high rate of glycolysis. Neoplastic cells and activated leukocytes have been shown to accumulate FDG. This characteristic feature enables the detection of various malignancies as well as acute and chronic inflammatory processes.[75,76] Increased uptake and retention of FDG in neoplastic and activated leukocytes are related to overexpression of the surface glucose transporter proteins and overproduction of glycolytic enzymes. The surface transporter proteins that are involved in the process of malignant transformation or stimulated leukocytes are mainly GLUT-1 and GLUT-3.[77–79] Intracellular concentration of hexokinase and glucose-6-phosphatase enzymes plays an important role in the mechanism of FDG accumulation. Once entering the cell, FDG is phosphorylated by hexokinase enzyme. In contrast to glucose, FDG will not continue in the glycolytic pathway. Glucose-6-phosphatase enzyme, can dephosphorylate FDG.[80] Malignant cells demonstrate overproduction of type II hexokinase and to a lesser extent type I hexokinase. Furthermore, tumoral microenvironment with its cellular content influences FDG uptake by neoplasms.[81,82] Stimulated leukocytes show overproduction of type II hexokinase.[65,83–85] Significant FDG uptake by inflammatory cells is, especially in neutrophils, a postmigratory phenomenon of activated cells and not dependent on chemotactic stimuli.[86–89]

FDG-PET has been shown to be useful in cases with FUO. According to the literature, a final diagnosis was possible, with the help of FDG-PET and PET/CT, in 25% to 91% of cases with FUO.[90–100] Furthermore, authors demonstrated high sensitivity and specificity for FDG-PET in detecting the source of FUO.[91,93,96,101] However, accurate calculation of sensitivity and specificity is difficult, as a substantial number of patients with FUO remain undiagnosed.[80]

Lorenzen and colleagues[96] studied 16 patients with FUO in whom diagnosis was not reached by conventional methods. FDG-PET led to the final diagnosis in 11 patients (69%). In another study, FDG-PET established the final diagnosis in 54% of the cases with FUO.[90] In a study that included 48 patients, the cause of FUO was explained in 91% of cases with the help of PET/CT.[93]

PATIENT PREPARATION

Appropriate preparation is the key to successful PET/CT imaging in pediatrics. Medical procedures can cause kids' distress. In addition, parents have increased interest and awareness to be fully informed about medical procedures. It is also important to be sure the child is informed at the appropriate level of understanding. Informed consent and ethical approval should be granted.[102]

Patients should fast for at least 4 hours before injection to reduce both glucose and insulin levels. Ideally, the glucose level before injection is less than 150 mg/dL.[103] Diabetic patients may need specialist consultation to adjust blood glucose level. Furthermore, insulin injection should be 1 hour or more before FDG administration.[103,104] All relevant clinical data and medications should be available.

Child cooperation must be evaluated before imaging and the need for sedation is assessed on an individual basis. Establishing suitable intravenous access before scanning is helpful to reduce the possibilities of extravasation.[70,105] A warm environment, minimal activity, and no talking are critical during the uptake time.[106] Voiding before scanning will reduce the urinary bladder uptake and ensure comfort during the scan time. Bladder catheterization can be used when anesthesia is required.[107]

Normally brain gray matter has intense FDG uptake. Myocardial uptake varies among subjects. FDG is seen through the urinary system. Physiologic mild to moderate uptake is noted in the liver, spleen, and growth epiphyseal plates. Other sites of normal uptake include salivary glands, thymus, digestive tract, genital system, and brown fat.[108,109]

INFECTIONS

Infection is the most critical cause of FUO in children.[8] FDG-PET imaging has been shown to be highly sensitive in patients at risk of infection even when the results of other diagnostic procedures were nonconclusive.[110,111]

FDG uptake is evident in cases with pneumonia (**Fig. 1**).[112–115] Mahfouz and colleagues[111] reported high sensitivity of FDG-PET in detecting 99 cases with respiratory infections at an early stage and the results of PET imaging influenced 28% of the management. Moreover, FDG-PET has been shown to detect acute bronchitis in the correct clinical settings (**Fig. 2**).[116]

PET/CT results are promising in the detection of abdominal infections and allow for precise anatomic localization (**Figs. 3** and **4**). A high sensitivity, up to 90%, has been reported for FDG-PET in revealing abdominal and pelvic abscesses, bacterial colitis, diverticulitis, and infected vascular grafts.[97,111,117] Furthermore, the

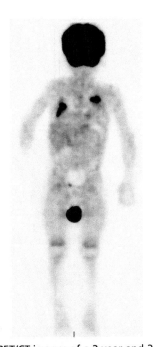

Fig. 1. The PET/CT images of a 2-year and 2-month-old nonspecified immunocompromised boy, who has known chronic lung disease and currently presented with fever, demonstrates multiple scattered regions of increased FDG uptake in both lungs, more prominent in the left upper lobe. The corresponding CT images reveal bilateral pulmonary parenchymal ground glass opacities. A week after PET/CT scan, lung biopsy in the left upper lobe was done and tissue culture revealed *Pneumocystis jiroveci*. Pneumocystis pneumonia was then established.

sensitivity and specificity of FDG-PET in cases of soft tissue infections were 96% and 70% as reported by Stumpe and colleagues.[118]

Sturm and colleagues[119] investigated 11 children with biliary cirrhosis who presented with FUO and were awaiting liver transplantation. Abnormal intrahepatic FDG uptake was detected in 5 cases. Generally, the presence of a localized intrahepatic infection does not render the patient unsuitable for transplantation, whereas a systemic infection is a relative contraindication and associated with increased risk of morbidity and mortality.[120,121]

In chronic osteomyelitis, the accuracy of FDG-PET in detecting and demonstrating the extent of disease was more than 90% **(Fig. 5)**.[122–124] FDG PET is especially useful in the evaluation of traumatic osteomyelitis because increased FDG activity in the site of an uncomplicated fracture lasts only a short period of time.[125] In malaria, using an animal model, FDG uptake by the spleen was found to be closely related to the blood-stage of malaria.[126]

It is common to notice normal colonic FDG activity in PET images in an adult patient. Therefore, evaluation of adult enterocolitis by FDG-PET can be challenging. However, such colonic FDG activity is rare or mild in infants and young children,[127] which makes it easy to use this modality to detect unexpected colitis. Ruf and colleagues[128] reported the use of FDG-PET in an 18-month-old boy and revealed unexpected infectious colitis after cardiac surgery, whereas all other imaging modalities, such as abdominal CT and ultrasound were normal. The diagnosis was confirmed by histopathological examination. The authors concluded that FDG-PET is a valuable tool in the detection of unknown inflammatory foci in children.

NONINFECTIOUS INFLAMMATION

Noninfectious inflammation comes next to infections as a cause for FUO in the pediatric group. It includes autoimmune and connective tissue diseases and granulomatous disorders, as well as miscellaneous diseases such as endocrine disorders.[6,129]

Although not investigated in children, FDG uptake by the synovium shows a significant correlation with the clinical evaluation of disease activity in patients with rheumatoid arthritis. Furthermore, PET imaging can delineate the extent of inflammation.[130–132] Systemic lupus erythematosus is another chronic inflammatory disease that affects multiple organ systems. The clinical course of the disease makes the management challenging. It has been found that PET in combination with MR imaging can be useful to differentiate functional from morphologic changes in the central nervous system involvement of systemic lupus erythematosus. These cases may show FDG hypometabolic areas in parietooccipital, cerebellar, or frontal regions.[133,134]

Childhood sarcoidosis is a disease with multisystem organ involvement, and the initial presentation as FUO is common. Patients with sarcoidosis frequently show an increased FDG uptake in mediastinal and hilar lymph nodes; the abnormal uptake may extend to the pulmonary parenchyma even in the absence of typical radiologic features.[90,92,97] Similarly, FDG avid lymphadenopathy can be the finding with tuberculosis, sarcoidlike disease, or Still's disease.[94,101] FDG-PET is known to be able to detect active sarcoid lesions undetected by Gallium scan.[135]

Crohn's disease is an inflammatory disorder of the digestive system and may cause extra-alimentary complications. Its atypical form may present as FUO.[136–138] Detection of disease activity is

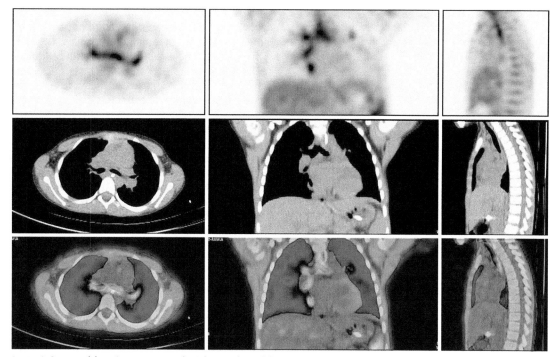

Fig. 2. A 6-year-old patient presented with cough and fever. Repeat chest x-rays were negative. Cervical, thoracic, abdominal, and pelvic contrast CT were normal. PET/CT imaging was performed to assess the source of the fever. The PET images showed intense activity in the chest, which corresponded well to all major airways on the CT and fused images and indicated bronchitis.

critical for management. FDG-PET has been able to show pathologic abnormalities within the digestive tract related to Chron's disease activity. In a study with 59 patients, FDG-PET detected 127 pathologic findings in the ileum, small bowel, and colon in 54 patients with sensitivity and specificity of 85.4% and 89.0%, respectively.[139]

Subacute thyroiditis is one of the causes of FUO in the absence of typical clinical features of thyroiditis.[129] FDG-PET imaging may demonstrate focal or diffuse FDG uptake of the thyroid in cases with subacute painless thyroiditis.[80,140,141]

Vasculitis, a condition of vessel inflammation associated with reactive mural destruction, can present as FUO. FDG-PET has been shown to be effective in cases of large-vessel vasculitis. In a study that included 26 patients with vasculitis, the degree of FDG uptake was significantly correlated to the laboratory results. The accuracy of FDG-PET in the detection of vasculitis was 78.6%.[142] In a different study, FDG-PET uptake was noted in three cases with vasculitis and three cases with pericarditis.[94]

Intravascular lymphomatosis is a rare systemic disease characterized by proliferation of lymphoid cells within the lumina of small arteries, veins, and capillaries. It has been reported that in patients

with biopsy-proven intravascular lymphomatosis who presented with FUO, diagnostic CT scan was negative but there were multiple sites of abnormal FDG activity on PET images.[143] Cystic fibrosis, another rare chronic multisystem disorder, is characterized by recurrent endobronchial infections, progressive obstructive pulmonary disease, and pancreatic insufficiency with intestinal malabsorption.[144,145] Chen and Schuster[146] in their study with 20 patients with cystic fibrosis concluded that the amount of FDG uptake by the lungs is correlated with the inflammatory burden in patients with cystic fibrosis.

MALIGNANCIES

Lymphoma, leukemia, sarcoma, and cancers of the liver, brain, kidney, colon, and pancreas can manifest as FUO.[147] PET/CT scanning in pediatric malignancies has been reported to have a high sensitivity reaching 95% and high specificity measuring up to 89%.[148]

FDG has been shown to accumulate in non-Hodgkin's and Hodgkin's lymphomas. Furthermore, FDG uptake is greater in the higher-grade lymphomas.[149–154] The incremental value of FDG-PET is the ability to demonstrate active scanning of the brain can be challenging because high FDG uptake by the gray matter can obscure pathologic lesions.[159] In spite of that, it has been shown that high-grade tumors have greater FDG uptake than low-grade tumors, which may appear isometabolic or hypometabolic in comparison with gray matter.[162–164] Furthermore, the degree of FDG uptake appears to correlate with survival.[165] Other tracers that are being evaluated to assess brain tumors that could be potentially valuable include [C-11]methionine, [F-18]3'-deoxy-3'-fluorothymidine, [C-11]methyl-L-tryptophan, and [F-18]fluoroethyl-L-tyrosine.[166–171] In neuroblastoma, another neoplasm occurring in the pediatric group, FDG, [C-11]hydroxyephedrine, and [C-11]epinephrine PET have been reported to be useful in establishing the diagnosis.[172,173]

Cases of bone sarcomas can be evaluated with PET/CT. FDG uptake in these cases helps to delineate the extent of the disease and identifies the presence of metastases.[174,175] On the other hand, rhabdomyosarcoma shows variable degree of FDG uptake, and the role of PET imaging is not established.[176–180]

Adrenocortical tumors and hepatoblastoma are examples of other tumors that can be diagnosed and monitored by PET imaging.[181,182]

Paraneoplastic syndromes are a group of clinical disorders involving nonmetastatic systemic effects that accompany malignant diseases. Fever is the most common presentation. FDG-PET is complimentary to MR imaging in assessing paraneoplastic limbic encephalitis, which is hypermetabolic on FDG-PET, and paraneoplastic cerebellar degeneration, which is hypometabolic by imaging. PET images have been shown to be able to detect abnormal brain metabolism caused by paraneoplastic encephalitis with normal brain MR images.[183] Furthermore, FDG-PET can detect occult malignant foci.[184,185]

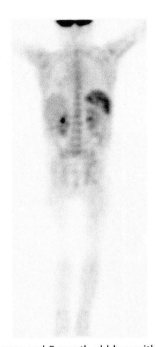

Fig. 3. A 3-year and 5-month-old boy with Di George Syndrome developed fever of unknown origin. PET images show diffusely increased FDG activity throughout the spleen without abnormality on the corresponding CT images. This finding is usually nonspecific; however, the subsequent workup found the abnormally increased splenic FDG activity was secondary to cytomegalovirus (CMV) infection.

disease sites that cannot be detected with other imaging modalities.[155–158] Currently, diagnostic PET/CT scanning is considered to have the highest accuracy among imaging modalities for evaluation of patients with lymphoma.[159–161]

Second to hematologic malignancies are neurologic tumors, which account for approximately 20% of pediatric cancers. Interpretation of PET

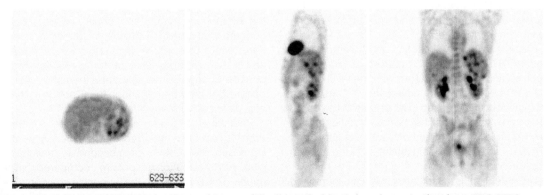

Fig. 4. This 10-year-old boy had a remote history of T-cell lymphoblastic lymphoma in the chest. FDG PET images showed no active lymphoma. However, FDG PET images found multiple hypermetabolic lesions in the liver and spleen. These lesions proved to be disseminated candidiasis.

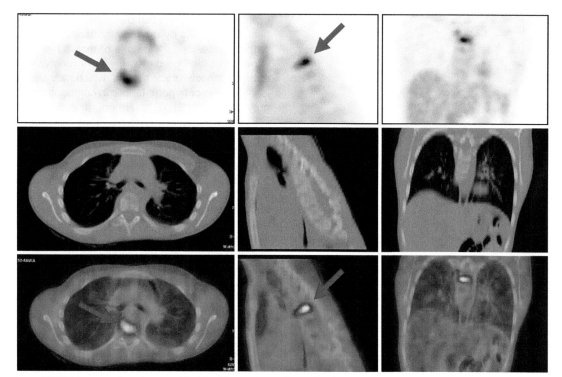

Fig. 5. PET/CT images of a 10-year-old girl with persistent lower back pain. PET images demonstrated intense FDG activity (*arrow*) in the upper thorax, which corresponded to a slightly compressed T6 vertebral body on CT and fused images. Subsequent bone biopsy proved that this patient suffered chronic osteomyelitis.

IMMUNOCOMPROMISED CHILDREN

FDG-PET is valuable in the diagnosis of infections in cases with neutropenia or lymphopenia. In a study that included seven immunocompromised children, FDG-PET imaging distinguished active from inactive lesions that appear equivocal on CT and revealed infective sites that could not be detected by CT. PET scanning allowed targeted biopsy and identification of the infective agents.[186] In another report of two immunocompromised neonates, PET imaging accurately localized the sites of invasive infections and was helpful in monitoring the management.[187]

Patients with HIV infection may demonstrate nodal FDG uptake and the pattern of uptake has been shown to be associated with the level of viral load.[188] Lucignani and colleagues[188] described multiple foci of increased FDG uptake in the upper torso mainly in the axillary nodes in patients with low viremia in comparison with axillary and inguinal increased nodal uptake in patients with high viremia.

HIV infection is associated with an increased risk of developing opportunistic infections and tumors that may produce FUO.[189] PET/CT imaging allows whole body evaluation and identification of sites of infections and tumors ability.[80,189] Furthermore, patients with HIV infection are susceptible to multicentric Castleman's disease, which is a rare lymphoproliferative disorder associated with infection by human herpesvirus 8 that occurs in patients with AIDS. In these patients, PET imaging detects pathologic lesions more frequently than CT scans.[190]

LIMITATIONS

Tissues with physiologic high FDG uptake such as the brain gray matter and urinary system may obscure pathologic FDG accumulation. In addition, focal FDG uptake in reactive lymph nodes and in the gastrointestinal tract may result in false positive scans. Conversely, false negative scans occur with disorders without focal abnormalities and diseases with small focal lesions.[191]

Radiation exposure is a growing concern in children. It has been reported that children have an increased risk of developing secondary malignancies from radiation exposure compared with adults. This is related to the longer life span of children.[73] Accordingly, radiation exposure to children should follow the ALARA principle (as low as is reasonably achievable).[192,193] The main source of overall radiation exposure in PET/CT is the diagnostic CT. The radiation exposure from a whole body PET/CT with diagnostic contrast-enhanced CT in pediatrics is approximately 15 mSv for a 10-kg, 1-year-old child and reaches about 21 mSv for a 55-kg, 15-year-old child. This radiation can be reduced by half with the use of low-dose CT.[148,194,195] Moreover, anesthesia, if required, carries the risk of adverse respiratory events.[196]

SUMMARY

The value of PET/CT imaging in cases with FUO is based on its capability of drawing a functional and anatomic map of the whole body. FDG is able to reveal most neoplasms, infections, and many inflammatory disorders that can present as FUO. The paramount value of PET/CT lies in the ability to provide early diagnosis in the absence of overt morphologic changes. Furthermore, functional imaging can discriminate active from silent lesions. Performing PET/CT imaging in patients with FUO may unveil the underlying pathology in a significant number of patients. Consequently, implementation of PET/CT scanning in the diagnostic algorithm helps to decrease the number of unsolved cases with FUO.

REFERENCES

1. Cunha BA. Fever of unknown origin: clinical overview of classic and current concepts. Infect Dis Clin North Am 2007;21:867–915, vii.
2. Cunha BA, Durie N, Selbs E, et al. Fever of unknown origin (FUO) due to Rosai-Dorfman disease with mediastinal adenopathy mimicking lymphoma: diagnostic importance of elevated serum ferritin levels and polyclonal gammopathy. Heart Lung 2009;38:83–8.
3. Powell K. Fever without a focus. In: Behrman R, Kleigman R, Arvin A, editors. Nelson textbook of pediatrics. Philadelphia: Saunders; 1996. p. 698–704.
4. Petersdorf RG, Beeson PB. Fever of unexplained origin: report on 100 cases. Medicine (Baltimore) 1961;40:1–30.
5. Durack DT, Street AC. Fever of unknown origin—reexamined and redefined. Curr Clin Top Infect Dis 1991;11:35–51.
6. Knockaert DC, Vanneste LJ, Bobbaers HJ. Recurrent or episodic fever of unknown origin. Review of 45 cases and survey of the literature. Medicine (Baltimore) 1993;72:184–96.
7. Knockaert DC. Recurrent fevers of unknown origin. Infect Dis Clin North Am 2007;21:1189–211, xi.
8. Akpede GO, Akenzua GI. Aetiology and management of children with acute fever of unknown origin. Paediatr Drugs 2001;3:169–93.
9. Knockaert DC, Vanneste LJ, Vanneste SB, et al. Fever of unknown origin in the 1980s. An update of the diagnostic spectrum. Arch Intern Med 1992;152:51–5.
10. Maytal J, Shinnar S. Febrile status epilepticus. Pediatrics 1990;86:611–6.
11. Shinnar S, Pellock JM, Berg AT, et al. Short-term outcomes of children with febrile status epilepticus. Epilepsia 2001;42:47–53.
12. Verity CM, Ross EM, Golding J. Outcome of childhood status epilepticus and lengthy febrile convulsions: findings of national cohort study. BMJ 1993; 307:225–8.
13. Drwal-Klein LA, Phelps SJ. Antipyretic therapy in the febrile child. Clin Pharm 1992;11:1005–21.
14. Murray KF, Hadzic N, Wirth S, et al. Drug-related hepatotoxicity and acute liver failure. J Pediatr Gastroenterol Nutr 2008;47:395–405.
15. Norris W, Paredes AH, Lewis JH. Drug-induced liver injury in 2007. Curr Opin Gastroenterol 2008; 24:287–97.
16. Zaffanello M, Brugnara M, Angeli S, et al. Acute non-oliguric kidney failure and cholestatic hepatitis induced by ibuprofen and acetaminophen: a case report. Acta Paediatr 2009;98:903–5.
17. McLellan D, Giebink GS. Perspectives on occult bacteremia in children. J Pediatr 1986;109:1–8.
18. Ross AC, Toltzis P, O'Riordan MA, et al. Frequency and risk factors for deep focus of infection in children with Staphylococcus aureus bacteremia. Pediatr Infect Dis J 2008;27:396–9.
19. Sureshkumar P, Jones M, Cumming RG, et al. Risk factors for urinary tract infection in children: a population-based study of 2856 children. J Paediatr Child Health 2009;45:87–97.
20. Wilson CB. Immunologic basis for increased susceptibility of the neonate to infection. J Pediatr 1986;108:1–12.
21. Daley CL. Tuberculosis recurrence in Africa: true relapse or re-infection? Lancet 1993;342:756–7.
22. Freifeld AG, Pizzo PA. The outpatient management of febrile neutropenia in cancer patients. Oncology (Williston Park) 1996;10:599–606, 611–2 [discussion: 615–6].
23. Friedland IR. Bacteraemia in severely malnourished children. Ann Trop Paediatr 1992;12:433–40.
24. Greenberg AE, Nsa W, Ryder RW, et al. Plasmodium falciparum malaria and perinatally acquired human immunodeficiency virus type 1 infection in Kinshasa, Zaire. A prospective, longitudinal cohort study of 587 children. N Engl J Med 1991;325:105–9.
25. Hayani A, Mahoney DH, Fernbach DJ. Role of bone marrow examination in the child with prolonged fever. J Pediatr 1990;116:919–20.

26. Karstaedt AS, Khoosal M, Crewe-Brown HH. Pneumococcal bacteremia during a decade in children in Soweto, South Africa. Pediatr Infect Dis J 2000; 19:454–7.

27. Maher D, Kumwenda J. Bacteraemia in Blantyre. Trop Doct 1994;24:82–3.

28. Spector SA, Gelber RD, McGrath N, et al. A controlled trial of intravenous immune globulin for the prevention of serious bacterial infections in children receiving zidovudine for advanced human immunodeficiency virus infection. Pediatric AIDS Clinical Trials Group. N Engl J Med 1994;331: 1181–7.

29. Wilimas JA, Flynn PM, Harris S, et al. A randomized study of outpatient treatment with ceftriaxone for selected febrile children with sickle cell disease. N Engl J Med 1993;329:472–6.

30. Zarkowsky HS, Gallagher D, Gill FM, et al. Bacteremia in sickle hemoglobinopathies. J Pediatr 1986;109:579–85.

31. Zwi KJ, Pettifor JM, Soderlund N. Paediatric hospital admissions at a South African urban regional hospital: the impact of HIV, 1992–1997. Ann Trop Paediatr 1999;19:135–42.

32. Steele RW, Jones SM, Lowe BA, et al. Usefulness of scanning procedures for diagnosis of fever of unknown origin in children. J Pediatr 1991;119: 526–30.

33. Lewis HM, Parry JV, Parry RP, et al. Role of viruses in febrile convulsions. Arch Dis Child 1979;54: 869–76.

34. Akpede GO, Abiodun PO, Sykes RM. Pattern of infections in children under-six years old presenting with convulsions associated with fever of acute onset in a children's emergency room in Benin City, Nigeria. J Trop Pediatr 1993;39:11–5.

35. Snow RW, Craig M, Deichmann U, et al. Estimating mortality, morbidity and disability due to malaria among Africa's non-pregnant population. Bull World Health Organ 1999;77:624–40.

36. Majeed HA. Differential diagnosis of fever of unknown origin in children. Curr Opin Rheumatol 2000;12:439–44.

37. Lohr JA, Hendley JO. Prolonged fever of unknown origin: a record of experiences with 54 childhood patients. Clin Pediatr (Phila) 1977;16:768–73.

38. Pizzo PA, Lovejoy FH Jr, Smith DH. Prolonged fever in children: review of 100 cases. Pediatrics 1975; 55:468–73.

39. de Kleijn EM, Vandenbroucke JP, van der Meer JW. Fever of unknown origin (FUO). I A. prospective multicenter study of 167 patients with FUO, using fixed epidemiologic entry criteria. The Netherlands FUO Study Group. Medicine (Baltimore) 1997;76: 392–400.

40. Durack D. Fever of unknown origin. In: Mackowiak P, editor. Fever basic mechanisms and management. 2nd edition. Philadelphia: Lippincott-Raven; 1997. p. 237–49.

41. Williams J, Bellamy R. Fever of unknown origin. Clin Med 2008;8:526–30.

42. Ishimine P. The evolving approach to the young child who has fever and no obvious source. Emerg Med Clin North Am 2007;25:1087–115, vii.

43. Ishimine P. Fever without source in children 0 to 36 months of age. Pediatr Clin North Am 2006;53: 167–94.

44. Hofer M, Mahlaoui N, Prieur AM. A child with a systemic febrile illness—differential diagnosis and management. Best Pract Res Clin Rheumatol 2006;20:627–40.

45. Baraff LJ. Management of infants and young children with fever without source. Pediatr Ann 2008; 37:673–9.

46. Gartner JC Jr. Fever of unknown origin. Adv Pediatr Infect Dis 1992;7:1–24.

47. Bramson RT, Meyer TL, Silbiger ML, et al. The futility of the chest radiograph in the febrile infant without respiratory symptoms. Pediatrics 1993;92: 524–6.

48. Crain EF, Bulas D, Bijur PE, et al. Is a chest radiograph necessary in the evaluation of every febrile infant less than 8 weeks of age? Pediatrics 1991; 88:821–4.

49. Heulitt MJ, Ablow RC, Santos CC, et al. Febrile infants less than 3 months old: value of chest radiography. Radiology 1988;167:135–7.

50. Patterson RJ, Bisset GS III, Kirks DR, et al. Chest radiographs in the evaluation of the febrile infant. AJR Am J Roentgenol 1990;155:833–5.

51. Bramson RT, Griscom NT, Cleveland RH. Interpretation of chest radiographs in infants with cough and fever. Radiology 2005;236:22–9.

52. Jasinski RW, Glazer GM, Francis IR, et al. CT and ultrasound in abscess detection at specific anatomic sites: a study of 198 patients. Comput Radiol 1987;11:41–7.

53. Roth AR, Basello GM. Approach to the adult patient with fever of unknown origin. Am Fam Physician 2003;68:2223–8.

54. Picus D, Siegel MJ, Balfe DM. Abdominal computed tomography in children with unexplained prolonged fever. J Comput Assist Tomogr 1984;8:851–6.

55. Kellenberger CJ, Epelman M, Miller SF, et al. Fast STIR whole-body MR imaging in children. Radiographics 2004;24:1317–30.

56. Bleeker-Rovers CP, van der Meer JW, Oyen WJ. Fever of unknown origin. Semin Nucl Med 2009; 39:81–7.

57. Knockaert DC, Mortelmans LA, De Roo MC, et al. Clinical value of gallium-67 scintigraphy in evaluation of fever of unknown origin. Clin Infect Dis 1994;18:601–5.

58. Palestro CJ. The current role of gallium imaging in infection. Semin Nucl Med 1994;24:128–41.

59. Kjaer A, Lebech AM. Diagnostic value of (111)In-granulocyte scintigraphy in patients with fever of unknown origin. J Nucl Med 2002;43:140–4.

60. Gratz S, Behr TM, Herrmann A, et al. Immunoscintigraphy (BW 250/183) in neonates and infants with fever of unknown origin. Nucl Med Commun 1998; 19:1037–45.

61. Maugeri D, Santangelo A, Abbate S, et al. A new method for diagnosing fever of unknown origin (FUO) due to infection of muscular-skeletal system in elderly people: leukoscan Tc-99m labelled scintigraphy. Eur Rev Med Pharmacol Sci 2001;5: 123–6.

62. Meller J, Ivancevic V, Conrad M, et al. Clinical value of immunoscintigraphy in patients with fever of unknown origin. J Nucl Med 1998;39:1248–53.

63. Oyen WJ, Claessens RA, Raemaekers JM, et al. Diagnosing infection in febrile granulocytopenic patients with indium-111-labeled human immunoglobulin G. J Clin Oncol 1992;10:61–8.

64. Keidar Z, Nitecki S. FDG-PET for the detection of infected vascular grafts. Q J Nucl Med Mol Imaging 2009;53:35–40.

65. Pauwels EK, Sturm EJ, Bombardieri E, et al. Positron-emission tomography with [18F]fluorodeoxyglucose. Part I. Biochemical uptake mechanism and its implication for clinical studies. J Cancer Res Clin Oncol 2000;126:549–59.

66. Petruzzi N, Shanthly N, Thakur M. Recent trends in soft-tissue infection imaging. Semin Nucl Med 2009;39:115–23.

67. Zhuang H, Yang H, Alavi A. Critical role of 18F-labeled fluorodeoxyglucose PET in the management of patients with arthroplasty. Radiol Clin North Am 2007;45:711–8, vii.

68. Zhuang H, Yu JQ, Alavi A. Applications of fluorodeoxyglucose-PET imaging in the detection of infection and inflammation and other benign disorders. Radiol Clin North Am 2005;43:121–34.

69. Zhuang H, Alavi A. 18-fluorodeoxyglucose positron emission tomographic imaging in the detection and monitoring of infection and inflammation. Semin Nucl Med 2002;32:47–59.

70. McQuattie S. Pediatric PET/CT imaging: tips and techniques. J Nucl Med Technol 2008;36:171–80.

71. Torigian DA, Huang SS, Houseni M, et al. Functional imaging of cancer with emphasis on molecular techniques. CA Cancer J Clin 2007;57: 206–24.

72. Chen YW, Huang MY, Chang CC, et al. FDG PET/CT findings of epithelioid sarcoma in a pediatric patient. Clin Nucl Med 2007;32:898–901.

73. Federman N, Feig SA. PET/CT in evaluating pediatric malignancies: a clinician's perspective. J Nucl Med 2007;48:1920–2.

74. Murphy JJ, Tawfeeq M, Chang B, et al. Early experience with PET/CT scan in the evaluation of pediatric abdominal neoplasms. J Pediatr Surg 2008; 43:2186–92.

75. Brown RS, Leung JY, Fisher SJ, et al. Intratumoral distribution of tritiated fluorodeoxyglucose in breast carcinoma: I. Are inflammatory cells important? J Nucl Med 1995;36:1854–61.

76. Vallabhajosula S. (18)F-labeled positron emission tomographic radiopharmaceuticals in oncology: an overview of radiochemistry and mechanisms of tumor localization. Semin Nucl Med 2007;37:400–19.

77. Chakrabarti R, Jung CY, Lee TP, et al. Changes in glucose transport and transporter isoforms during the activation of human peripheral blood lymphocytes by phytohemagglutinin. J Immunol 1994; 152:2660–8.

78. Miyamoto M, Sato EF, Nishikawa M, et al. Effect of endogenously generated nitric oxide on the energy metabolism of peritoneal macrophages. Physiol Chem Phys Med NMR 2003;35:1–11.

79. Sorbara LR, Maldarelli F, Chamoun G, et al. Human immunodeficiency virus type 1 infection of H9 cells induces increased glucose transporter expression. J Virol 1996;70:7275–9.

80. Meller J, Sahlmann CO, Scheel AK. 18F-FDG PET and PET/CT in fever of unknown origin. J Nucl Med 2007;48:35–45.

81. Kubota R, Yamada S, Kubota K, et al. Intratumoral distribution of fluorine-18-fluorodeoxyglucose in vivo: high accumulation in macrophages and granulation tissues studied by microautoradiography. J Nucl Med 1992;33:1972–80.

82. Whiteside TL. The tumor microenvironment and its role in promoting tumor growth. Oncogene 2008; 27:5904–12.

83. Ak I, Stokkel MP, Pauwels EK. Positron emission tomography with 2-[18F]fluoro-2-deoxy-D-glucose in oncology. Part II. The clinical value in detecting and staging primary tumours. J Cancer Res Clin Oncol 2000;126:560–74.

84. Mellanen P, Minn H, Grenman R, et al. Expression of glucose transporters in head-and-neck tumors. Int J Cancer 1994;56:622–9.

85. Merrall NW, Plevin R, Gould GW. Growth factors, mitogens, oncogenes and the regulation of glucose transport. Cell Signal 1993;5:667–75.

86. Gamelli RL, Liu H, He LK, et al. Augmentations of glucose uptake and glucose transporter-1 in macrophages following thermal injury and sepsis in mice. J Leukoc Biol 1996;59:639–47.

87. Fukuzumi M, Shinomiya H, Shimizu Y, et al. Endotoxin-induced enhancement of glucose influx into murine peritoneal macrophages via GLUT1. Infect Immun 1996;64:108–12.

88. Jacobs DB, Lee TP, Jung CY, et al. Mechanism of mitogen-induced stimulation of glucose transport

in human peripheral blood mononuclear cells. Evidence of an intracellular reserve pool of glucose carriers and their recruitment. J Clin Invest 1989; 83:437–43.

89. Malide D, Davies-Hill TM, Levine M, et al. Distinct localization of GLUT-1, -3, and -5 in human monocyte-derived macrophages: effects of cell activation. Am J Physiol 1998;274:E516–26.

90. Bleeker-Rovers CP, de Kleijn EM, Corstens FH, et al. Clinical value of FDG PET in patients with fever of unknown origin and patients suspected of focal infection or inflammation. Eur J Nucl Med Mol Imaging 2004;31:29–37.

91. Blockmans D, Knockaert D, Maes A, et al. Clinical value of [(18)F]fluoro-deoxyglucose positron emission tomography for patients with fever of unknown origin. Clin Infect Dis 2001;32:191–6.

92. Buysschaert I, Vanderschueren S, Blockmans D, et al. Contribution of (18)fluoro-deoxyglucose positron emission tomography to the work-up of patients with fever of unknown origin. Eur J Intern Med 2004;15:151–6.

93. Ferda J, Ferdova E, Zahlava J, et al. Fever of unknown origin: a value of (18)F-FDG-PET/CT with integrated full diagnostic isotropic CT imaging. Eur J Radiol 2009, in press.

94. Keidar Z, Gurman-Balbir A, Gaitini D, et al. Fever of unknown origin: the role of 18F-FDG PET/CT. J Nucl Med 2008;49:1980–5.

95. Kjaer A, Lebech AM, Eigtved A, et al. Fever of unknown origin: prospective comparison of diagnostic value of 18F-FDG PET and 111In-granulocyte scintigraphy. Eur J Nucl Med Mol Imaging 2004;31:622–6.

96. Lorenzen J, Buchert R, Bohuslavizki KH. Value of FDG PET in patients with fever of unknown origin. Nucl Med Commun 2001;22:779–83.

97. Meller J, Altenvoerde G, Munzel U, et al. Fever of unknown origin: prospective comparison of [18F]FDG imaging with a double-head coincidence camera and gallium-67 citrate SPET. Eur J Nucl Med 2000;27:1617–25.

98. Meller J, Sahlmann CO, Gurocak O, et al. FDG-PET in patients with fever of unknown origin: the importance of diagnosing large vessel vasculitis. Q J Nucl Med Mol Imaging 2009;53:51–63.

99. Meller J, Sahlmann CO, Lehmann K, et al. [F-18-FDG hybrid camera PET in patients with postoperative fever]. Nuklearmedizin 2002;41:22–9 [in German].

100. Skoura E, Giannopoulou C, Keramida G, et al. A case of fever of unknown origin: (18)F-FDG-PET/CT findings in Takayasu's arteritis. Hell J Nucl Med 2008;11:172–4.

101. Federici L, Blondet C, Imperiale A, et al. Value of (18)F-FDG-PET/CT in patients with fever of unknown origin and unexplained prolonged inflammatory syndrome: a single centre analysis experience. Int J Clin Pract 2008, in press.

102. Quinn M, Carraccio C, Sacchetti A. Pain, punctures, and pediatricians. Pediatr Emerg Care 1993;9:12–4.

103. Hamblen SM, Lowe VJ. Clinical 18F-FDG oncology patient preparation techniques. J Nucl Med Technol 2003;31:3–7, quiz 8–10.

104. Kaste SC. Issues specific to implementing PET-CT for pediatric oncology: what we have learned along the way. Pediatr Radiol 2004;34:205–13.

105. Nadel HR, Shulkin B. Pediatric positron emission tomography-computed tomography protocol considerations. Semin Ultrasound CT MR 2008; 29:271–6.

106. Kim S, Krynyckyi BR, Machac J, et al. Temporal relation between temperature change and FDG uptake in brown adipose tissue. Eur J Nucl Med Mol Imaging 2008;35:984–9.

107. Gordon BA, Flanagan FL, Dehdashti F. Whole-body positron emission tomography: normal variations, pitfalls, and technical considerations. AJR Am J Roentgenol 1997;169:1675–80.

108. Abouzied MM, Crawford ES, Nabi HA. 18F-FDG imaging: pitfalls and artifacts. J Nucl Med Technol 2005;33:145–55, quiz 162–143.

109. Kostakoglu L, Hardoff R, Mirtcheva R, et al. PET-CT fusion imaging in differentiating physiologic from pathologic FDG uptake. Radiographics 2004;24: 1411–31.

110. Bleeker-Rovers CP, Vos FJ, Wanten GJ, et al. 18F-FDG PET in detecting metastatic infectious disease. J Nucl Med 2005;46:2014–9.

111. Mahfouz T, Miceli MH, Saghafifar F, et al. 18F-fluorodeoxyglucose positron emission tomography contributes to the diagnosis and management of infections in patients with multiple myeloma: a study of 165 infectious episodes. J Clin Oncol 2005;23: 7857–63.

112. Jones HA, Sriskandan S, Peters AM, et al. Dissociation of neutrophil emigration and metabolic activity in lobar pneumonia and bronchiectasis. Eur Respir J 1997;10:795–803.

113. Vinson AE, Solis V, Williams HT, et al. F-18-FDG-PET/CT leads to diagnosis of cryptococcal pneumonia where recurrent metastatic rhabdomyosarcoma was suspected. Clin Nucl Med 2007;32:401–3.

114. Sojan SM, Chew G. *Pneumocystis carinii* pneumonia on F-18 FDG PET. Clin Nucl Med 2005;30: 763–4.

115. Yu JQ, Kumar R, Xiu Y, et al. Diffuse FDG uptake in the lungs in aspiration pneumonia on positron emission tomographic imaging. Clin Nucl Med 2004;29:567–8.

116. Kicska G, Zhuang H, Alavi A. Acute bronchitis imaged with F-18 FDG positron emission tomography. Clin Nucl Med 2003;28:511–2.

117. Sugawara Y, Braun DK, Kison PV, et al. Rapid detection of human infections with fluorine-18 fluorodeoxyglucose and positron emission tomography: preliminary results. Eur J Nucl Med 1998; 25:1238–43.

118. Stumpe KD, Dazzi H, Schaffner A, et al. Infection imaging using whole-body FDG-PET. Eur J Nucl Med 2000;27:822–32.

119. Sturm E, Rings EH, Scholvinck EH, et al. Fluordeoxyglucose positron emission tomography contributes to management of pediatric liver transplantation candidates with fever of unknown origin. Liver Transpl 2006;12:1698–704.

120. Sharma P, Rakela J. Management of pre-liver transplantation patient—part 2. Liver Transpl 2005;11: 249–60.

121. Sharma P, Rakela J. Management of pre-liver transplantation patients—part 1. Liver Transpl 2005;11: 124–33.

122. Chacko TK, Zhuang H, Nakhoda KZ, et al. Applications of fluorodeoxyglucose positron emission tomography in the diagnosis of infection. Nucl Med Commun 2003;24:615–24.

123. Guhlmann A, Brecht-Krauss D, Suger G, et al. Chronic osteomyelitis: detection with FDG PET and correlation with histopathologic findings. Radiology 1998;206:749–54.

124. Zhuang H, Duarte PS, Pourdehand M, et al. Exclusion of chronic osteomyelitis with F-18 fluorodeoxyglucose positron emission tomographic imaging. Clin Nucl Med 2000;25:281–4.

125. Zhuang H, Sam JW, Chacko TK, et al. Rapid normalization of osseous FDG uptake following traumatic or surgical fractures. Eur J Nucl Med Mol Imaging 2003;30:1096–103.

126. Kawai S, Ikeda E, Sugiyama M, et al. Enhancement of splenic glucose metabolism during acute malarial infection: correlation of findings of FDG-PET imaging with pathological changes in a primate model of severe human malaria. Am J Trop Med Hyg 2006;74:353–60.

127. El-Haddad G, Alavi A, Mavi A, et al. Normal variants in [18F]-fluorodeoxyglucose PET imaging. Radiol Clin North Am 2004;42:1063–81, viii.

128. Ruf J, Griebenow B, Stiller B, et al. Detection of infectious colitis by 18F-fluorodeoxyglucose-positron emission tomography in a child receiving intensive care after cardiac surgery. Pediatr Radiol 2005;35:702–5.

129. Vanderschueren S, Knockaert D, Adriaenssens T, et al. From prolonged febrile illness to fever of unknown origin: the challenge continues. Arch Intern Med 2003;163:1033–41.

130. Goerres GW, Forster A, Uebelhart D, et al. F-18 FDG whole-body PET for the assessment of disease activity in patients with rheumatoid arthritis. Clin Nucl Med 2006;31:386–90.

131. Ju JH, Kang KY, Kim IJ, et al. Visualization and localization of rheumatoid knee synovitis with FDG-PET/CT images. Clin Rheumatol 2008; 27(Suppl 2):S39–41.

132. Vogel WV, van Riel PL, Oyen WJ. FDG-PET/CT can visualise the extent of inflammation in rheumatoid arthritis of the tarsus. Eur J Nucl Med Mol Imaging 2007;34:439.

133. Radu CG, Shu CJ, Shelly SM, et al. Positron emission tomography with computed tomography imaging of neuroinflammation in experimental autoimmune encephalomyelitis. Proc Natl Acad Sci U S A 2007;104:1937–42.

134. Weiner SM, Otte A, Schumacher M, et al. Diagnosis and monitoring of central nervous system involvement in systemic lupus erythematosus: value of F-18 fluorodeoxyglucose PET. Ann Rheum Dis 2000;59:377–85.

135. Xiu Y, Yu JQ, Cheng E, et al. Sarcoidosis demonstrated by FDG PET imaging with negative findings on gallium scintigraphy. Clin Nucl Med 2005;30: 193–5.

136. Barbado FJ, Vazquez JJ, Pena JM, et al. Pyrexia of unknown origin: changing spectrum of diseases in two consecutive series. Postgrad Med J 1992;68: 884–7.

137. Larson EB, Featherstone HJ, Petersdorf RG. Fever of undetermined origin: diagnosis and follow-up of 105 cases, 1970–1980. Medicine (Baltimore) 1982; 61:269–92.

138. Lonardo A, Tondelli E, Selmi I, et al. Isolated jejunal Crohn's disease in a young adult presenting as fever of unknown origin. Am J Gastroenterol 1998;93:2285–7.

139. Neurath MF, Vehling D, Schunk K, et al. Noninvasive assessment of Crohn's disease activity: a comparison of 18F-fluorodeoxyglucose positron emission tomography, hydromagnetic resonance imaging, and granulocyte scintigraphy with labeled antibodies. Am J Gastroenterol 2002;97:1978–85.

140. Salvatori M, Melis L, Castaldi P, et al. Clinical significance of focal and diffuse thyroid diseases identified by (18)F-fluorodeoxyglucose positron emission tomography. Biomed Pharmacother 2007;61: 488–93.

141. Chen YK, Chen YL, Cheng RH, et al. The significance of FDG uptake in bilateral thyroid glands. Nucl Med Commun 2007;28:117–22.

142. Walter MA, Melzer RA, Schindler C, et al. The value of [18F]FDG-PET in the diagnosis of large-vessel vasculitis and the assessment of activity and extent of disease. Eur J Nucl Med Mol Imaging 2005;32: 674–81.

143. Hoshino A, Kawada E, Ukita T, et al. Usefulness of FDG-PET to diagnose intravascular lymphomatosis presenting as fever of unknown origin. Am J Hematol 2004;76:236–9.

144. Amin R, Ratjen F. Cystic fibrosis: a review of pulmonary and nutritional therapies. Adv Pediatr 2008; 55:99–121.

145. Chen DL, Ferkol TW, Mintun MA, et al. Quantifying pulmonary inflammation in cystic fibrosis with positron emission tomography. Am J Respir Crit Care Med 2006;173:1363–9.

146. Chen DL, Schuster DP. Imaging pulmonary inflammation with positron emission tomography: a biomarker for drug development. Mol Pharm 2006;3:488–95.

147. Sorensen HT, Mellemkjaer L, Skriver MV, et al. Fever of unknown origin and cancer: a population-based study. Lancet Oncol 2005;6:851–5.

148. Kleis M, Daldrup-Link H, Matthay K, et al. Diagnostic value of PET/CT for the staging and restaging of pediatric tumors. Eur J Nucl Med Mol Imaging 2009;36:23–36.

149. Barrington SF, Carr R. Staging of Burkitt's lymphoma and response to treatment monitored by PET scanning. Clin Oncol (R Coll Radiol) 1995; 7:334–5.

150. Delbeke D. Oncological applications of FDG PET imaging: brain tumors, colorectal cancer, lymphoma and melanoma. J Nucl Med 1999;40: 591–603.

151. Hines-Thomas M, Kaste SC, Hudson MM, et al. Comparison of gallium and PET scans at diagnosis and follow-up of pediatric patients with Hodgkin lymphoma. Pediatr Blood Cancer 2008;51: 198–203.

152. Hudson MM, Krasin MJ, Kaste SC. PET imaging in pediatric Hodgkin's lymphoma. Pediatr Radiol 2004;34:190–8.

153. Okada J, Yoshikawa K, Imazeki K, et al. The use of FDG-PET in the detection and management of malignant lymphoma: correlation of uptake with prognosis. J Nucl Med 1991;32:686–91.

154. Rodriguez M, Rehn S, Ahlstrom H, et al. Predicting malignancy grade with PET in non-Hodgkin's lymphoma. J Nucl Med 1995;36:1790–6.

155. Hernandez-Pampaloni M, Takalkar A, Yu JQ, et al. F-18 FDG-PET imaging and correlation with CT in staging and follow-up of pediatric lymphomas. Pediatr Radiol 2006;36:524–31.

156. Moog F, Bangerter M, Kotzerke J, et al. 18-F-fluorodeoxyglucose-positron emission tomography as a new approach to detect lymphomatous bone marrow. J Clin Oncol 1998;16:603–9.

157. Newman JS, Francis IR, Kaminski MS, et al. Imaging of lymphoma with PET with 2-[F-18]-fluoro-2-deoxy-D-glucose: correlation with CT. Radiology 1994;190:111–6.

158. Paul R. Comparison of fluorine-18-2-fluorodeoxyglucose and gallium-67 citrate imaging for detection of lymphoma. J Nucl Med 1987;28: 288–92.

159. Jadvar H, Connolly LP, Fahey FH, et al. PET and PET/CT in pediatric oncology. Semin Nucl Med 2007;37:316–31.

160. Larsson P, Holzgraefe B, Kalzen H, et al. PET/CT examination in an anaplastic malignant lymphoma with extensive reactive involvement. Clin Nucl Med 2008;33:619–20.

161. Yang DH, Min JJ, Jeong YY, et al. The combined evaluation of interim contrast-enhanced computerized tomography (CT) and FDG-PET/CT predicts the clinical outcomes and may impact on the therapeutic plans in patients with aggressive non-Hodgkin's lymphoma. Ann Hematol 2008;88:425–32.

162. Borgwardt L, Hojgaard L, Carstensen H, et al. Increased fluorine-18 2-fluoro-2-deoxy-D-glucose (FDG) uptake in childhood CNS tumors is correlated with malignancy grade: a study with FDG positron emission tomography/magnetic resonance imaging coregistration and image fusion. J Clin Oncol 2005;23:3030–7.

163. Francavilla TL, Miletich RS, Di Chiro G, et al. Positron emission tomography in the detection of malignant degeneration of low-grade gliomas. Neurosurgery 1989;24:1–5.

164. Schifter T, Hoffman JM, Hanson MW, et al. Serial FDG-PET studies in the prediction of survival in patients with primary brain tumors. J Comput Assist Tomogr 1993;17:509–61.

165. Patronas NJ, Di Chiro G, Kufta C, et al. Prediction of survival in glioma patients by means of positron emission tomography. J Neurosurg 1985;62: 816–22.

166. Choi SJ, Kim JS, Kim JH, et al. [18F]3'-deoxy-3'-fluorothymidine PET for the diagnosis and grading of brain tumors. Eur J Nucl Med Mol Imaging 2005; 32:653–9.

167. Floeth FW, Pauleit D, Wittsack HJ, et al. Multimodal metabolic imaging of cerebral gliomas: positron emission tomography with [18F]fluoroethyl-L-tyrosine and magnetic resonance spectroscopy. J Neurosurg 2005;102:318–27.

168. Juhasz C, Chugani DC, Muzik O, et al. In vivo uptake and metabolism of alpha-[11C]methyl-L-tryptophan in human brain tumors. J Cereb Blood Flow Metab 2006;26:345–57.

169. Langen KJ, Hamacher K, Weckesser M, et al. O-(2-[18F]fluoroethyl)-L-tyrosine: uptake mechanisms and clinical applications. Nucl Med Biol 2006;33: 287–94.

170. Pauleit D, Floeth F, Hamacher K, et al. O-(2-[18F]fluoroethyl)-L-tyrosine PET combined with MRI improves the diagnostic assessment of cerebral gliomas. Brain 2005;128:678–87.

171. Weckesser M, Langen KJ, Rickert CH, et al. O-(2-[18F]fluorethyl)-L-tyrosine PET in the clinical evaluation of primary brain tumours. Eur J Nucl Med Mol Imaging 2005;32:422–9.

172. Jaramillo D, Laor T, Gebhardt MC. Pediatric musculoskeletal neoplasms. Evaluation with MR imaging. Magn Reson Imaging Clin N Am 1996;4:749–70.

173. Shulkin BL, Wieland DM, Baro ME, et al. PET hydroxyephedrine imaging of neuroblastoma. J Nucl Med 1996;37:16–21.

174. Gyorke T, Zajic T, Lange A, et al. Impact of FDG PET for staging of Ewing sarcomas and primitive neuroectodermal tumours. Nucl Med Commun 2006;27:17–24.

175. Huang TL, Liu RS, Chen TH, et al. Comparison between F-18-FDG positron emission tomography and histology for the assessment of tumor necrosis rates in primary osteosarcoma. J Chin Med Assoc 2006;69:372–6.

176. Franzius C, Juergens KU, Vormoor J. PET/CT with diagnostic CT in the evaluation of childhood sarcoma. AJR Am J Roentgenol 2006;186:581 [author reply 581–2].

177. McCarville MB, Christie R, Daw NC, et al. PET/CT in the evaluation of childhood sarcomas. AJR Am J Roentgenol 2005;184:1293–304.

178. Seshadri N, Wright P, Balan KK. Rhabdomyosarcoma with widespread bone marrow infiltration: beneficial management role of F-18 FDG PET. Clin Nucl Med 2007;32:787–9.

179. Ben Arush MW, Israel O, Kedar Z, et al. Detection of isolated distant metastasis in soft tissue sarcoma by fluorodeoxyglucose positron emission tomography: case report. Pediatr Hematol Oncol 2001;18:295–8.

180. Peng F, Rabkin G, Muzik O. Use of 2-deoxy-2-[F-18]-fluoro-D-glucose positron emission tomography to monitor therapeutic response by rhabdomyosarcoma in children: report of a retrospective case study. Clin Nucl Med 2006;31:394–7.

181. Mackie GC, Shulkin BL, Ribeiro RC, et al. Use of [18F]fluorodeoxyglucose positron emission tomography in evaluating locally recurrent and metastatic adrenocortical carcinoma. J Clin Endocrinol Metab 2006;91:2665–71.

182. Mody RJ, Pohlen JA, Malde S, et al. FDG PET for the study of primary hepatic malignancies in children. Pediatr Blood Cancer 2006;47:51–5.

183. Dadparvar S, Anderson GS, Bhargava P, et al. Paraneoplastic encephalitis associated with cystic teratoma is detected by fluorodeoxyglucose positron emission tomography with negative magnetic resonance image findings. Clin Nucl Med 2003;28:893–6.

184. Linke R, Voltz R. FDG-PET in paraneoplastic syndromes. Recent Results Cancer Res 2008; 170:203–11.

185. Suzuki H, Hasegawa T, Higuchi M, et al. Usefulness of [18F] fluoro-2-deoxyglucose-positron emission tomography-computed tomography (FDG-PET-CT) in the detection of lung cancer recurrence with paraneoplastic neurological syndrome. Clin Oncol (R Coll Radiol) 2006;18:636–7.

186. Gungor T, Engel-Bicik I, Eich G, et al. Diagnostic and therapeutic impact of whole body positron emission tomography using fluorine-18-fluoro-2-deoxy-D-glucose in children with chronic granulomatous disease. Arch Dis Child 2001;85: 341–5.

187. Depas G, Decortis T, Francotte N, et al. F-18 FDG PET in infectious diseases in children. Clin Nucl Med 2007;32:593–8.

188. Lucignani G, Orunesu E, Cesari M, et al. FDG-PET imaging in HIV-infected subjects: relation with therapy and immunovirological variables. Eur J Nucl Med Mol Imaging 2009;36:640–7.

189. O'Doherty MJ, Barrington SF, Campbell M, et al. PET scanning and the human immunodeficiency virus-positive patient. J Nucl Med 1997;38: 1575–83.

190. Barker R, Kazmi F, Stebbing J, et al. FDG-PET/CT imaging in the management of HIV-associated multicentric Castleman's disease. Eur J Nucl Med Mol Imaging 2009;36:648–52.

191. Bleeker-Rovers CP, Vos FJ, Mudde AH, et al. A prospective multi-centre study of the value of FDG-PET as part of a structured diagnostic protocol in patients with fever of unknown origin. Eur J Nucl Med Mol Imaging 2007;34:694–703.

192. Willis CE, Slovis TL. The ALARA concept in pediatric CR and DR: dose reduction in pediatric radiographic exams—a white paper conference. AJR Am J Roentgenol 2005;184:373–4.

193. Frush DP, Frush KS. 'Sleeping with the enemy?' Expectations and reality in imaging children in the emergency setting. Pediatr Radiol 2008;38(Suppl 4):S633–8.

194. Brix G, Lechel U, Glatting G, et al. Radiation exposure of patients undergoing whole-body dual-modality 18F-FDG PET/CT examinations. J Nucl Med 2005;46:608–13.

195. Byrne A, Nadel H. Whole body low dose 18F-FDG PET/CT in pediatric oncology. J Nucl Med 2007; 48(suppl 2):118P [abstract].

196. Sanborn PA, Michna E, Zurakowski D, et al. Adverse cardiovascular and respiratory events during sedation of pediatric patients for imaging examinations. Radiology 2005;237:288–94.

FDG PET and PET/CT in the Management of Pediatric Lymphoma Patients

Gang Cheng, MD, Sabah Servaes, MD,
Abass Alavi, MD, MD (Hon), PhD (Hon), DSc (Hon),
Hongming Zhuang, MD, PhD*

KEYWORDS

• FDG • PET • PET/CT • Lymphoma • Pediatric

Lymphoma is the seventh most common malignancy in the United States and is the third most common malignancy in children. Lymphoma accounts for about 12% of all childhood cancers. About 1700 children in the United States are diagnosed yearly with lymphoma; approximately 40% of these cases are Hodgkin's disease. Non-Hodgkin's lymphoma (NHL) is more common than Hodgkin's lymphoma (HD) and contributes to the most mortality from lymphoma.[1]

It is critical to assess a patient with lymphoma accurately. Local radiation may be sufficient for stage I follicular lymphoma; however, systemic therapy has to be employed for advanced stages of disease. Historically, staging was determined surgically. This type of staging was replaced by cross-sectional imaging modalities, mainly computed tomography (CT) scanning, which has been the standard practice for many years. Ga-67 scan had some roles, especially in the assessment of residual malignancy. Now, positron emission tomography (PET) with fluorine-18 fluoro-deoxy-glucose (FDG) has emerged as a powerful imaging modality in the clinical practice of lymphoma and many other cancers. Fluorine-18 fluorodeoxyglucose positron emission tomography (FDG PET) uses an F-18–labeled glucose analog (ie, FDG) that is transported into cells but cannot be metabolized. The "trapped" F-18–labeled FDG within cells thus serves as a marker of hypermetabolic tissues, such as neoplastic tissues, in the body.

FDG PET imaging has had an ever-increasing role in the clinical practice of oncology since the U.S. Health Care Administration approved whole-body FDG PET imaging for several oncological indications in the late 1990s. Use of FDG PET or PET/CT in HD or NHL in adults has become a routine and is widely used for pretreatment staging, assessment of response during therapy, and response assessment after completion of therapy.[2–4] In contrast to extensive publications in the adult population, only a limited number of studies have investigated the role of FDG PET in children and adolescents with lymphoma. This article reviews the currently available literature on the clinical application of FDG PET in the management of childhood lymphoma, including its significance in initial diagnosis, response assessment, post-therapy residual evaluation and follow-up studies. A common problem in these studies is that histopathological verifications are not available, and neither CT nor FDG PET results can be compared with any reference standard. Discordant findings are generally solved by long-term clinical follow-up.

Department of Radiology, Division of Nuclear Medicine, Children's Hospital of Pennsylvania, 34th and Civic Center Blvd, Philadelphia, PA 19104, USA
* Corresponding author.
E-mail address: zhuang@email.chop.edu (H. Zhuang).

PET Clin 3 (2009) 621–634
doi:10.1016/j.cpet.2009.04.004

FDG PET VERSUS CONVENTIONAL IMAGING STUDY

Conventional imaging modalities (CIMs) such as CT, magnetic resonance (MR) imaging, ultrasonography and gallium scan are often used to delineate the extent of disease involvement in lymphoma patients. CT staging has been the first choice for a long time in lymphoma staging because of its high sensitivity and accuracy, as well as its wide availability and relatively low cost. Now, accumulating evidence indicates FDG PET is superior to traditional imaging modalities for the evaluation of lymphoma. Analysis of multiple clinical studies shows that FDG PET has both higher sensitivity and specificity than either CT or gallium scan.[5] Similar findings have been reported in pediatric lymphoma patients.[1,6–8]

FDG PET Versus CT

Current CT machines produce excellent quality of images with submillimeter resolution and provide high sensitivity and specificity in pretreatment staging. Because of its spatial resolution, CT scan has been the gold standard for decades in the evaluation of lymphoma patients. However, the specificity of CT is low in lymphoma patients in response assessment following therapy because residual mass often persists for a long time after treatment, and only 20% of the patients with residual mass post therapy have persistent disease.[3,9] Although CT is excellent in determination of the size and location of tumor tissues, CT is frequently not able to differentiate viable tumors from necrotic or fibrotic tissues. Another reason for the low specificity of CT imaging is that CT diagnosis is heavily dependent on the "size criteria." One × one centimeter is most commonly used as a limit for a normal-sized lymph node. Sometimes location-specific size criteria are employed (eg, 12 mm in the para-aortic region and 8 mm in the gastrohepatic ligament or porta hepatis).[9] Nevertheless, CT often cannot detect a malignant lesion in a small node. Also, as previously described, lymph nodes may remain enlarged in size following therapy but may not necessarily reflect active disease. In addition, CT has a low sensitivity for evaluation of bone marrow infiltration by lymphoma because bone marrow involvement causes minimal structural/morphologic changes and may appear normal on CT images.

In contrast, FDG PET scan examines "functional changes" that are relatively independent of morphologic changes. Because of its superior signal-to-noise contrast, FDG PET has been shown to be more sensitive than CT in the detection of even tumor of small dimension or metabolically active normal-sized lymph nodes, although CT imaging has better spatial resolution in delineating anatomic changes. Direct comparison of FDG PET and CT findings in patients with lymphoma suggests that FDG PET contributes substantially to accurate staging in patients with lymphoma.[10] Enlarged lymph nodes on CT are not necessary caused by lymphoma (Fig. 1). In addition, PET images are more sensitive than CT in the detection of bone marrow involvement (Fig. 2). Furthermore, FDG PET images can detect lesions in lymph nodes with a normal size (Fig. 3). In 81 consecutive and previously untreated patients with malignant NHL (n = 43) or HD (n = 38), FDG PET outperformed contrast-enhanced CT and provided more information about extranodal lymphoma than CT, and led to changes in tumor staging in 13/81 patients.[11] Similarly, FDG PET was found to be more sensitive than CIMs for staging and restaging of pediatric HD and NHL.

Ga-67 Imaging Versus FDG PET

Whole-body Ga-67 citrate (Ga-67) imaging had been used for a long time for functional imaging in lymphoma. Before PET scan became available, the primary role of Ga-67 imaging was to evaluate the effectiveness of therapy. However, the spatial resolution of Ga-67 imaging is poor and the sensitivity and specificity are low. PET outperformed both CT and Ga-67 scan with superior accuracy in staging and in restaging of lymphoma in adult patients.[12] Lin and colleagues[13] reported from 46 cases of new and recurrent lymphoma that FDG PET was superior to Ga-67 imaging in nodal site positivity rate (97% versus 79%) and in detecting more abnormal sites in 48% of patients. Mody and colleagues examined the value of FDG PET in the care of pediatric patients with lymphomas (8–19 years of age). In both pediatric HD and NHL, FDG PET had higher sensitivity and specificity than gallium scanning.[14] FDG PET is valuable especially for detecting infradiaphragmatic lesions in children, such as those in the spleen.[15] More recently, Hines-Thomas and colleagues compared the value of FDG PET and gallium and CT scans on 44 pediatric HD patients at diagnosis, early response, off chemotherapy, and off-therapy evaluations. They found that FDG PET upstaged four patients at diagnosis but did not lead to a change in therapy in any of them. At early response evaluation, FDG PET changed the response category in two patients and led to a change in radiation dose for one patient. In contrast, gallium did not change the stage of treatment for any patient.[16] Radiation exposure from Ga-67 scan is higher than most other nuclear medicine scans including PET/CT.

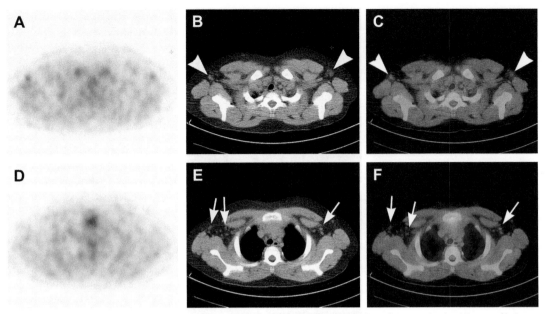

Fig. 1. This PET/CT study was done on an 8-year-old boy with lymphoblastic lymphoma who had been off chemotherapy for 4 years. The study was done because recent diagnostic CT scan showed adenopathy in the bilateral neck and axilla. However, PET/CT scan did not reveal hypermetabolic lesions characteristic of lymphoma recurrence. Transaxial sections at two different levels are presented here, showing mildly enlarged bilateral axillary nodes with minimal FDG uptake (*A–C, arrowheads*) and multiple smaller axillary nodes at lower levels (*D–F, arrows*). Diffuse, mildly increased FDG uptake in the anterior mediastinum was caused by thymus activity (*D–F*).

Now, Ga-67 scan is seldom performed because of wider adoption of PET/CT imaging. Despite of the lack of pediatric study of comparison between Ga-67 and PET/CT, it is conceivable that information obtained from adult patients is very likely also applicable to children.

FDG PET Versus FDG PET/CT

FDG PET is a functional study that is relatively independent of tumor size. It has a high tumor-to-background contrast and thus a high sensitivity in visualization of hypermetabolic diseases. FDG PET has relatively poor spatial resolution in visualization of normal organs and tissues, and thus lesion localization is suboptimal. This disadvantage is significantly corrected by hybrid PET-CT scanning, which clearly enhances its diagnostic abilities in lymphoma patients. PET/CT combines a PET scanner with a multidetector helical CT scanner to obtain fused PET and CT images so that precise localization of abnormal lesions can be determined with high confidence. With the benefit of current technologies, there is little additional dose from the CT.

A combined PET/CT system allows accurate spatial localization of abnormal tracer uptake. The current literature suggests that combined

PET/CT imaging offers a diagnostic advantage over FDG PET.[17] Recently, Raanani and colleagues[18] have shown in a retrospective study of 103 consecutive adult patients with newly diagnosed NHL (n = 68) and HD (n = 35) that in comparison to the assessment by CT alone, PET/CT upstaged 31% in NHL and 32% in HD (most in stages I and II) patients, and changed the management decisions in approximately a quarter of NHL and a third of HD patients. The authors concluded that PET/CT as the initial staging procedure may obviate the need for additional diagnostic CT in the majority of patients.[18] No significant differences were found between unenhanced low-dose PET/CT, contrast-enhanced low-dose PET/CT and contrast-enhanced full-dose PET/CT for lymph node and extranodal disease in lymphomas,[19,20] although full-dose PET/CT yielded more precise lesion delineation, it showed fewer indeterminate findings and showed a higher number of extranodal sites affected than did unenhanced low-dose PET/CT.

As in the adult population, PET/CT increases the diagnostic accuracy in pediatric cancer patients. In a study involving a total of 118 FDG PET/CT studies of 46 pediatric patients, 324 sites of increased FDG uptake were detected. Discordant PET and PET/CT interpretations were found in 97

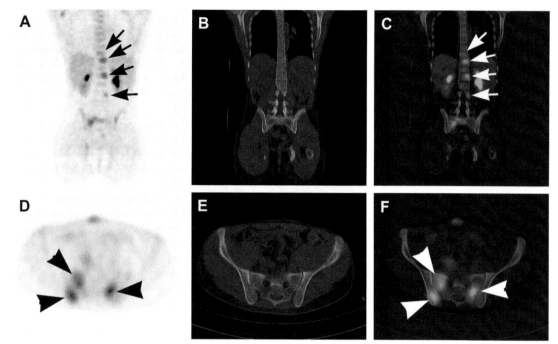

Fig. 2. This patient was a 20-year-old male who had Hodgkin's lymphoma. PET/CT scan on initial staging showed abnormally increased FDG uptake in T10, T11, L1, L3 (*arrows* in *A* and *C*) and in the right iliac and bilateral sacral bones (*arrowheads* in *D* and *F*) but no corresponding abnormal findings on the CT images (*B* and *E*).

sites (30%). PET alone had a significantly higher proportion of equivocal and a lower proportion of benign lesion than PET/CT (*P*<.001). PET/CT had significantly improved characterization of abnormal FDG foci in children who had cancer than PET alone by avoiding misinterpretation of increased tracer uptake in brown fat (39%), bowel

(17%), muscle (8%) and thymus (7%), and thus decreased false-positive PET findings.[21]

INITIAL STAGING

It is critically important that lymphoma patients be staged accurately to direct the treatment plan.

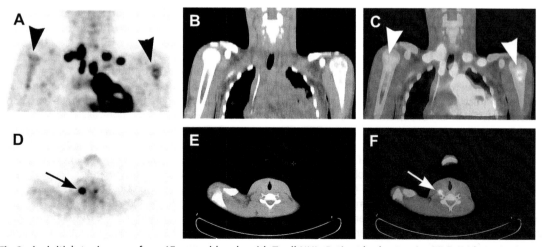

Fig. 3. An initial staging scan for a 15-year old male with T cell NHL. Patient had extensive FDG-avid tumor tissues in the mediastinum and bilateral thoracic inlets (*A* to *C*). However, lesions in the right lower neck were missed on diagnostic CT scans because of their small size (*D* to *F*). The abnormal bone marrow activity in bilateral humeri (*arrowheads* in *A* and *C*) was also missed by CT.

This assertion is especially true for HD and for early stage patients, as any change in staging may necessitate modification of disease management and the possibility of avoiding intensive treatment and less long term side effects. Traditionally, the Ann Arbor staging system was used to determine whether focal radiation or systemic treatment should be used. In the last three decades, CT scan has been the choice for lymphoma staging. Since its introduction as an initial staging option in the mid-1990s, FDG PET scanning has proved to be of high sensitivity in detecting localized or generalized lymphoma (both HD and NHL). Most common types of lymphoma (HD and aggressive NHL, such as diffuse large B-cell NHL, follicular NHL, and mantle cell NHL) are FDG-avid.[22,23] There are a plethora of studies demonstrating that FDG PET has higher sensitivity and specifictity in staging HD and high-grade NHL than CT imaging in the adult population, with an accuracy of 85%–98% (see reviews[3,24]). Especially in the detection of bone marrow involvement, FDG PET has significantly outperformed CT in the assessment of disease involvement.[22] Although the literature is more limited in the pediatric population of lymphoma patients, the available studies are generally compatible with the discoveries in the adult population. The reported impact of FDG PET staging on the management of adult lymphoma patients ranged from 8%–45% in prospective and retrospective studies,[25] and ranged from 10%–23% in studies conducted in pediatric patients.[1,6,26] Fused PET/CT imaging has further improved FDG PET performance in lymphoma (modification of staging in 32.3% of patients as in a recent report[8]).

In an early study including seven pediatric HD patients, FDG PET revealed more extensive disease than CIMs, leading to upstaging in four patients and modified clinical management in one patient. The impact of FDG PET on lymphoma is obvious despite the small sample size in this study.[6] Amthauer and colleagues[27] reported FDG PET in the initial staging of pediatric NHL patients resulted in upstaging followed by an intensified poly-chemotherapy in one of ten patients. Depas and colleagues reviewed the value of FDG PET in 19 children with HD (n = 14) or NHL (n = 5). FDG PET downstaged one patient from stage IV to stage II and upstaged one patient from stage III to stage IV, thereby changing the disease stage and treatment in 10.5% of the cases at initial evaluation.[1] Hermann and colleagues compared whole-body FDG-PET with CT scans in 25 children with histologically proven HD (n = 18) and NHL (n = 7). In each patient, 30 regions were analyzed (22 nodal, 8 extranodal), with 662 regions (470

nodal, 192 extranodal) compared in the study. FDG-PET and CT scans had concordant positive findings in 91 regions (14%) and had concordant negative findings in 517 regions (78%). Discrepancies were mainly observed in cervical/abdominal lymph nodes, the spleen and the skeleton. As compared with CT, FDG-PET scan resulted in modification of staging in five of 25 children with lymphoma (a higher staging in four and a lower staging in two of 25 patients).[26]

Only a few prospective studies are available in the literature evaluating the role of FDG PET in the management of pediatric lymphoma patients.[28,29] A prospective, blinded study compared FDG-PET with conventional staging methods (CSMs), including CT, ultrasound, bone scanning and bone marrow examination, for initial staging of 55 children and adolescents with HD (mean age 15.5 years, range 3.9–18.9 years). It was found that FDG PET correctly changed the staging in 15% of patients (seven up-stagings and two down-stagings). FDG PET had a significantly higher sensitivity for nodal staging but a similar sensitivity for extranodal staging. FDG PET identified significantly more positive lymphoma sites (34%) that were negative on CSMs, while CSMs revealed only 5% additional lesions. The sensitivity of FDG PET and CSMs for pretreatment staging was 96.5% and 87.5%, respectively; specificity was 100% and 60%, and accuracy, 96.7% and 85.2%, respectively. In 5% of patients, radiation regime was modified based on FDG PET findings.[28] FDG-PET was inferior to CT for the detection of small lung metastases (often < 5 mm) because of its limited spatial resolution, which was the major cause of its false negative findings in the study. Nowadays, this shortcoming has been largely overcome with wider adoption of hybrid PET/CT in most clinical practice.

The impact of FDG PET on lymphoma staging is greater with fused PET/CT scan. A prospective study by Furth and colleagues further demonstrated the value of integrated FDG PET/CT in the initial staging of pediatric HL versus conventional imaging modalities (CIM: with CT and MRI) in 33 patients (4–18 years of age) with histologically proven HL. The accuracy of CIM, FDG PET, side-by-side and image-fused FDG PET and CIM was: 86%, 89%, 94%, and 97% respectively for lymph node regions above the diaphragm; 94%, 94%, 97%, and 98% respectively for lymph node regions below the diaphragm; and the accuracy was 96%, 96%, 100%, and 100%, respectively in extranodal regions.[29] Miller and colleagues[8] evaluated the role of 18F-Fluorodeoxyglucose (18F-FDG) PET/CT in 31 pediatric patients (mean age 12.9) with HL (n = 24) and NHL (n = 7) and found that PET/CT findings resulted in a change in staging in approximately one out of three (32.3%) pediatric patients with HL and NHL, with upstaging in seven (22.6%) and downstaging in three (9.6%) patients. This finding is consistent with the authors' own clinical experience: among 18 pediatric HL patients who had a PET/CT scan at diagnosis with a diagnostic contrast CT within one week of PET/CT before any therapy, PET/CT scan detected more positive lesions than diagnostic CT scan (especially in extranodal lesions). Six patients (33.3%) were upstaged using PET/CT as compared with diagnostic CT (one from stage II to III; two from stage II to IV; two from stage III to IV, and one stage II case on PET/CT, which was negative on diagnostic CT) (Cheng G, unpublished data, 2008). Image fusion not only increased the sensitivity and specificity, but more importantly, it significantly improved the reviewers' confidence.

INTERIM TREATMENT MONITORING

A combined modality approach of multi-agent chemotherapy and selected field radiotherapy is the current widely accepted treatment strategy, which has yielded excellent results in children and adolescents with lymphomas. However, current therapy has many major late side effects, including infections such as the overwhelming post-splenectomy infection syndrome, gonad dysfunction (sterility in men and premature onset of menopause in women), and other late complications involving the heart, lungs and thyroid gland. In addition, some patients develop secondary malignancies 15–30 years after the initial diagnosis and treatment, which is associated with the treatment of the primary disease. With the high cure rate, the current focus in lymphoma treatment is to avoid late side effects while maintaining effectiveness of current therapy.

There is much interest in the potential value of FDG PET as an early response indicator to guide the therapeutic strategy in lymphoma patients. It has been advocated that patients who respond poorly to therapy should be identified promptly and be treated more aggressively, while patients who had a favorable response to therapy may avoid aggressive treatment. For example, early stage HD patients with complete response or a negative FDG-PET at the end of chemotherapy might not receive radiotherapy to reduce the risk of a secondary malignancy and other long-term side effects while maintaining a high cure rate.[30–32] Before the introduction of FDG PET scan, it was often difficult to evaluate clinical response in children with lymphoma, especially with mediastinal involvement. Response assessment by CIMs depends on visualization of tumor size regression in the involved regions, which is often slow and protracted, and metabolic activity of a residual tumor mass cannot be evaluated by CT. One of the major advantages of FDG PET study is that FDG PET detects biochemical changes in tumor tissues, which are relatively independent of anatomic changes. FDG PET is able to differentiate fibrosis/necrosis from viable tumor. This functional information is particularly useful in determining response to therapy (**Fig. 4**). If patient responds well to the therapy, decrease or normalization in FDG uptake in tumor tissues occurs soon after the initiation of treatment, preceding shrinkage of tumor tissues. This information allows early response assessment in the treatment of lymphoma patients and therapeutic strategies can be adjusted accordingly (response-adapted therapy), even before the completion of therapy. For this purpose, the specific lymphoma entity has to be FDG-avid, which is generally achieved by obtaining a baseline scan to assess the extent of disease and the degree of FDG uptake in lymphoma sites in a given patient.

Numerous studies demonstrate that interim FDG PET scans predict clinical outcome in adult lymphoma patients.[9,33] The value of early response assessment with FDG PET is well established in adults with either HD or histologically aggressive NHL, and interim evaluation of response to therapy by FDG PET is becoming a routine part of patient care in the adult population to guide treatment. The current literature indicates that interim FDG PET in adult lymphoma patients is superior to CT scan in predicting complete response rate, event-free survival and overall survival, and provides important and independent prognostic information in certain aggressive lymphomas.[34–36] FDG PET imaging after a few cycles of chemotherapy cycles is superior to CT scan in predicting progression-free survival and is as reliable as definitive response assessment at the end of therapy (see review[37]). FDG PET has strong potential to identify favorably responding patients accurately so that overly aggressive treatments can be spared, and to identify unfavorably responding patients so that the physician can adjust management accordingly and in a timely manner.

A few available studies in pediatric lymphoma patients also demonstrate the usefulness of FDG PET in the evaluation of early response to therapy. Amthauer and colleagues[27] reported that in five pediatric NHL patients with uncertain residual masses on conventional imaging during therapy, FDG PET correctly detected viable residual tumors

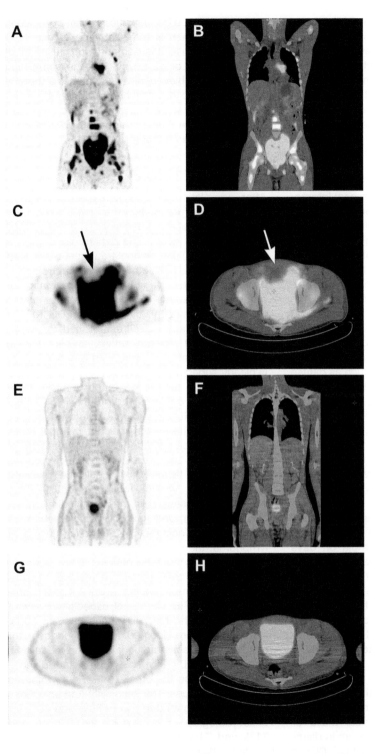

Fig. 4. This patient was a 19-year-old female with large B cell lymphoma. PET/CT scan on initial staging showed abnormally increased FDG uptake in the mediastinum and bilateral hila, mesenteric nodes, pelvis soft tissues, and multiple bone marrow involvements (*A–D*). The patient was admitted because of acute urinary retention and had a Foley catheter in place when imaged. The extensive FDG uptake in the pelvis is because of lymphoma tissues while the urinary bladder was pushed forward with minimal tracer activity (*arrows* in *C–D*). Repeat study was done 7 days later after a single cycle of chemotherapy (*E–H*), which showed complete metabolic response to therapy. In this repeat study, Foley catheter was removed and full bladder with radioactive urine was present (*G–H*). This patient received additional chemotherapy after that, and had been followed for 26 months with no evidence of tumor recurrence.

in one case, which was confirmed during follow-up, while the remaining four FDG-PET negative patients remained tumor-free. In a study of 48 patients who had aggressive lymphoma (24 HD, 24 NHL), mid-treatment PET scan was shown to be associated with later remission: 61% (for NHL) and 65% (for HD) achieved complete remission in PET-negative patients, while only 50% (for NHL) and 25% (for HD) achieved complete remission in PET-positive patients.[38] Miller and colleagues examined the value of FDG PET/CT imaging in 31 pediatric patients with HD (n = 24) and NHL (n = 7). It was found that PET/CT had a negative predictive value of 96% and when used for monitoring response to treatment, a negative study was generally associated with disease-free period (mean 15.4 ± 8.8 months), even when residual mass was detected. The positive predictive value (PPV) of persistent increased 18F-FDG uptake was 100% in three patients with active disease, significantly higher than the PPV of residual CT mass, which was 14%,[8] but this sample size is small.

The important role of FDG PET imaging in lymphoma is also evidenced by the recent International Harmonization Project recommendations, which has developed guidelines for performing and interpreting FDG PET imaging for treatment assessment in patients with lymphoma both in clinical practice and in clinical trials, based on published FDG PET literature and the collective expertise of its members in the use of FDG PET in lymphoma.[39,40] The recommendations should principally apply in the pediatric population and include the following several important points:[1] pretherapy FDG PET is recommended strongly with routinely FDG avid lymphoma such as diffuse large B cell lymphoma, follicular lymphoma, or (HD), and is recommended as mandatory for variably FDG-avid lymphomas (if FDG PET is used to assess their response to therapy).[2] For response assessment at the conclusion of therapy, FDG PET should be performed at least 3 weeks (preferably at 6–8 weeks) after chemotherapy or chemo-immunotherapy, and at 8–12 weeks after radiation or chemoradiotherapy. If an interim FDG PET is to be obtained for response assessment, it should be performed as closely as possible (ie, within 4 days) to the subsequent cycle; for example on days 17–21 of a 21-day cycle or days 10–14 of a 14-day cycle.[3] Visual assessment alone is sufficient to assess treatment response as positive or negative after completion of therapy.[4] For response assessment at the conclusion of therapy, mediastinal blood pool activity is recommended as the reference level to define FDG PET positivity for a residual mass ≥ 2 cm in greatest transverse diameter, regardless of its location, while surrounding background activity is recommended as the reference level to define FDG PET positivity for a smaller residual mass or a normal sized lymph node (≤ 1 × 1 cm in diameter).[5] Use of attenuation-corrected FDG PET is strongly encouraged.

Although it sounds appealing that the treatment strategy may be adjusted early, based on the interim FDG PET findings, there is lack of clinical evidence that such adjusted treatment strategy will lead to improved survival and/or decreased rate of late stage complications. Many questions still remain: when is the best time to use FDG PET for response assessment after initiation of therapy (7 day or 42 days)? Will the same high cure rate be achieved with less intensive therapy in patients who have favorable early response? Can clinicians achieve a higher cure rate with more aggressive therapy in patients who have an unfavorable interim response?

END OF THERAPY EVALUATION

After completion of several cycles of chemotherapy or chemoradiation therapy, it is critically important to make the decision: (1) if the therapy has reached its goal (if the patient has complete response); or (2) if additional treatment is required (if the patient has a residual mass of lymphoma); or (3) if second-line salvage treatment or radiation or others are needed. In contrast to the interim response assessment, the value of FDG PET at the end of therapy is well established for determining residual disease activity and in guiding the management of patients with lymphoma, and is clearly superior to CT scan.

Many efforts have been made to predict the likely treatment outcome and prognosis of patient with HD and NHL[41,42] and imaging studies play an important role here. A significant residual mass may form and persist after definitive treatment of HL or NHL. It could be composed of necrotic tissue, fibrous tissue, or it could be resistant residual tumor. Various imaging modalities are available to assess this mass, including radiograph, CT scan, and gallium scan. Although CT scan has high accuracy in the initial staging of lymphoma, the specificity of positive CT findings in the treated lymphoma patients is low because many patients have persistent residual masses and enlarged lymph nodes that are not necessarily viable tumors (**Fig. 5**). In a retrospective review of 256 children who had HD during 1985 to 2003, 26 patients were deemed to be of concern for residual disease by traditional imaging modalities, although only 10 (38%) showed resistant disease upon biopsy and the other 16 (62%) had fibrotic or necrotic tissues. The sensitivity and specificity of each imaging modality were 60% and 38% for chest radiograph, 67% and 8% for CT scan, and 71% and 71% for gallium scan.[43] These CIMs are not sufficiently sensitive or specific to differentiate residual resistant tumor tissues from nontumor tissues, and surgical biopsy is still needed to rule out any harboring resistant tumor cells in these residual masses. Being a functional imaging modality, FDG PET has a unique role in the post-therapy evaluation of lymphoma patients.

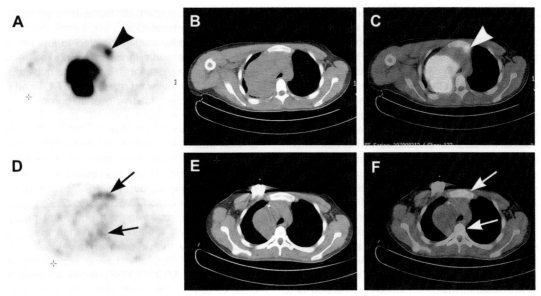

Fig. 5. This patient was a 17-year-old female with Hodgkin's lymphoma. PET/CT scan on initial staging showed abnormally increased FDG uptake in a large right mediastainal mass (*A–C*) and a smaller focus of FDG uptake in a prevascular lymph node (*arrowhead*). Five weeks after chemotherapy, no abnormally increased FDG uptake was visualized, while significant mediastinal mass persisted (*E* and *F*). Mildly increased FDG uptake in the bone marrow is consistent with recent chemotherapy (*arrows*).

The role of FDG PET in the characterization of residual masses of lymphoma after completion of chemotherapy is well documented in adult lymphoma patients. In general, FDG PET has a high negative predictive value and variable positive predictive value. Zijlstra and colleagues in a meta-analysis reviewed 15 studies (705 patients) up to January 2004, using histology or follow-up of at least 12 months as a valid reference test. They found that FDG PET had reasonable sensitivity and high specificity for evaluation of post-therapy residual disease in HD and in NHL. The pooled sensitivity and specificity for detection of residual disease in HD were 84% (95% CI 71%–92%) and 90% (95% CI 84%–94%), respectively. For NHL, pooled sensitivity and specificity were 72% (95% CI 61%–82%), and 100% (95% CI 97%–100%), respectively.[44] In a more recent meta-analysis, Terasawa and colleagues[45] analyzed cases with HD or aggressive NHL for patients who completed first-line chemotherapy, radiotherapy, or combined-modality therapy (with or without residual disease) and underwent conventional imaging tests such as CT, ultrasonography, or MRI for post-treatment restaging just before or after undergoing FDG PET. They found good overall diagnostic accuracy irrespective of the presence of any visible residual mass on CIMs.[45]

Several studies have examined FDG PET for post-treatment evaluation in the pediatric population of lymphoma patients. A negative FDG PET at the end of treatment of HD and NHL is often predictive of long-term remission.[7,8,46]

In pediatric HD and NHL patients, FDG PET was also very accurate for characterization of post-therapy residual masses. Depas and colleagues reported that FDG PET had very high specificity at end of therapy evaluation in 16 children with lymphoma (8 HD and 8 NHL). FDG PET resulted in a true negative in 15/16 patients with one false positive in a HD patient because muscle activity was reported as possible malignancy. This confusion should not occur if hybrid PET/CT is employed. Overall, FDG PET had a specificity of 94% at the end of treatment (versus 54% for conventional methods, including physical examination, laboratory studies, chest radiograph, CT, MRI, ultrasonography and bone scan when available).[1] Amthauer and colleagues also reported that FDG PET correctly revealed in one out of five pediatric NHL patients persistent tumor metabolism after completion of initial therapy. The patient had disease progression and died shortly after restaging.[27] In a review of twelve FDG PET scans in ten pediatric lymphoma patients, it was found that FDG PET and CT scans were concordant in seven cases. In all five cases with discordant findings, FDG PET was negative while diagnostic CT scans were positive. All adenopathy detected by CT scans eventually disappeared during follow-up studies, indicating false positive CT findings.[7] More recently, in a study of 26 pediatric patients

(8–19 years of age) with lymphoma, FDG PET provided incremental information in 21% of HD cases and 33% of NHL cases in comparison with conventional imaging studies (CT/MRI), and was especially useful in distinguishing scar tissue from residual disease at the end of therapy.[14]

In a prospective study with 26 pediatric patients with newly diagnosed mediastinal HD (n = 16) and NHL (n = 10), FDG PET was used to evaluate residual mediastinal disease following completion of therapy (the median interval between the end of therapy to imaging was 17.5 days for NHL and was 72 days for HD). Edeline and colleagues[46] reported that none of the 11 FDG PET negative patients with HD relapsed (and remained in their first remission for at least 28 months after the end of therapy), even though they all had residual mass on CT scan. For patients with NHL, four out of five patients with negative FDG PET findings (all with residual mass) remained in remission for at least 45 months, and the only exception was a patient with anaplastic lymphoma with negative evaluation on FDG PET scan.

SURVEILLANCE IMAGING DURING FOLLOW-UP

After completion of treatment for HD and complete remission has been achieved, children with lymphoma are commonly followed-up for 5 years or so with regular surveillance imaging studies to identify evidence of residual disease and to monitor for relapse of disease. The most challenging issue is again the residual mass, which is common and may persist in children who have completed treatment for lymphoma. CT surveillance during follow up to assess disease status is unsatisfactory. In adult HD patients, the sensitivity and specificity of FDG PET were reported as 87.5% and 94.4% respectively, in contrast to 25% and 56% for CT scans. The positive and negative predictive values of PET (versus CT scans) were 87.5% and 94.4% (versus 20% and 62.5%), respectively.[47]

A few retrospective clinical studies addressed this issue in pediatric lymphoma patients. It was reported that FDG PET revealed more extensive disease than CIMs and led to upstaging in 2/4 pediatric HD patients, because of clinical evidence of recurrence (mean: 19 months after completion of initial therapy).[6] In a long-term follow-up study of 19 pediatric lymphoma patients who had achieved complete remission, 59 FDG PET studies were performed (38 HD and 21 NHL) in 19 children (13 HD, 6 NHL), with a mean interval between the end of therapy and the first follow-up study of 9 months. There were no false negatives in HD patients but 3/21 studies in NHL patients were false positives. Overall, FDG PET had a specificity of 95% during the systematic follow-up (versus 66% for conventional methods).[1]

However, some studies pointed to low PPV of FDG PET as a surveillance of lymphoma recurrence in pediatric patients. Rhodes and colleagues retrospectively reviewed results of PET/CT and CT scan alone during follow-up after completion of therapy in 41 children with HD and NHL, with a median follow-up of 2.3 years. FDG uptake higher than that of the liver was considered positive. They found that PET/CT scan is more sensitive than diagnostic CT (with a sensitivity of 95% and 79%, respectively), but the PPV of PET/CT is similar to diagnostic CT (53% and 52%, respectively). Also no children with equivocal positive PET/CT findings (uptake higher than the background but less than in the liver) developed recurrent disease.[48] Similarly, Levine and colleagues reviewed 255 FDG PET scans on 47 pediatric patients (age 3–26 years) with HD. Among 156 FDG PET scans obtained on 34 patients as routine surveillance after completion of therapy, 128 scans were accurate with no false negative. However, among the 28 positive FDG PET scans, only three of the scans were true positives (in two patients), and 25 scans were demonstrated to be false positives (in 12 patients). The PPV for FDG PET scans obtained in that study during routine follow-up was 11%, with a false positive rate of 16%, in contrast to 100% negative predictive value in the same settings.[49] The contributing factors to false positive studies include fibrosis, appendicitis, transformation of germinal centers, abdominal wall hernia, normal thymus and HIV associated lymphadenopathy.[49] Separately, in a retrospective study, 23 consecutive pediatric HD patients were reviewed with FDG PET scan for post-treatment evaluation. It was found that FDG PET is highly sensitive with a strong negative predictive value (100%), but its specificity is low (57.1%). Twenty-two of the 23 patients had a negative FDG PET scan at the end of therapy and 12 (52.2%) of them had consistent negative FDG PET scans within 6–42 months following completion of therapy. However, in 11 patients who had a positive FDG PET scan within 6–9 months after the end of therapy, only two patients had relapsed HD confirmed by biopsy. The low PPV (18.2%) compares with a concurrent CT study.[50] The authors concluded that a negative FDG PET scan is more accurately representative of disease remission than a positive FDG PET is for relapsed HD. Correlation of CT results performed at the time of a positive FDG PET scan did not consistently predict disease relapse. The authors further stated that FDG PET scan positive solely at sites other than the original tumor sites at diagnosis rarely indicates relapsed HD.[50] It should be noted that in both studies of Levine and Meany and colleagues PET alone (not PET/CT) was employed, which is associated with much higher false-positive findings. With the advent and wider application of combined PET/CT, the ability to correlate PET data with more precise anatomic location is well established, and many false positive studies can be avoided or minimized. It is reported that using dual-time point imaging technique is potentially helpful in distinguishing benign lesions from some types of malignancies.[51–56] However, there is little experience in the evaluation of lymphomas and more clinical studies (especially well-designed, prospective studies with a large patient population) are needed to evaluate the true value of FDG PET for early detection of tumor recurrence and the clinical impact of PET on patient management and outcome.

In short, the role of FDG PET in post-treatment surveillance of lymphoma is not proven. Follow-up FDG PET scans that are performed after completion of therapy in pediatric lymphoma patients have a very high negative predictive value, but the PPV is low and false positive rate is high. Generally, any positive FDG PET scans after treatment should be interpreted cautiously and biopsy correlation should be considered before any therapeutic decisions are made. Follow-up PET/CT scan may be indicated if patients develop new clinical signs of tumor recurrence or any abnormal findings using conventional staging methods.

BONE MARROW EVALUATION

An important aspect and also a major limitation of CT imaging in the management of lymphoma is the evaluation of bone marrow involvement, and accumulating evidence demonstrates that FDG PET and bone marrow biopsy are complementary in the evaluation of bone marrow involvement (**Figs. 2** and **3**). Retrospective analysis of 106 consecutive patients with confirmed diagnosis of lymphoma (18 HD and 88 NHL) found that FDG PET and bone marrow biopsy are complementary in assessing the presence of bone marrow involvement.[57] FDG PET was more sensitive than bone marrow biopsy in HD and NHL but not in follicular lymphoma. In a study of 50 patients with HD (n = 12) and NHL (n = 38), FDG PET scans were analyzed in comparison with unilateral iliac crest marrow aspirates and biopsies. The FDG PET scan and marrow histology agreed in 39 patients (78%), being concordant positive in 26% and concordant negative in 52% of patients. Bone marrow biopsy missed four patients who were

correctly diagnosed by FDG PET. Among the three patients who were missed by FDG PET, two of them had NHL whose malignant cells did not take up FDG at lymph node or marrow disease sites.[58] Excluding the cases of non–FDG-avid lymphoma, FDG PET seemed superior to biopsy for evaluation of bone marrow involvement in lymphoma, and may reduce the need for staging marrow biopsy. FDG PET versus bone marrow biopsy in the detection of bone marrow involvement was reviewed in 194 consecutive adult patients with HD or aggressive NHL. The sensitivity, specificity, accuracy, positive and negative predictive value for FDG PET were 65.3%, 98.6%, 90.2%, 94.1% and 89.3%, respectively. The sensitivity, specificity, accuracy, positive and negative predictive value for bone marrow biopsy were 55.1%, 100%, 88.7%, 100% and 86.8%, respectively. Although FDG PET and bone marrow biopsy had similar specificity and accuracy, both had relatively low sensitivity in detecting bone marrow disease with concordant positive findings in only 10 out of 49 patients. A significant amount of bone marrow disease missed by bone marrow biopsy was detected by FDG-PET, and the treatment regimen was changed in 12 patients based on FDG-PET findings.[59] Similar findings were reported in pediatric lymphoma patients. In a prospective, blinded study with 55 children and adolescents with HD, the value of FDG PET was compared with other conventional staging methods, including bone marrow examination for initial staging; FDG PET correctly changed the staging in 15% of patients (mostly upstagings).[28]

SUMMARY

Since its introduction, FDG PET has demonstrated substantial impact on patient management of HD and aggressive NHL. PET/CT imaging is superior for lymphoma staging to FDG PET or CT alone and is becoming the modality of choice for staging and restaging of nodal and extranodal involvement of lymphoma, for evaluating therapeutic response, and for establishing patient prognosis. It should be kept in mind that many of the data in pediatric lymphoma patients reviewed here were obtained with FDG PET alone without direct CT correlation, and available data had shown nothing but significant contribution to the management of lymphoma in pediatric as well as in adult patients. Now with wide-spread availability and acceptance of combined PET/CT devices, which collect the information of tumor metabolism and tumor size simultaneously, and which lead to higher sensitivity and specificity for staging, restaging, and treatment monitoring, FDG PET will be an essential and integrated part of the management of lymphoma patients throughout the treatment process.[4,31]

REFERENCES

1. Depas G, De Barsy C, Jerusalem G, et al. 18F-FDG PET in children with lymphomas. Eur J Nucl Med Mol Imaging 2005;32:31–8.
2. Jerusalem G, Hustinx R, Beguin Y, et al. Evaluation of therapy for lymphoma. Semin Nucl Med 2005; 35:186–96.
3. Seam P, Juweid ME, Cheson BD. The role of FDG-PET scans in patients with lymphoma. Blood 2007; 110:3507–16.
4. Kasamon YL, Jones RJ, Wahl RL. Integrating PET and PET/CT into the risk-adapted therapy of lymphoma. J Nucl Med 2007;48(S1):19–27S.
5. Kirby AM, Mikhaeel NG. The role of FDG PET in the management of lymphoma: what is the evidence base? Nucl Med Commun 2007;28:335–54.
6. Montravers F, McNamara D, Landman-Parker J, et al. [(18)F]FDG in childhood lymphoma: clinical utility and impact on management. Eur J Nucl Med Mol Imaging 2002;29:1155–65.
7. Hernandez-Pampaloni M, Takalkar A, Yu JQ, et al. F-18 FDG-PET imaging and correlation with CT in staging and follow-up of pediatric lymphomas. Pediatr Radiol 2006;36:524–31.
8. Miller E, Metser U, Avrahami G, et al. Role of 18F-FDG PET/CT in staging and follow-up of lymphoma in pediatric and young adult patients. J Comput Assist Tomogr 2006;30:689–94.
9. Hampson FA, Shaw AS. Response assessment in lymphoma. Clin Radiol 2008;63:125–35.
10. Tatsumi M, Cohade C, Nakamoto Y, et al. Direct comparison of FDG PET and CT findings in patients with lymphoma: initial experience. Radiology 2005; 237:1038–45.
11. Moog F, Bangerter M, Diederichs CG, et al. Extranodal malignant lymphoma: detection with FDG PET versus CT. Radiology 1998;206:475–81.
12. Foo SS, Mitchell PL, Berlangieri SU, et al. Positron emission tomography scanning in the assessment of patients with lymphoma [see comment]. Intern Med J 2004;34:388–97.
13. Lin P, Chu J, Kneebone A, et al. Direct comparison of 18F-fluorodeoxyglucose coincidence gamma camera tomography with gallium scanning for the staging of lymphoma. Intern Med J 2005;35:91–6.
14. Mody RJ, Bui C, Hutchinson RJ, et al. Comparison of (18)F Flurodeoxyglucose PET with Ga-67 scintigraphy and conventional imaging modalities in pediatric lymphoma. Leuk Lymphoma 2007;48:699–707.
15. Rini JN, Nunez R, Nichols K, et al. Coincidence-detection FDG-PET versus gallium in children and young adults with newly diagnosed Hodgkin's disease. Pediatr Radiol 2005;35:169–78.
16. Hines-Thomas M, Kaste SC, Hudson MM, et al. Comparison of gallium and PET scans at diagnosis and follow-up of pediatric patients with Hodgkin lymphoma. Pediatr Blood Cancer 2008;51:198–203.
17. Allen-Auerbach M, Quon A, Weber WA, et al. Comparison between 2-deoxy-2-[18F]fluoro-D-glucose positron emission tomography and positron emission tomography/computed tomography hardware fusion for staging of patients with lymphoma. Mol Imaging Biol 2004;6:411–6.
18. Raanani P, Shasha Y, Perry C, et al. Is CT scan still necessary for staging in Hodgkin and non-Hodgkin lymphoma patients in the PET/CT era? Ann Oncol 2006;17:117–22.
19. Rodriguez-Vigil B, Gomez-Leon N, Pinilla I, et al. PET/CT in lymphoma: prospective study of enhanced full-dose PET/CT versus unenhanced low-dose PET/CT. J Nucl Med 2006;47:1643–8.
20. la Fougere C, Pfluger T, Schneider V, et al. Restaging of patients with lymphoma. Comparison of low dose CT (20 mAs) with contrast enhanced diagnostic CT in combined [18F]-FDG PET/CT. Nucl Med 2008;47:37–42.
21. Bar-Sever Z, Keidar Z, Ben-Barak A, et al. The incremental value of 18F-FDG PET/CT in paediatric malignancies. [see comment]. Eur J Nucl Med Mol Imaging 2007;34:630–7.
22. Buchmann I, Reinhardt M, Elsner K, et al. 2-(fluorine-18)fluoro-2-deoxy-D-glucose positron emission tomography in the detection and staging of malignant lymphoma. A bicenter trial. Cancer 2001;91:889–99.
23. Buchmann I, Neumaier B, Schreckenberger M, et al. [18F]3'-deoxy-3'-fluorothymidine-PET in NHL patients: whole-body biodistribution and imaging of lymphoma manifestations–a pilot study. Cancer Biother Radiopharm 2004;19:436–42.
24. Hicks RJ, Mac Manus MP, Seymour JF. Initial staging of lymphoma with positron emission tomography and computed tomography. Semin Nucl Med 2005; 35:165–75.
25. Allen-Auerbach M, de Vos S, Czernin J. The impact of fluorodeoxyglucose-positron emission tomography in primary staging and patient management in lymphoma patients. Radiol Clin North Am 2008;46: 199–211.
26. Hermann S, Wormanns D, Pixberg M, et al. Staging in childhood lymphoma: differences between FDG-PET and CT. Nucl Med 2005;44:1–7.
27. Amthauer H, Furth C, Denecke T, et al. FDG-PET in 10 children with non-Hodgkin's lymphoma: initial experience in staging and follow-up. Klin Padiatr 2005;217:327–33.
28. Kabickova E, Sumerauer D, Cumlivska E, et al. Comparison of 18F-FDG-PET and standard procedures for the pretreatment staging of children and adolescents with Hodgkin's disease. Eur J Nucl Med Mol Imaging 2006;33:1025–31.

29. Furth C, Denecke T, Steffen I, et al. Correlative imaging strategies implementing CT, MRI, and PET for staging of childhood Hodgkin disease. J Pediatr Hematol Oncol 2006;28:501–12.

30. Korholz D, Kluge R, Wickmann L, et al. Importance of F18-fluorodeoxy-D-2-glucose positron emission tomography (FDG-PET) for staging and therapy control of Hodgkin's lymphoma in childhood and adolescence - consequences for the GPOH-HD 2003 protocol. Onkologie 2003;26: 489–93.

31. Korholz D, Claviez A, Hasenclever D, et al. The concept of the GPOH-HD 2003 therapy study for pediatric Hodgkin's disease: evolution in the tradition of the DAL/GPOH studies. Klin Padiatr 2004;216:150–6.

32. Sweetenham JW. Minimizing late effects in children and adults with Hodgkin lymphoma - the beginning of the end for radiation therapy [comment]. Leuk Lymphoma 2008;49:839–40.

33. Schoder H, Moskowitz C. PET imaging for response assessment in lymphoma: potential and limitations. Radiol Clin North Am 2008;46:225–41.

34. Haioun C, Itti E, Rahmouni A, et al. [18F]fluoro-2-deoxy-D-glucose positron emission tomography (FDG-PET) in aggressive lymphoma: an early prognostic tool for predicting patient outcome. Blood 2005;106:1376–81.

35. Hutchings M, Loft A, Hansen M, et al. FDG-PET after two cycles of chemotherapy predicts treatment failure and progression-free survival in Hodgkin lymphoma. Blood 2006;107:52–9.

36. Kasamon YL, Wahl RL. FDG PET and risk-adapted therapy in Hodgkin's and non-Hodgkin's lymphoma. Curr Opin Oncol 2008;20:206–19.

37. MacManus MP, Seymour JF, Hicks RJ. Overview of early response assessment in lymphoma with FDG-PET. Cancer Imaging 2007;7:10–8.

38. Querellou S, Valette F, Bodet-Milin C, et al. FDG-PET/CT predicts outcome in patients with aggressive non-Hodgkin's lymphoma and Hodgkin's disease. Ann Hematol 2006;85:759–67.

39. Cheson BD, Pfistner B, Juweid ME, et al. Revised response criteria for malignant lymphoma. J Clin Oncol 2007;25:579–86.

40. Juweid ME, Stroobants S, Hoekstra OS, et al. Use of positron emission tomography for response assessment of lymphoma: consensus of the Imaging Subcommittee of International Harmonization Project in Lymphoma. J Clin Oncol 2007;25: 571–8.

41. Hasenclever D, Diehl V. A prognostic score for advanced Hodgkin's disease. International Prognostic Factors Project on Advanced Hodgkin's Disease [see comment]. N Engl J Med 1998;339: 1506–14.

42. A predictive model for aggressive non-Hodgkin's lymphoma. The International Non-Hodgkin's Lymphoma Prognostic Factors Project [see comment]. N Engl J Med 1993;329:987–94.

43. Nasr A, Stulberg J, Weitzman S, et al. Assessment of residual posttreatment masses in Hodgkin's disease and the need for biopsy in children. J Pediatr Surg 2006;41:972–4.

44. Zijlstra JM, Lindauer-van der Werf G, Hoekstra OS, et al. 18F-fluoro-deoxyglucose positron emission tomography for post-treatment evaluation of malignant lymphoma: a systematic review. Haematologica 2006;91:522–9.

45. Terasawa T, Nihashi T, Hotta T, et al. 18F-FDG PET for posttherapy assessment of Hodgkin's disease and aggressive Non-Hodgkin's lymphoma: a systematic review [see comment]. J Nucl Med 2008;49: 13–21.

46. Edeline V, Bonardel G, Brisse H, et al. Prospective study of 18F-FDG PET in pediatric mediastinal lymphoma: a single center experience. Leuk Lymphoma 2007;48:823–6.

47. Dittmann H, Sokler M, Kollmannsberger C, et al. Comparison of 18FDG-PET with CT scans in the evaluation of patients with residual and recurrent Hodgkin's lymphoma. Oncol Rep 2001;8:1393–9.

48. Rhodes MM, Delbeke D, Whitlock JA, et al. Utility of FDG-PET/CT in follow-up of children treated for Hodgkin and non-Hodgkin lymphoma. J Pediatr Hematol Oncol 2006;28:300–6.

49. Levine JM, Weiner M, Kelly KM. Routine use of PET scans after completion of therapy in pediatric Hodgkin disease results in a high false positive rate [see comment]. J Pediatr Hematol Oncol 2006;28:711–4.

50. Meany HJ, Gidvani VK, Minniti CP. Utility of PET scans to predict disease relapse in pediatric patients with Hodgkin lymphoma. Pediatr Blood Cancer 2007;48:399–402.

51. Kubota K, Itoh M, Ozaki K, et al. Advantage of delayed whole-body FDG-PET imaging for tumour detection. Eur J Nucl Med 2001;28:696–703.

52. Xiu Y, Bhutani C, Dhurairaj T, et al. Dual-time point FDG PET imaging in the evaluation of pulmonary nodules with minimally increased metabolic activity. Clin Nucl Med 2007;32:101–5.

53. Zhuang H, Pourdehnad M, Lambright ES, et al. Dual time point 18F-FDG PET imaging for differentiating malignant from inflammatory processes. J Nucl Med 2001;42:1412–7.

54. Conrad GR, Sinha P. Narrow time-window dual-point 18F-FDG PET for the diagnosis of thoracic malignancy. Nucl Med Commun 2003;24:1129–37.

55. Lai CH, Huang KG, See LC, et al. Restaging of recurrent cervical carcinoma with dual-phase [18F]fluoro-2-deoxy-D-glucose positron emission tomography. Cancer 2004;100:544–52.

56. Zytoon AA, Murakami K, El-Kholy MR, et al. Positron emission tomography and breast lesions: low FDG

activity in early phase imaging is not essentially benign. Clin Nucl Med 2008;33:931–3.

57. Fuster D, Chiang S, Andreadis C, et al. Can [18F]fluorodeoxyglucose positron emission tomography imaging complement biopsy results from the iliac crest for the detection of bone marrow involvement in patients with malignant lymphoma? Nucl Med Commun 2006;27:11–5.

58. Carr R, Barrington SF, Madan B, et al. Detection of lymphoma in bone marrow by whole-body positron emission tomography. Blood 1998;91:3340–6.

59. Pelosi E, Penna D, Deandreis D, et al. FDG-PET in the detection of bone marrow disease in Hodgkin's disease and aggressive non-Hodgkin's lymphoma and its impact on clinical management. Q J Nucl Med Mol Imaging 2008;52:9–16.

Index

Note: Page numbers of article titles are in **boldface** type.

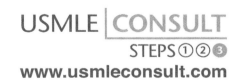

Moving?

Make sure your subscription moves with you!

To notify us of your new address, find your **Clinics Account Number** (located on your mailing label above your name), and contact customer service at:

E-mail: elspcs@elsevier.com

800-654-2452 (subscribers in the U.S. & Canada)
314-453-7041 (subscribers outside of the U.S. & Canada)

Fax number: 314-523-5170

Elsevier Periodicals Customer Service
11830 Westline Industrial Drive
St. Louis, MO 63146

*To ensure uninterrupted delivery of your subscription, please notify us at least 4 weeks in advance of move.

ELSEVIER

Printed and bound by CPI Group (UK) Ltd, Croydon, CR0 4YY

03/10/2024

01040352-0009